STRESS-INDUCED AND FEAR CIRCUITRY DISORDERS

Advancing the Research Agenda for DSM-V

STRESS-INDUCED AND FEAR CIRCUITRY DISORDERS

Advancing the Research Agenda for DSM-V

Edited by

Gavin Andrews, M.D.
Dennis S. Charney, M.D.
Paul J. Sirovatka, M.S.
Darrel A. Regier, M.D., M.P.H.

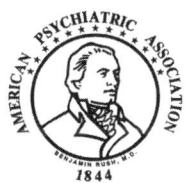

Published by the
American Psychiatric Association
Arlington, Virginia

Note: The authors have worked to ensure that all information in this book is accurate at the time of publication and consistent with general psychiatric and medical standards, and that information concerning drug dosages, schedules, and routes of administration is accurate at the time of publication and consistent with standards set by the U.S. Food and Drug Administration and the general medical community. As medical research and practice continue to advance, however, therapeutic standards may change. Moreover, specific situations may require a specific therapeutic response not included in this book. For these reasons and because human and mechanical errors sometimes occur, we recommend that readers follow the advice of physicians directly involved in their care or the care of a member of their family.

The findings, opinions, and conclusions of this report do not necessarily represent the views of the officers, trustees, or all members of the American Psychiatric Association. The views expressed are those of the authors of the individual chapters.

Copyright © 2009 American Psychiatric Association
ALL RIGHTS RESERVED

Manufactured in the United States of America on acid-free paper
12 11 10 09 08   5 4 3 2 1
First Edition

Typeset in Adobe's Frutiger and AGaramond.

American Psychiatric Association
1000 Wilson Boulevard
Arlington, VA 22209-3901
www.psych.org

Library of Congress Cataloging-in-Publication Data
Stress-induced and fear circuitry disorders : advancing the research agenda for DSM-V / edited by Gavin Andrews ... [et al.]. — 1st ed.
 p. ; cm.
Includes bibliographical references and index.
ISBN 978-0-89042-344-8 (pbk. : alk. paper)
 1. Anxiety disorders—Diagnosis. 2. Anxiety disorders—Classification. 3. Panic disorders—Diagnosis. 4. Panic disorders—Classification. 5. Post-traumatic stress disorder—Diagnosis. 6. Post-traumatic stress disorder—Classification. 7. Diagnostic and statistical manual of mental disorders. I. Andrews, Gavin.
[DNLM: 1. Diagnostic and statistical manual of mental disorders. 2. Stress Disorders, Traumatic—classification. 3. Phobic Disorders—classification. 4. Phobic Disorders—diagnosis. 5. Stress Disorders, Traumatic—diagnosis. WM 172 S9151 2009]
 RC531.S764 2009
 616.85'22—dc22

2008024613

British Library Cataloguing in Publication Data
A CIP record is available from the British Library.

CONTENTS

CONTRIBUTORS vii
DISCLOSURE STATEMENT xi
PREFACE xv
    Dennis S. Charney, M.D., and Gavin Andrews, M.D.

PART 1
Stress-Induced and Fear Circuitry Disorders

1 POSTTRAUMATIC STRESS DISORDER 3
    Matthew J. Friedman, M.D., and Elie G. Karam, M.D.

2 PANIC DISORDER 31
    *Carlo Faravelli, M.D., Toshi A. Furukawa, M.D., Ph.D., and
    Elisabetta Truglia, M.D.*

3 SOCIAL PHOBIA 59
    *Susan Bögels, Ph.D., and Murray B. Stein, M.D., FRCPC,
    M.P.H.*

4 SPECIFIC PHOBIAS 77
    *Paul M. G. Emmelkamp, Ph.D., and
    Hans-Ulrich Wittchen, Ph.D.*

PART 2
Course and Classification

5 CONTINUITY AND ETIOLOGY OF ANXIETY DISORDERS:
ARE THEY STABLE ACROSS THE LIFE COURSE? 105
    *Richie Poulton, Ph.D., Daniel S. Pine, M.D., and
    HonaLee Harrington, B.A.*

6 STRESS-INDUCED AND FEAR CIRCUITRY ANXIETY DISORDERS:
ARE THEY A DISTINCT GROUP? 125
    Abby J. Fyer, M.D., and Timothy A. Brown, Ph.D.

PART 3
Special Topics

7 ANXIETY DISORDERS IN AFRICAN AMERICANS AND
OTHER ETHNIC MINORITIES 139
   William B. Lawson, M.D., Ph.D.

8 THE GENETIC BASIS OF ANXIETY DISORDERS 145
   Thalia C. Eley, Ph.D.

9 SEROTONIN, SENSITIVE PERIODS, AND ANXIETY 159
   Mark D. Alter, M.D., Ph.D., and Rene Hen, Ph.D.

10 ROLE OF COGNITION IN STRESS-INDUCED AND
FEAR CIRCUITRY DISORDERS 175
   *Jonathan D. Huppert, Ph.D., Edna B. Foa, Ph.D.,
   Richard J. McNally, Ph.D., and Shawn P. Cahill, Ph.D.*

11 STRESS AND PSYCHOSOCIAL FACTORS IN ONSET OF
FEAR CIRCUITRY DISORDERS 195
   Ronald M. Rapee, Ph.D., and Richard A. Bryant, Ph.D.

12 NEUROIMAGING AND NEUROANATOMY OF STRESS-INDUCED
AND FEAR CIRCUITRY DISORDERS 215
   Scott L. Rauch, M.D., and Wayne C. Drevets, M.D.

13 ROLE OF NEUROCHEMICAL AND NEUROENDOCRINE MARKERS
OF FEAR IN CLASSIFICATION OF ANXIETY DISORDERS 255
   Rachel Yehuda, Ph.D.

14 ANXIETY AND SUBSTANCE ABUSE: IMPLICATIONS FOR
PATHOPHYSIOLOGY AND DSM-V 265
   Edward V. Nunes, M.D., and Carlos Blanco, M.D., Ph.D.

15 CONCLUDING REMARKS 283
   *Gavin Andrews, M.D., Peter McEvoy, Ph.D., and
   Tim Slade, Ph.D.*

INDEX 301

CONTRIBUTORS

Mark D. Alter, M.D., Ph.D.
Assistant Professor, Divisions of Child Psychiatry and Integrative Neuroscience, Department of Psychiatry, Columbia University College of Physicians and Surgeons, New York, New York

Gavin Andrews, M.D.
Scientia Professor of Psychiatry and Director, Clinical Research Unit for Anxiety and Depression, School of Psychiatry, University of New South Wales, Darlinghurst, Australia

Carlos Blanco, M.D., Ph.D.
Associate Professor of Clinical Psychiatry, Columbia University College of Physicians and Surgeons, New York State Psychiatric Institute, New York, New York

Susan Bögels, Ph.D
Professor of Psychiatry and Family and Preventive Medicine, University of California, San Diego; Director, Anxiety and Traumatic Stress Program, UCSD and Department of Veterans Affairs San Diego Healthcare System, San Diego, California

Timothy A. Brown, Ph.D.
Professor, Department of Psychology, Center for Anxiety and Related Disorders, Boston, Massachusetts

Richard A. Bryant, Ph.D.
Scientia Professor, School of Psychology, University of New South Wales, Sydney, Australia

Shawn P. Cahill, Ph.D.
Assistant Professor of Clinical Psychology in Psychiatry, Center for the Treatment and Study of Anxiety, University of Pennsylvania, Philadelphia, Pennsylvania

Dennis S. Charney, M.D.
Dean of the Mount Sinai School of Medicine, Executive Vice President of Academic Affairs of the Mount Sinai Medical Center; Professor in the Departments of Psychiatry, Neuroscience, and Pharmacology & Systems Therapeutics, Mount Sinai School of Medicine, New York, New York

Wayne C. Drevets, M.D.
Senior Investigator and Chief, Section on Neuroimaging in Mood and Anxiety Disorders, Division of Intramural Research Programs, National Institutes of Health/National Institute of Mental Health, Bethesda, Maryland

Thalia C. Eley, Ph.D.
Senior Lecturer and MRC Fellow, Social, Genetic, and Developmental Psychiatry Centre, Institute of Psychiatry, King's College, London, United Kingdom

Paul M. G. Emmelkamp, Ph.D.
Academy Professor, Royal Netherlands Academy of Arts and Sciences, University of Amsterdam, The Netherlands

Carlo Faravelli, M.D.
Professor of Psychiatry, Department of Psychology, University of Florence, Firenze, Italy

Edna B. Foa, Ph.D.
Professor of Clinical Psychology in Psychiatry; Director, Center for the Treatment and Study of Anxiety, University of Pennsylvania, Philadelphia, Pennsylvania

Matthew J. Friedman, M.D.
Executive Director, National Center for PTSD, VA Medical Center, White River Junction, Vermont; Professor of Psychiatry and of Pharmacology, Department of Psychiatry, Dartmouth Medical School, Hanover, New Hampshire

Toshi A. Furukawa, M.D., Ph.D.
Professor and Chair, Department of Psychiatry and Cognitive-Behavioral Medicine, Nagoya City University Graduate School of Medical Sciences, Nagoya, Japan

Abby J. Fyer, M.D.
Professor of Clinical Psychiatry, Columbia University College of Physicians and Surgeons; Director, Anxiety Genetics Unit, New York, New York

HonaLee Harrington, B.A.
Associate in Research, Department of Psychology and Neuroscience, Duke University, Durham, North Carolina

Rene Hen, Ph.D.
Professor, Division of Integrative Neuroscience, Department of Psychiatry, Neuroscience, and Pharmacology, Columbia University College of Physicians and Surgeons, New York, New York

Contributors

Jonathan D. Huppert, Ph.D.
Associate Professor, Department of Psychology, The Hebrew University of Jerusalem, Mt. Scopus, Jerusalem; Adjunct Associate Professor of Psychology in Psychiatry, Center for the Treatment and Study of Anxiety, Department of Psychiatry, University of Pennsylvania, Philadelphia, Pennsylvania

Elie G. Karam, M.D.
Professor and Head, Department of Psychiatry and Clinical Psychology, St. George Hospital University Medical Center, Faculty of Medicine, Balamand University; Institute for Development, Research, Advocacy, and Applied Care (IDRAAC); Medical Institute for Neuropsychological Disorders (MIND), Beirut, Achrafieh, Lebanon

William B. Lawson, M.D., Ph.D.
Professor and Chair, Department of Psychiatry and Behavioral Sciences, Howard University College of Medicine and Hospital, Washington, D.C.

Peter McEvoy, Ph.D.
Clinical Director, Clinical Research Unit for Anxiety and Depression, St. Vincent's Hospital, Darlinghurst, Australia

Richard J. McNally, Ph.D.
Professor, Department of Psychology, Harvard University, Cambridge, Massachusetts

Edward V. Nunes, M.D.
Professor of Clinical Psychiatry, Columbia University College of Physicians and Surgeons, New York State Psychiatric Institute, New York, New York

Daniel S. Pine, M.D.
Chief of Developmental Studies, Mood and Anxiety Disorders Program, National Institute of Mental Health, Bethesda, Maryland

Richie Poulton, Ph.D.
Professor and Director, Dunedin Multidisciplinary Health and Development Research Unit, Department of Preventative and Social Medicine, Dunedin School of Medicine; Co-Director, National Centre for Lifecourse Research, University of Otago, Dunedin, New Zealand

Ronald M. Rapee, Ph.D.
Director, Centre for Emotional Health, Department of Psychology, Macquarie University, Sydney, Australia

Scott L. Rauch, M.D.
Chair, Partners Psychiatry Mental Health; President and Psychiatrist in Chief, McLean Hospital, Belmont, Massachussetts; Professor of Psychiatry, Harvard Medical School, Boston, Massachussetts

Darrel A. Regier, M.D., M.P.H.
Executive Director, American Psychiatric Institute for Research and Education; Director, Division of Research, American Psychiatric Association, Arlington, Virginia

Paul J. Sirovatka, M.S. (1947–2007)
Director, Research Policy Analysis, Division of Research and American Psychiatric Institute for Research and Education, American Psychiatric Association, Arlington, Virginia

Tim Slade, Ph.D.
Postdoctoral Fellow, Clinical Research Unit for Anxiety and Depression, University of New South Wales, Darlinghurst, Australia

Murray B. Stein, M.D., FRCPC, M.P.H.
Professor, Department of Developmental Psychopathology, University of Amsterdam, The Netherlands

Elisabetta Truglia, M.D.
Psychiatrist, Department of Psychiatry and Neurology, University of Florence, Firenze, Italy

Hans-Ulrich Wittchen, Ph.D.
Director, Institute of Clinical Psychology and Psychotherapy, Technische Universität Dresden, Dresden, Germany

Rachel Yehuda, Ph.D.
Professor of Psychiatry and Neurobiology, Psychiatry Department, and Director, Traumatic Stress Studies Division, Mt. Sinai School of Medicine, New York, New York; Director, PTSD Clinic and Research Lab, James J. Peters Veterans Affairs Hospital, Bronx, New York

DISCLOSURE STATEMENT

The research conference series that produced this monograph was supported with funding from the U.S. National Institutes of Health (NIH) Grant U13 MH067855 (Principal Investigator: Darrel A. Regier, M.D., M.P.H.). The National Institute of Mental Health (NIMH), the National Institute on Drug Abuse (NIDA), and the National Institute on Alcohol Abuse and Alcoholism (NIAAA) jointly supported this cooperative research planning conference project. The conference series was not part of the official revision process for *Diagnostic and Statistical Manual of Mental Disorders, Fifth Edition* (DSM-V), but rather was a separate, rigorous research planning initiative meant to inform revisions of psychiatric diagnostic classification systems. No private-industry sources provided funding for this research review.

Coordination and oversight of the overall research review, publicly titled "The Future of Psychiatric Diagnosis: Refining the Research Agenda," were provided by an Executive Steering Committee composed of representatives of the several entities that cooperatively sponsored the NIH-funded project. Members of the Executive Steering Committee included:

- *American Psychiatric Institute for Research and Education*—Darrel A. Regier, M.D., M.P.H. (P.I.), Michael B. First, M.D. (co-P.I.; consultant)
- *World Health Organization*—Benedetto Saraceno, M.D., and Norman Sartorius, M.D., Ph.D. (consultant)
- *National Institutes of Health*—Bruce Cuthbert, Ph.D., Wayne S. Fenton, M.D. (NIMH; consultant), Michael Kozak, Ph.D. (NIMH), Bridget F. Grant, Ph.D. (NIAAA), and Wilson M. Compton, M.D. (NIDA)
- NIMH grant project officers were Lisa Colpe, Ph.D., Karen H. Bourdon, M.A., and Mercedes Rubio, Ph.D.
- APIRE staff were William E. Narrow, M.D., M.P.H. (co-P.I.), Emily A. Kuhl, Ph.D., Maritza Rubio-Stipec, Sc.D. (consultant), Paul J. Sirovatka, M.S., Jennifer Shupinka, Erin Dalder-Alpher, Kristin Edwards, Leah Engel, Seung-Hee Hong, and Rocio Salvador

The following contributors to this book have indicated financial interests in other affiliations with a commercial supporter, a manufacturer of a commercial product, a provider of a commercial service, a nongovernmental organization, and/or government agency, as listed below:

Dennis S. Charney, M.D.—The author has been a consultant for AstraZeneca, Bristol-Myers Squibb, Cyberonics, Neurogen, Neuroscience Education Institute, Novartis, Orexigen, and Unilever UK Central Resources Limited. The author holds a patent on the drug ketamine.

Matthew J. Friedman, M.D.—The author has received an honorarium from AstraZeneca.

Toshi A. Furukawa, M.D., Ph.D.—The author has received research funds and speaking fees from Asahi Kasei, Astellas, Dai-Nippon, Sumitomo, Eisai, Eli Lilly, GlaxoSmithKline, Janssen, Kyowa Hakko, Meiji, Nikken Kagaku, Organon, Otsuka, Pfizer, and Yoshitomi. The author has received research funding from the Japanese Ministry of Education, Science, and Technology and the Japanese Ministry of Health, Labor, and Welfare.

Edward V. Nunes, M.D.—The author has received research support from Pfizer and GlaxoSmithKline.

Scott L. Rauch, M.D.—The author has received research funds through Massachusetts General Hospital from Medtronic, Inc., Cyberonics, and Cephalon. The author received honoraria from Novartis, Neurogen, Sepracor, and Medtronic, Inc. The author is a trustee at McLean Hospital and serves on the Board of the Massachusetts Society for Medical Research, as well as on the National Foundation of Mental Health Board.

Darrel A. Regier, M.D., M.P.H.—The author, as Executive Director of American Psychiatric Institute for Research and Education, oversees all federal and industry-sponsored research and research training grants in APIRE but receives no external salary funding or honoraria from any government or industry.

Murray B. Stein, M.D., FRCPC, M.P.H.—The author has received research support from Eli Lilly and GlaxoSmithKline. The author has been in a consultant for AstraZeneca, Avera Pharmaceuticals, BrainCells Inc., Bristol-Myers Squibb, Eli Lilly, EPI-Q Inc., Forest, Hoffmann-La Roche Pharmaceuticals, Integral Health Decisions Inc., Jazz Pharmaceuticals, Johnson & Johnson, Mindsite, Sanofi-Aventis, Transcept Pharmaceuticals, and Virtual Reality Medical Center.

The following contributors to this book do not have any conflicts of interest to disclose:

Mark D. Alter, M.D., Ph.D.
Gavin Andrews, M.D.
Carlos Blanco M.D., Ph.D.
Susan Bögels, Ph.D.
Timothy A. Brown, M.D.
Richard A. Bryant, Ph.D.
Shawn Cahill, Ph.D.
Wayne C. Drevets, M.D.
Thalia C. Eley, Ph.D.
Paul M.G. Emmelkamp, Ph.D.
Carlo Faravelli, M.D.
Edna B. Foa, Ph.D.
Abby J. Fyer, M.D.
HonaLee Harrington, B.A.
Rene Hen, Ph.D.
Jonathan D. Huppert, Ph.D.
Elie G. Karam, M.D.
William B. Lawson, M.D., Ph.D.
Peter McEvoy, Ph.D.
Richard J. McNally, Ph.D.
Daniel S. Pine, M.D.
Richie Poulton, Ph.D.
Ronald M. Rapee, Ph.D.
Tim Slade, Ph.D.
Elisabetta Truglia, M.D.
Hans-Ulrich Wittchen, Ph.D.
Rachel Yehuda, Ph.D.

PREFACE

Dennis S. Charney, M.D.
Gavin Andrews, M.D.

For more than half a century, the *Diagnostic and Statistical Manual of Mental Disorders* has both guided and spurred treatment and research on disorders of the mind, emotions, and behaviors. This resource has remained a vital force for all this time because it has continued to incorporate new knowledge, stemming both from the experiences of psychiatric clinicians as they work with patients in changing societies and cultures and from advances in the rapidly expanding neurological and behavioral sciences. DSM is now in one of its renewal periods. A broad cross-section of the psychiatric and scientific community—organized into workgroups by expertise—is working together to develop the fifth iteration, DSM-V.

Historically, psychiatric classifications have been organized around prevailing etiological theories of the times. However, the utility of this approach is limited by the validity of the etiological assumptions. Whereas DSM-III (American Psychiatric Association 1980) and DSM-IV (American Psychiatric Association 1994) were strictly atheoretical and descriptive, a major question now being asked is whether it might be time to explore linking DSM to developing etiological knowledge (Charney et al. 2002).

The American Psychiatric Association Pathophysiology Workgroup considered that although a diagnostic classification linked to etiology might improve treatment and prognostication, it probably would be years, even decades, before such linkage would be possible across the majority of psychiatric disorders. Yet might it be possible to link classification to etiology across a small number of related disorders?

One apparently related grouping of disorders consists of those disorders in which stress or fear appear to be contributory factors. These disorders also represent an increasingly urgent need for psychiatric care in populations and cultures around the world.

The Stress-Induced and Fear Circuitry Disorders Workgroup undertook to explore the possibility of linking classification and etiology along with other challenges for addressing treatment needs, and gaps in knowledge, for these disorders.

This workgroup met in Arlington, Virginia, on June 22–24, 2005. This monograph details the discussions of this international group, of which 11 of the 26 contributors were from countries outside the United States.

This workgroup focused on four disorders of interest, as covered in Part 1 of this volume: posttraumatic stress disorder (Friedman and Karam, Chapter 1); panic disorder and agoraphobia (Faravelli and colleagues, Chapter 2); social phobia (Bögels and Stein, Chapter 3); and specific phobias (Emmelkamp and Wittchen, Chapter 4). For these four types of disorders, two questions were asked (Part 2): whether the disorders were stable across the lifespan (Poulton and colleagues, Chapter 5), and whether the disorders formed a cohesive and distinct group (Fyer and Brown, Chapter 6). Discussions then focused, in Part 3, on how these disorders might affect minority populations differently (Lawson, Chapter 7); the etiology of the disorders, including gene–environment interactions (Eley, Chapter 8); neural mechanisms of normal fear and anxiety (Alter and Hen, Chapter 9); the role of cognitions (Huppert and colleagues, Chapter 10); the contributions of stress and psychosocial factors to these disorders (Rapee and Bryant, Chapter 11); neural structure and function (Rauch and Drevets, Chapter 12); neurochemistry and neuroendocrinology of the disorders (Yehuda, Chapter 13); and the roles and contributions of substance abuse to these disorders (Nunes, Chapter 14).

In the concluding chapter, insights gained from this workgroup, and the relevance of these insights to developing a research agenda for DSM-V that might, among other things, begin to link classification of these disorders to their underlying etiology, are discussed by Andrews and colleagues.

References

American Psychiatric Association: Diagnostic and Statistical Manual of Mental Disorders, 3rd Edition. Washington, DC, American Psychiatric Association, 1980

American Psychiatric Association: Diagnostic and Statistical Manual of Mental Disorders, 4th Edition. Washington, DC, American Psychiatric Association, 1994

Charney DS, Barlow DH, Botteron K, et al: A neuroscience research agenda to guide development of a pathophysiologically based classification system, in A Research Agenda for DSM-V. Edited by Kupfer DJ, First MB, Regier DE. Washington, DC, American Psychiatric Association, 2002, pp 31–84

PART 1

STRESS-INDUCED AND FEAR CIRCUITRY DISORDERS

1

POSTTRAUMATIC STRESS DISORDER

Matthew J. Friedman, M.D.
Elie G. Karam, M.D.

As we move toward a joint revision of DSM-IV-TR (American Psychiatric Association 2000) and ICD-10 (World Health Organization 1992), it will be important to examine what we have learned about posttraumatic stress disorder (PTSD) during the past 25 years. Such a review will provide a basis and guidance for any revisions in the diagnostic criteria for PTSD. To that end, we here consider these topics:

1. Might PTSD be a stress-related fear circuitry disorder?
2. What are the important differences between DSM-IV (American Psychiatric Association 1994) and ICD-10 relevant to PTSD?
3. What facts would support a change to any diagnostic criterion for PTSD?
4. What other diagnostic factors, such as categorical versus dimensional issues, should we consider?
5. How should we assess the contributions of comorbid disorders to PTSD?
6. What are the influences of cross-cultural factors on PTSD?
7. What are the contributions of developmental issues to PTSD?

It should be noted that this chapter does not address acute posttraumatic reactions, including acute stress disorder, a complex topic beyond the scope of the present review.

PTSD as a Stress-Related Fear Circuitry Disorder?

Animal research, fortified by brain imaging studies in humans, has identified neurocircuitry that mediates processing of threatening or fearful stimuli. Such stimuli activate the amygdala, which, in turn, produces outputs to the hippocampus (to mediate memory consolidation and spatial learning); orbital frontal cortex (to process memory of emotional events and choice behaviors); locus coeruleus/thalamus/hypothalamus (to mediate autonomic and fear reactions); and dorsal/ventral striatums (to instigate instrumental approach or avoidance behavior) (Davis and Whalen 2001).

In PTSD, the normal restraining influence of the medial prefrontal cortex, especially the anterior cingulate gyrus and orbitofrontal cortex, has been severely disrupted (Charney 2004; Vermetten and Bremner 2002). Furthermore, significant reduction in anterior cingulate gyrus volume has recently been detected in combat veterans with PTSD (Woodward et al. 2006). The resulting disinhibition of the amygdala increases the likelihood of recurrent fear conditioning because ambiguous stimuli are more likely to be misinterpreted as threatening; normal counterbalancing inhibitory prefrontal cortex restraint is nullified; and sensitization of key limbic nuclei may occur, thereby lowering the threshold for fearful reactivity (Charney 2004; Charney et al. 1993).

In addition to animal and brain imaging studies, Pavlovian fear conditioning has been repeatedly proposed as a model for PTSD in and of itself (Kolb 1989), as a component of a two-factor theory model (Keane et al. 1985), and within a cognitive context of activated fear networks (Foa and Kozak 1986; Lang 1977).

The great body of data on the human stress response has also provided a major theoretical and clinical context through which to explicate the pathophysiology of PTSD, with respect to both adrenergic hyperreactivity and hypothalamic-pituitary-adrenal (HPA) dysregulation (Charney 2004; Friedman and McEwen 2004; Southwick et al. 2007). In short, PTSD may exemplify the prototypical stress-related fear circuitry disorder.

This model has important implications for future, non-self-report diagnostic assessment and for understanding risk and protective factors for PTSD. Excellent recent reviews of non-self-report diagnostic assessment have addressed psychophysiological (Orr et al. 2004), neuropsychological (Knight and Taft 2004), neuroimaging (Kaufman et al. 2004a), and psychobiological (Friedman 2004) laboratory approaches. A comprehensive discussion of this topic is beyond the scope of this chapter; however, a few illustrative examples are provided.

POTENTIAL NONVERBAL DIAGNOSTIC IMPLICATIONS OF THE STRESS-RELATED FEAR CIRCUITRY MODEL

A major goal of all psychiatric diagnostic procedures has been to augment self-report assessment techniques (e.g., structured clinical interviews and questionnaires) with independent nonverbal laboratory procedures. That goal has not been achieved so far. There are two promising laboratory approaches that may, potentially, evolve into useful clinical techniques: a) PTSD symptoms can be triggered by exposing affected individuals to trauma-related stimuli; and b) several pharmacological probes have distinguished individuals with PTSD from those without the disorder.

In stimulus-driven paradigms, subjects are exposed to traumatic reminders. These may be trauma-related auditory or visual stimuli or brief individualized autobiographical narratives (e.g., "script driven imagery") of their unique traumatic experiences. The most robust results have been from studies in which psychophysiological measures have been obtained. After exposure to such stimuli, PTSD subjects exhibit greater cardiovascular, electrodermal, and electromyographic activity than non-PTSD comparison subjects (Blanchard et al. 1982; Malloy et al. 1983; Pitman et al. 1987). As summarized by Orr et al. (2004), tests of psychophysiological reactivity have successfully identified individuals with PTSD, with sensitivity values in the range of 60%–90% and specificity values of 80%. In general, subjects with greatest PTSD symptom severity were those who tended to exhibit the greatest physiological hyperreactivity (Keane et al. 1998; Orr et al. 2004). Thus, this approach had good sensitivity, but specificity was problematic because of a high number of false negatives.

Stimulus-driven protocols have also been used in brain imaging studies. In general, PTSD subjects exhibited greater amygdala activation and reduced activation of hippocampus and prefrontal cortex (Kaufman et al. 2004a). Although we are far from a routine clinical utilization of this approach for independent, nonverbal diagnostic assessment, stimulus-driven protocols hold promise for the future. They are also an elegant approach designed to activate psychobiological fear circuits through exposure to trauma-related stimuli.

A number of pharmacological probes have generated intriguing findings with PTSD subjects. Yehuda et al. (1993) tested their theory of enhanced negative feedback in the HPA system with the dexamethasone suppression test (DST). In contrast to subjects with major depression, in which challenge with the glucocorticoid dexamethasone produces nonsuppression of HPA activity, PTSD subjects exhibit supersuppression during the DST. This finding appears to be unique to PTSD patients, but it has not been tested widely enough to warrant endorsement as a clinical diagnostic test at this time (Friedman 2004).

A second pharmacological probe that has been evaluated is the α_2-adrenergic receptor antagonist yohimbine, whose action on these inhibitory receptors produces adrenergic disinhibition. As in patients with panic disorder, yohimbine can produce panic attacks in 60% of PTSD patients. In addition, it can produce PTSD flashbacks in approximately 40% of PTSD patients (Southwick et al. 1993). Furthermore, yohimbine has been shown to alter cerebral blood flow in PTSD patients in a manner consistent with excessive activation of the adrenergic system (Bremner et al. 1997).

Taken together, these findings, and others, suggest the possibility of translating laboratory protocols into practical, clinical diagnostic tests.

POTENTIAL GENETIC, COGNITIVE, AND NEUROSCIENTIFIC RISK FACTORS FOR THE DEVELOPMENT OF PTSD

Most pre-, peri-, and posttraumatic risk factors are derived from verbal reports. However, there are some intriguing genetic, cognitive, and neuroscientific risk factors to consider with respect to PTSD.

Genetic Factors

Genetic research with the Vietnam Era Twin Registry has shown that there are two heritable factors that predict PTSD. First, there are heritable differences in the likelihood that an individual will be exposed to a traumatic stressor. Second, there are heritable differences with regard to the likelihood that an individual exposed to a criterion A event will develop PTSD (Koenen et al. 2002; True et al. 1993). In addition, a genetically mediated shared familial vulnerability also contributes to PTSD itself as well as to the comorbidity of PTSD and major depression and the comorbidity of PTSD and dysthymia (Koenen et al. 2003).

Recent interest in the psychobiology of resilience has suggested a number of psychobiological mechanisms that might mediate resilience or vulnerability to developing PTSD after traumatic exposure (Charney 2004; Friedman 2002). One genetic mediator might be the serotonin transporter gene. Although it has not been demonstrated in PTSD, there is good evidence for a gene–environment interaction with respect to onset of depressive symptoms. In comparisons of large cohorts of individuals exposed to stressful environmental events, persons homozygous for the long allele of this gene tended to be resistant to depression, whereas those homozygous for the short allele tended to be most vulnerable to that disorder (Caspi et al. 2003; Kaufman et al. 2004b).

Cognitive Factors

Cognitive factors may also contribute to resilience or vulnerability. Given the fear conditioning model, it has been proposed that people who develop PTSD after traumatic exposure are those who are more susceptible to fear conditioning, more aroused by threatening stimuli, and more resistant to extinction after the danger has passed (Orr et al. 2000).

Neuroscientific Risk Factors

Three potential neuroscientific risk factors have emerged from recent research on structural magnetic resonance imaging and neurohormonal studies under stressful conditions. The first possible risk factor is suggested by magnetic resonance imaging findings from monozygotic twins recruited from the Vietnam Era Twin Registry and concerns hippocampal volume. This study compared Vietnam combat veterans with and without PTSD with their twin brothers who did not see military action in Vietnam. Whereas veterans with PTSD had smaller hippocampal volumes than veterans without PTSD, non-exposed twins of the PTSD cohort also had smaller hippocampal volumes, whereas non-exposed twin brothers of the non-PTSD combat veterans had larger hippocampal volumes. These results suggest that smaller hippocampal volume may be a risk factor for PTSD rather than a consequence of the disorder (Gilbertson et al. 2002).

The second finding comes from research with U.S. Special Forces troops exposed to an extremely stressful training experience during which sequential neurohormonal samples were obtained. Troops who had the greatest capacity to mobilize neuropeptide Y and to sustain such elevated levels throughout the training coped with the severe stress and performed much better than non–Special Forces troops who were unable to mobilize and sustain neuropeptide Y levels to the same extent (Morgan et al. 2000, 2001).

The third finding comes from research on firefighters from Australia on the auditory startle response, measured through orbicularis oculi (eyeblink) electromyograms and skin conductance responses to delivered acoustic stimuli. Initial findings from this prospective study (pre- and posttrauma) point to the possibility that elevated startle response could be a vulnerability factor for posttraumatic stress responses (Guthrie and Bryant 2005).

Differences Between DSM-IV and ICD-10

There are significant differences in the diagnostic criteria for PTSD in ICD-10 and DSM-IV (Table 1–1). Most notably, ICD-10 includes neither criterion A2 (discussed later) nor any of the numbing symptoms (criteria C4 through C7). On the other hand, psychogenic amnesia is much more prominent in ICD-10 than in DSM-IV. Neither diagnostic scheme includes dissociation, although dissociative symptoms are decisive in acute stress disorder. The two systems also differ with regard to onset of PTSD symptoms (criterion E): in ICD-10 onset must occur within 6 months of the trauma, whereas in DSM-IV, it cannot occur within the first month after trauma but may have its onset at any time (including many years) after the traumatic event—as in delayed-onset PTSD. Finally, the F criterion, functional impairment, found in all DSM-IV diagnoses is not included in ICD-10.

TABLE 1–1. Comparison between ICD-10 and DSM-IV diagnostic criteria for posttraumatic stress disorder (PTSD)

ICD-10	DSM-IV
A. Exposure to stressor	A1. Exposure to stressor
	A2. Emotional reaction to stressor
B. Persistent remembering of the stressor in one of the following: intrusive flashbacks, vivid memories or recurring dreams, experiencing distress when reminded of the stressor	Requires one or more of
	B1. Intrusive recollections
	B2. Distressing dreams
	B3. Acting/feeling as though event were recurring
	B4. Psychological distress when exposed to reminders
	B5. Physiological reactivity when exposed to reminders
C. Requires only one symptom of actual or preferred avoidance	Requires three or more of
	C1. Avoidance of thoughts, feelings, or conversations associated with the stressor
	C2. Avoidance of activities, places, or people associated with the stressor
	C3. Inability to recall
	C4. Diminished interest in significant activities
	C5. Detachment from others
	C6. Restricted affect
	C7. Sense of foreshortened future

TABLE 1–1. Comparison between ICD-10 and DSM-IV diagnostic criteria for posttraumatic stress disorder (PTSD) *(continued)*

ICD-10	DSM-IV

Either of D1 or D2:
  D1. inability to recall
  D2. two or more of
    Sleep problems
    Irritability
    Concentration problems
    Hypervigilance
    Exaggerated startle
	Two or more of
	  D1. Sleep problems
	  D2. Irritability
	  D3. Concentration problems
	  D4. Hypervigilance
	  D5. Exaggerated startle response

E. Onset of symptoms within 6 months of the stressor	E. Duration of the disturbance is at least 1 month
	F. Requires distress or impairment

Source. Reprinted from Peters L, Slade T, Andrews G. "A comparison of ICD-10 and DSM-IV criteria for posttraumatic stress disorder." *Journal of Traumatic Stress* 1999; 12: 335–343. Used with permission.

Peters et al. (1999) gathered data on 1,364 participants, utilizing the Composite International Diagnostic Interview (World Health Organization 1992) to diagnose PTSD according to both ICD-10 and DSM-IV criteria. DSM-IV was more restrictive, with only 3% of participants meeting the diagnostic criteria, in contrast to 7% meeting the ICD-10 criteria. This discrepancy was primarily attributable to criteria C and F. Among the 59 participants whose symptoms met the ICD-10 criteria for PTSD, 33 denied numbing of responsiveness (criterion C) and 35 denied clinically significant distress or impairment (criterion F). Surprisingly differences in criterion A (e.g., A2) and criterion E (onset) accounted for relatively few discrepancies.

These findings underscore the importance of developing a unified set of diagnostic criteria for PTSD for DSM-V and ICD-11.

Facts That Would Support a Change to Any Diagnostic Criterion

THE A (STRESSOR) CRITERION

ICD-10 criterion A defines *traumatic stress* as a "stressful event or situation…of an exceptional threatening or catastrophic nature…likely to cause pervasive distress in almost anyone" (World Health Organization 1992, p.344). For DSM-IV, significant changes were made in criterion A; it was divided into objective (A1) and subjective (A2) components in which the A1 criterion resembled the DSM-III-R (American Psychiatric Association 1987) criterion A, except that a greater number of events were approved as stressor events. Also, in DSM-IV, in addition to exposure to an A1 event, it was necessary that an exposed individual experience an intense emotional reaction (criterion A2) characterized as "fear, helplessness, or horror."

The A1 Criterion

As noted by Kilpatrick et al. (1998) in summarizing findings from the DSM-IV field trials, discussions over how to operationalize the A criterion boiled down to a debate over how broad versus how narrow criterion A should be. Proponents of a broad definition argued that criterion A should include any event that can produce PTSD symptoms, whereas advocates for a more restrictive definition feared that such a broad definition would trivialize the PTSD diagnosis and defeat the purpose of the original DSM-III (American Psychiatric Association 1980) PTSD construct by permitting people exposed to less stressful events to meet the A criterion. The DSM-IV field trials appeared to allay this concern, because few people developed PTSD unless they experienced extremely stressful life events. As a result, the DSM-IV A criterion expanded from the DSM-III definition of an experience that "would be markedly distressing to almost anyone" to that of a person having "experienced," "witnessed," or "been confronted by" a threat to physical integrity (O'Brien 1998). Breslau and Kessler (2001) tested the implications of this change in criterion A1 in a representative sample of 2,181 individuals in southeast Michigan who were interviewed about lifetime history of traumatic events and PTSD diagnosis. Lifetime exposure to traumatic events was 68.1% when estimated by a narrow set of qualifying A1 events that included seven events of "assaultive violence" (e.g., combat, rape, assault) and seven "other injury events" (e.g., serious accident, natural disaster, witnessing death/serious injury). When the A1 criterion was expanded to include "learning about" traumatic events to close relatives (e.g., rape, assault, accident), lifetime prevalence of exposure to traumatic events increased to 89.6%. These investigators concluded that there was a 59.2% increase in lifetime exposure to a traumatic event due to the expanded A1 criterion. These lifetime exposure estimates are considerably higher than estimates obtained from other studies (Kessler et al. 1995), indicating a problem with the expanded definition.

Other researchers have argued that it does not matter whether a broad or narrow definition is set for A1, suggesting that what really matters is whether people meet the other criteria (B, C, D, E, F) for PTSD and that it would make no difference if the A1 criterion were completely eliminated. For example, a recent study of 1,543 adults exposed to one of four Florida hurricanes found a PTSD prevalence of 11.2% (179 out of 1,543) with no A1 (or A2) requirement and 11.2% (173 out of 1,543) with requirement for A1 (but not A2) (Acierno et al. 2006). More extensive data on this question are currently being gathered by Ronald Kessler and collaborators, within the context of both the National Comorbidity Lifetime Study and a World Health Organization survey (Demyttenaere et al. 2004).

Complete elimination of criterion A was discussed by the DSM-IV PTSD Task Force. Although this group acknowledged the possibility that someone might meet the B, C, and D criteria without meeting the A criterion, the option was rejected for fear "that the loosening of Criterion A may lead to widespread and frivolous use of the concept" (Davidson and Foa 1991, p. 347).

Two more recent articles indicate that the full PTSD syndrome may be expressed after nontraumatic events. In a random sample of 2,997 Dutch adults, those ($n=519$) reporting adverse nontraumatic life events (such as chronic illness, marital discord, or unemployment) had higher average PTSD (B, C, and D) symptom severity scores than the 284 participants who met DSM-IV diagnostic criteria for PTSD (Mol et al. 2005). Similarly, among 454 American college undergraduates, PTSD symptom severity was higher among participants with nontraumatic stressors (such as death or illness of a loved one) than among those who met the full PTSD diagnostic criteria (Gold et al. 2005).

The A2 Criterion

Recognizing that traumatic stress, like pain, cannot be objectified because it has a major subjective component, the DSM-IV Task Force stipulated that exposure to an A1 event, per se, was not a sufficient condition for meeting the stressor criterion. Instead, the A2 criterion was introduced to ensure that exposure to an A1 event was associated with an intense subjective reaction characterized as "fear, helplessness, or horror." It was expected that imposition of the A2 criterion would ensure that people would not be eligible for a PTSD diagnosis unless they had reacted strongly to a threatening event. It was also expected that imposition of the A2 criterion would minimize any "frivolous" PTSD diagnoses that might result from broadening the A1 criterion. Finally, on the basis of data from the DSM-IV field trials (Kilpatrick et al. 1998) it was expected that few people exposed to low magnitude (nontraumatic) events would meet the A2 criterion and therefore would not be eligible for the PTSD diagnosis.

There are few studies to guide us concerning the utility of the A2 criterion. Brewin et al. (2000) found that intense levels of immediate post-exposure fear, helplessness, and horror were weakly predictive of PTSD 6 months later. They also found evidence that other posttraumatic emotional reactions (such as anger or shame) also predicted PTSD. There were, however, a small number of people in this study who denied post-exposure A2 emotions but met PTSD criteria at 6 months. Creamer et al. (2005) examined a community sample of 6,104 adults with a history of trauma exposure and found that most (76% males and 81% females) had symptoms that met criterion A2. In a study of PTSD symptomatology among undergraduate participants, Roemer et al. (1998) reported that only helplessness, and not fear or horror, correlated with posttraumatic symptoms. These authors also reported that peritraumatic emotional numbing predicted subsequent PTSD.

There are currently two negative studies about the utility of the A2 criterion. Kilpatrick et al. (1998), reporting on results from the DSM-IV field trials, found no effect of A2 on PTSD prevalence. Likewise, Schnurr et al. (2002) surveyed a sample of 436 older male military veterans and also found that presence or absence of A2 had no effect on PTSD prevalence. However, although the presence of A2 did not predict PTSD diagnosis, it did predict PTSD severity.

On the other hand, a consistent finding from three studies (Brewin et al. 2000; Kilpatrick et al. 1998; Schnurr et al. 2002) concerns the negative predictive value of A2. In other words, people who do not exhibit an intense posttraumatic emotional reaction are unlikely to develop PTSD. Schnurr et al. (2002) suggested that A2 may be most useful in screening out individuals unlikely to develop PTSD. Whereas this may be useful in postdisaster screening, it does not appear to have a major bearing on improving diagnostic accuracy.

In the DSM-IV field trials, Kilpatrick et al. (1998) reported that, rather than correlating with A2 symptoms, most of the variance of posttraumatic distress was accounted for by a panic reaction consisting of two components: "panic-physiological arousal" and "other panic symptoms" (such as trembling, shaking, tachycardia, and fear of dying). Other investigators have emphasized the positive predictive value of a fright reaction (Tarquinio et al. 2003; Vaiva et al. 2003) or peritraumatic autonomic activation (Bracha et al. 2004).

Taken together, these findings suggest that more research is needed to determine 1) the positive predictive value of a posttraumatic emotional/physiological response for the later development of PTSD and 2) the degree to which the nature of such a response conforms to the current A2 definition of "fear, helplessness, and horror."

Summarizing A1 and A2 Criteria

The few published studies that have addressed this matter have not validated the reconfiguration of the stressor criterion by the DSM-IV PTSD Task Force. Although an expanded A1 criterion has permitted more events to qualify as catastrophic stressors, it is not clear that the expansion has substantially increased PTSD prevalence estimates, despite some arguments to the contrary (Breslau and Kessler 2001). Nor does it appear that introduction of the A2 criterion has affected PTSD prevalence as originally intended. Furthermore, the major discrepancies between DSM-IV and ICD-10 PTSD prevalence appear to be related to absence of C (numbing) and F (functional status) criteria rather than to different definitions of the stressor criterion.

This review of the A criterion is based on the very few studies available. Hopefully, soon-to-be released findings from the National Comorbidity Lifetime Study and World Health Organization survey will help us sort out these questions with more confidence. However, the present evidence cannot refute recommendations to abolish the A or A1/A2 criterion entirely. We can expect that this question will be debated once again as we move closer to developing joint DSM-V/ICD-11 diagnostic criteria for PTSD.

THE B, C, AND D CRITERIA: FACTOR STRUCTURE OF PTSD AND OCCURRENCE OF SYMPTOMS

Factor Structure of PTSD

The DSM-IV PTSD construct consists of three symptom clusters, as represented by criteria B (re-experiencing), C (avoidant/numbing), and D (hyperarousal). Questions have been raised about how well this construct has held together in practice. In other words, are there three distinct symptom clusters? Are these three clusters subsumed by an overarching construct, the PTSD diagnosis?

A number of studies have utilized confirmatory factor analysis to examine whether the three DSM-IV symptom clusters are valid or whether other models might provide a better fit to the data. With this method, it has been possible to test a number of different models. Different investigators have found two-, three-, or four-factor models as the best fit for their data. As we review these findings, it is important to note that different PTSD assessment instruments were used by different investigators and that these instruments were administered to individuals whose PTSD developed from different types of traumatic experiences.

To our knowledge, there is only one study supporting the DSM-IV three-factor model. Foy et al. (1997), utilizing the Los Angeles Symptom Checklist with a variety of adult trauma populations, identified three highly correlated factors representing the DSM-IV symptom categories of reexperiencing, avoidance/numbing, and arousal. A second study with 5,664 child and adolescent survivors of Hurricane Hugo who were assessed with the PTSD Reaction Index suggested a different three-factor model: reexperiencing/active avoidance, numbing/passive avoidance, and arousal (Anthony et al. 1999).

Five studies have supported a four-factor model. Reexperiencing, avoidance, and arousal were distinct clusters in all five studies. The fourth factor, "numbing," was identified in four studies: Asmundson et al. (2000), utilizing the PTSD Checklist with referrals to a primary care clinic; King et al. (1998), utilizing the Clinician Administered PTSD Scale with male military veterans; Marshall (2004), utilizing the PTSD Checklist with young adult survivors of community violence after hospitalization for physical injuries; and McWilliams et al. (2005), utilizing the National Institute of Mental Health Diagnostic Interview Schedule with a PTSD-positive subsample from the National Comorbidity Survey. In a fifth study that utilized the PTSD Checklist with deployed Gulf War veterans, the fourth factor (in addition to reexperiencing, avoidance, and arousal) characterized as "dysphoria" (in which "numbing" was nested) provided a better fit than four-factor models in which numbing was the fourth factor (Simms et al. 2002). The authors acknowledged that dysphoria may represent a nonspecific component of disorders comorbid with PTSD.

Finally, three studies have supported a two-factor solution, although the specific factors were somewhat different. In two studies, the factors were characterized as reexperiencing/avoidance and hyperarousal/numbing. The first study utilized the PTSD Symptom Scale with both motor vehicle accident survivors and United Nations peacekeepers (Taylor et al. 1998), whereas the second survey utilized the Clinician Administered PTSD Scale to assess motor vehicle accident survivors (Buckley et al. 1998). The third study, which utilized the PTSD Checklist with Australian Vietnam veterans, found that a two-factor model, which included intrusion/hyperarousal and an avoidance factor, offered the best solution (Creamer et al. 2003).

Taken together, most confirmatory factor analyses do not support the three-factor DSM-IV model. They also suggest that serious consideration should be given to including a fourth, "numbing" symptom cluster in DSM-V and ICD-11.

It is noteworthy that we were unable to find any confirmatory factor analysis studies that tested the ICD-10 model. Because lack of numbing symptoms in ICD-10 was one of the major reasons for observed discrepancies between ICD-10 and DSM-IV (Peters et al. 1999), and given that a numbing factor has been detected in most of the studies testing the DSM-IV three-factor model, it would seem that numbing symptoms should be included in ICD-11.

Frequency of Occurrence of Symptoms

The definition of a threshold of frequency for occurrence of symptoms (once or less vs. twice or more per week) doubled the prevalence of PTSD in a study on war and non-war trauma in an epidemiological study (Karam et al. 1996). Thus, adoption of frequency criteria for the three PTSD symptom clusters could have a major impact on prevalence estimates. Replication of this finding in other settings could help clarify this issue further. This issue is of practical importance in structured interviews and potentially of importance in biological research. When considering a dimensional approach, assessing symptom frequency could be helpful in characterizing different spectra of PTSD symptom expression and might have a bearing on explication of subsyndromal clinical presentations.

THE E (DURATION) CRITERION

A major difference between DSM-IV and ICD-10 concerns the E criterion. In DSM-IV, PTSD may be diagnosed at any time after a traumatic event, except during the first month. In ICD-10, PTSD can only be diagnosed within 6 months of exposure to the stressful event.

The DSM-IV rationale is that a 1-month window must be allowed before diagnosing PTSD in order to permit normal recovery to occur and to avoid pathologizing normal acute posttraumatic distress. A more significant, and controversial, difference between the two diagnostic systems is that DSM-IV recognizes delayed-onset PTSD, whereas ICD-10 does not. Sometimes the interval between trauma and positive diagnosis may be of many years' duration.

This aspect of DSM-IV has had a significant impact in compensation claims in which the claimant may not have exhibited PTSD symptoms for many years. As reviewed by Bryant and Harvey (2002), delayed onset may represent unrecognized PTSD, subsyndromal PTSD that later escalates to the full syndrome, or a true delay of syndrome onset. These authors conducted a prospective study with 103 motor vehicle accident survivors among whom five patients who had not met the PTSD criteria at 6 months, met the full criteria 2 years after the accident. Similar findings have been reported with American Gulf War veterans who did not exhibit PTSD at the time of demobilization but who did so 18–24 months later (Wolfe et al. 1999).

These findings suggest that delayed-onset PTSD does occur. It is unclear whether it is more likely to occur following military, civilian-accident, or natural-disaster trauma (it appears to be very uncommon in the last-mentioned [Norris et al. 2003]). The preponderance of evidence suggests that DSM-V and ICD-11 should retain DSM-IV's capacity to diagnose delayed-onset PTSD.

THE F (FUNCTIONAL IMPAIRMENT) CRITERION

The biggest discrepancy between PTSD-positive individuals as diagnosed by ICD-10 and DSM-IV, respectively, is due to the importance of functional capacity, the F criterion, which is absent from the former and present in the latter. As stated previously, among 59 individuals who met the ICD-10 PTSD criteria, 35 failed to meet the DSM-IV criteria because they denied clinically significant distress or impairment. This issue not only concerns PTSD but applies globally to all psychiatric diagnoses classified within the two systems. Within the PTSD context, however, it is particularly pertinent because of ongoing concern about how to set a diagnostic threshold that is high enough to filter out normal posttraumatic distress but low enough to identify people with posttraumatic symptomatology that is clinically significant and potentially responsive to evidence-based treatments for PTSD, and with an underlying pathophysiology that conforms to the best biopsychosocial model of this disorder.

Some recent evidence from the postdisaster field suggests that acute posttraumatic functional impairment is a better prognostic indicator of subsequent PTSD than symptom severity (Norris et al. 2002a, 2002b; North and Westerhaus 2003). Norris et al. (2003) have shown that functional impairment is the best single predictor of duration of PTSD symptoms. Furthermore, because we consider posttraumatic stress as a dimensional state, spanning a spectrum of reactions from normal distress to PTSD, one can make a good argument that we should draw the diagnostic line at the point of functional incapacity or immobilization.

If we take such a step, however, we will need to do a much better job operationalizing "functional incapacity" than is currently done by using the 0–100 Global Assessment of Function (GAF) scale. Our suggestion is that a separate DSM-V/ICD-11 task force be charged to develop hard and fast criteria for assessing functional capacity across many pertinent domains in which it is clinically significant, including marriage, family, interpersonal/social, vocational/scholastic, self-care, dangerousness to self or others, disability status, activities of daily living, and quality of life. Thorp and Stein (2005) have recently written an excellent guide to the published literature on PTSD and functioning.

Greater emphasis on a well-operationalized F criterion would also address many concerns discussed previously with respect to the narrowness or breadth of the A criterion. Such complicated discussions may become moot if the focus shifts from qualifying versus nonqualifying (e.g., "traumatic") stressors to the symptom severity and functional impact due to exposure to such events. This argument was first proposed by Kilpatrick et al. (1998) after the DSM-IV field trials. It is also a line of reasoning that supports the proposal to completely abolish the A criterion. Should that occur in DSM-V and ICD-11, PTSD would take its place alongside almost all other psychiatric diagnoses where the focus is on symptomatic and functional clinical significance rather than on causal factors.

On the other hand, one of us (E.G.K.) feels that there is much to be gained from considering impairment as a separate dimensional attribute of PTSD (and other DSM-V psychiatric diagnoses). Although this author agrees that a threshold is needed for public health, medicolegal, and epidemiologic studies, he believes that the available research evidence suggests that although dysfunction is a clear marker for psychopathology, it should not be a sine qua non criterion for a diagnosis, and that the nonrecognition, by the subject, of dysfunction (in its present definition) is not necessarily equal to normality. For example, if comorbidity of depression is considered a clear marker of abnormality (regardless of subjective assessment of dysfunction), subjects with PTSD who report little or no dysfunction still exhibit two to three times the prevalence of comorbid depression when compared with subjects with no PTSD (Karam 1997). This author therefore suggests changing the current PTSD F (functional impairment) criterion to a dimensional assessment of level of impairment (e.g., not present, some, and a lot) and possibly defining specific thresholds for scientific or for clinical purposes. Thus, when diagnosing PTSD (and the other psychiatric diagnoses), one would first determine presence of the full syndrome (vs. partial: see subsection "Partial/Subsyndromal PTSD" below) and then rate the degree of impairment would be rated as absent or present (with two or three degrees of severity).

The first author (M.J.F.) does not share this view and believes that it is essential to keep the impairment criterion as a necessary criterion for making the diagnosis.

Categorical Versus Dimensional Issues
PARTIAL/SUBSYNDROMAL PTSD

If one reviews the number of accepted depressive diagnoses between DSM-I (American Psychiatric Association 1952) and DSM-IV, it is notable that there has been a substantial increase in such disorders over time. In DSM-I, only two diagnoses, psychotic depression and manic-depressive disorder, were admissible. Many more have been added since that time, including dysthymia, depression not otherwise specified, and depressive character disorder.

For PTSD, the situation is quite different. Rather than a spectrum of diagnostic options that characterize the variety of clinical presentations in which dysphoria and anhedonia are cardinal features, there is only one official diagnosis for people with intrusion, avoidant/numbing, and hyperarousal symptoms after exposure to an extremely stressful event. Either you have PTSD or you do not, and if you do not, you may not be eligible for clinical services or third-party reimbursement because you do not fit into any official diagnostic category. Adjustment disorders do not meet this diagnostic need because, by definition, they are transient, not chronic problems.

In recent years, more than 50 publications have reported on the prevalence or morbidity of "partial" or "subsyndromal" PTSD. Findings from population surveys and clinical samples have identified a cohort of individuals who had been exposed to an extremely stressful event; failed to meet full PTSD criteria; exhibited a number of B, C, and D symptoms; met the F criterion for functional impairment; and exhibited clinically significant symptoms. Generally, the partial PTSD cohort has exhibited less symptom severity and functional impairment than the full PTSD group but more symptom severity than a comparison group that met neither full nor partial PTSD diagnostic criteria (Breslau et al. 2004; Carlier and Gersons 1995; Lipschitz et al. 2000; Mylle and Maes 2004; Schnurr et al. 2000; Stein et al. 1997; Taylor and Koch 1995; Weiss et al. 1992; Zlotnick et al. 2004).

One problem with this literature is that different criteria have been used from one study to the next, ranging from an individualized adjudication process (Weiss et al. 1992) to hard-and-fast criteria that vary from one investigation to the next (e.g., see Breslau et al. 2004; Schnurr et al. 2000). Zlotnick et al. (2004) cautioned that, when considering partial PTSD, it may be important to distinguish between individuals who previously met full PTSD criteria and are now in partial remission from those who have never met full diagnostic criteria.

Mylle and Maes (2004) argued that subthreshold and partial PTSD syndromes that meet the F criterion should be regarded as specific nosological categories. We agree that the F criterion should be an important component of any partial/subthreshold PTSD diagnosis. We also think that strict diagnostic criteria are necessary.

COMPLEX PTSD/DISORDERS OF EXTREME STRESS NOT OTHERWISE SPECIFIED

Many clinicians who have worked with individuals exposed to severe and protracted traumatic exposure (most notably childhood sexual abuse and torture within the context of political incarceration) argue that the most significant clinical sequelae are not delineated by the PTSD construct. Although such individuals often do meet DSM-IV/ICD-10 PTSD criteria, the most debilitating symptoms include behavioral difficulties (such as impulsivity, aggression, sexual acting out, alcohol/drug misuse, and self-destructive actions); emotional difficulties (such as affective lability, rage, depression, and panic); cognitive difficulties (such as dissociation, amnesia, and pathological changes in personal identity [dissociative identity disorder]); interpersonal difficulties; and somatization (Herman 1992; Linehan et al. 1994).

There was a spirited discussion by the DSM-IV Task Force about whether to include complex PTSD/disorders of extreme stress not otherwise specified (DES-

NOS) in DSM-IV. This proposal was not adopted because results from the DSM-IV field trials indicated that 92% of individuals with complex PTSD/DESNOS also met criteria for PTSD. Under the circumstances, it was decided that there was little scientific support for this new diagnosis and that it would be superfluous to include it as a separate nosological category. For purposes of the present discussion, we mention complex PTSD/DESNOS as a posttraumatic syndrome that does not necessarily conform to the PTSD construct but might merit its own niche within a dimensional PTSD construct.

OTHER POSTSTRESS (TRAUMATIC/NONTRAUMATIC STRESS) SYNDROMES

If we shift from a psychiatric to a medical focus, it is noteworthy that, in medicine, the major emphasis is on "stress," per se, rather than "traumatic stress." Indeed, there is a rich literature, dating back to the seminal work of Selye (1946) and reiterated by Chrousos and Gold (1992) and McEwen (1998), showing how chronic stress might produce medical illness. McEwen and Stellar (1993) proposed the concept of "allostatic load" as an explanatory model for how the biological alterations associated with chronic stress (especially the downstream consequences of heightened HPA axis function) might increase the risk for medical illness. Friedman and McEwen (2004) later illustrated the applicability of the allostatic load model to PTSD. They showed that there was considerable, but not complete, overlap between biological alterations observed in chronic stress syndromes and those detected in PTSD. Such a theoretical orientation integrates a wealth of scientific evidence showing that prevalence of medical illness is greater among people with PTSD than among those without the disorder (Schnurr and Green 2004).

For purposes of the present discussion, these observations raise two diagnostic questions: 1) Should there be a category of posttraumatic medical disorders? and 2) Should there be a psychiatric chronic stress disorder in which "chronic stress" is not restricted to "traumatic stress" as defined by the A criterion?

With regard to the first question, there are emerging data showing higher prevalence of cardiovascular, gastrointestinal, endocrinological, musculoskeletal, and immunological disorders associated with PTSD (Schnurr and Green 2004). Furthermore, there are recognized diseases such as chronic fatigue syndrome and fibromyalgia that defy traditional mind–body distinctions between medical and psychiatric diagnoses, in which exposure to stress is clearly a precipitating factor and the syndrome exhibits a combination of traditional medical and traditional psychiatric symptoms. As we consider poststress (traumatic or nontraumatic stress) syndromes within a dimensional context, it is important to recognize that two different dimensions are under consideration: 1) the dimensionality of the stressor (e.g., traumatic vs. nontraumatic); and 2) how such stress exposure might be expressed: PTSD, partial PTSD, complex PTSD/DESNOS, medical illness, and so on. One difference between adverse medical outcomes associated with PTSD and those associated with chronic stress might have to do with the duration of exposure. Whereas chronic stress syndrome results from protracted exposure, PTSD-related medical disorders might require only a brief period of traumatization that is sufficient to precipitate a full-fledged PTSD syndrome.

The second question concerns the legitimacy of nontraumatic stress as a precipitant for a psychiatric syndrome that might be called "post–severe stress syndrome." There is evidence to support such a proposal. First, as discussed previously, two recent studies have reported higher PTSD symptom severity among individuals with nontraumatic life events (such as chronic illness, death of a loved one, marital discord, or unemployment) than among individuals with PTSD (Gold et al. 2005; Mol et al. 2005). Furthermore, the full PTSD syndrome has been observed in medical patients in whom the stressful event was a nontraumatic illness, such as AIDS (Martinez et al. 2002), breast cancer (Amir and Ramati 2002), cancer (Redd et al. 2001), and lymphoma (Geffen et al. 2003).

Comorbidity

Data from the National Comorbidity Study indicate that 80% of individuals with PTSD will meet criteria for at least one other psychiatric disorder (Kessler et al. 1995). The most common coexisting disorders with PTSD include major depressive disorder (MDD), dysthymia, simple phobia, social phobia, panic disorder, generalized anxiety disorder (GAD), alcohol abuse/dependence, and drug abuse/dependence. It is noteworthy that the three other Axis I disorders proposed for the stress-related fear circuitry disorder category—panic disorder, simple phobia, and social phobia—are on this list.

One reason for so much comorbidity is the overlap in symptoms that characterize different psychiatric disorders. For example, PTSD shares symptoms of autonomic arousal with panic disorder and GAD and impaired concentration and insomnia with GAD and depression. It has been suggested previously that extensive comorbidity is an artifact of a diagnostic system that relies entirely on phenomenology.

On the other hand, a reason for this high comorbidity might simply reside not only in the setting and nature of the traumata but also in the specifics of the recipient (subject); these and a plethora of distal factors could lead not only to a "true" comorbidity of MDD and PTSD but also to MDD without PTSD as evidenced in epidemiological studies. Independent laboratory assessment procedures are needed to move beyond our current phenomenological nosological system. For example, the DST indicates that depression comorbid with PTSD (e.g., PTSD/MDD) may have a different underlying pathophysiology than true melancholia (MDD). Whereas the former is often associated with DST supersuppression, the latter is generally associated with DST nonsuppression (Friedman and Yehuda 1995). Given these divergent DST results, we must consider whether comorbid PTSD/MDD is really a depressive subtype of PTSD rather than the co-occurrence of two distinct diagnostic entities, PTSD and MDD.

Cross-Cultural Factors

The PTSD diagnosis has been criticized from a cross-cultural perspective as a Euro-American construct that has little relevance to posttraumatic syndromes encountered in traditional societies (Summerfield 2004). Furthermore, two cardinal symptoms of posttraumatic reactions in traditional societies, somatization and dissociation (Kirmayer 1996), are missing from both DSM-IV and ICD-10 diagnostic criteria for PTSD. Although there may be culture-specific idioms of distress that provide a better characterization of chronic posttraumatic distress syndromes found in one ethnocultural context or another (Marsella et al. 1996), PTSD has been documented throughout the world (Green et al. 2003). In multiple studies, de Jong et al. (2001) and Karam et al. (2006, 2008) have documented a high prevalence of PTSD in non-Western nations subjected to war or internal conflict such as Algeria, Cambodia, Lebanon, Palestine, and the former Yugoslavia. One difficulty with this issue is that it has been difficult to find similar traumatic events affecting people from widely different cultures. North et al. (2005) recently reported on a comparison between Kenyan survivors of the bombing of the American embassy in Nairobi and American survivors of the bombing of the federal building in Oklahoma City. Both events were remarkably similar with respect to death, injury, destruction, and other consequences. Similar too was PTSD prevalence among Africans and Americans exposed to each traumatic event, respectively.

As proposed by Osterman and de Jong (2007), the time has come for the fields of mental health and anthropology to end the debate about the validity of the PTSD diagnosis. These authors argued that what is needed is a "culturally competent model of traumatic stress" that addresses how culture may differentially influence explanatory models of traumatic stress, how it is implicated in the appraisal of risk/protective factors, and how such understanding might contribute to diagnosis and treatment.

Developmental Issues

A thorough discussion of PTSD, within a developmental context, is beyond the scope of the present paper. This topic refers to changes in appraisal and reaction to traumatic events as well as to differences in expression of posttraumatic distress at either end of the life span. For understanding the problems of children who have experienced traumatic events, a developmental context must incorporate the dynamic and evolving relationship among experience, neurological processing, and brain development. It must also address self-regulation from a developmental perspective because it appears to be a central problem for children with traumatic stress (Saxe et al. 2007). For older individuals, a developmental approach must seek to understand age-specific psychosocial, behavioral, and neurobiological factors that mediate and moderate trauma-related symptom expression and clinical course (Cook and Niederehe 2007).

A comprehensive, longitudinal developmental approach is also needed to explicate how memories for traumatic events are differentially encoded, stored, and retrieved by the immature and developing brain.

Conclusion

A stress-related fear-circuitry disorders model appears to provide an excellent context within which to conceptualize PTSD. Such a model has important implications for non-self-report diagnostic assessment strategies and for understanding risk and protective factors for PTSD. (It should be noted that this overview has only addressed the applicability of this model to PTSD and not to acute stress reactions or acute stress disorder.)

1. There are important differences between DSM-IV and ICD-10 that will need to be reconciled in DSM-V and ICD-11. Major inconsistencies appear to involve the lack of criterion C (numbing) and functional capacity (criterion E) in ICD-10.
2. Any revisions in PTSD diagnostic criteria need to address the following: a) discrepancies in the A criterion between the two systems; b) apparent failure of the A2 criterion to improve diagnostic precision in DSM-IV; c) omission of numbing symptoms from ICD-10; d) discrepancies in the E (onset) criterion between the two systems; and e) lack of the F (functional capacity) criterion in ICD-10. The suggestion that impairment should become an independent dimension rather than a diagnostic criterion is the opinion of one of the authors (E.G.K.).
3. There is substantial evidence suggesting that posttraumatic and post-nontraumatic stress syndromes should be understood as dimensional rather than categorical disorders. This applies especially to partial/subsyndromal PTSD, for which the data are strongest, and could apply also to the severity/frequency of occurrence of symptoms and the accompanying impairment/dysfunction.
4. Extensive comorbidity found in DSM-IV and ICD-10 may be an artifact of a diagnostic system that relies entirely on phenomenology. An alternative scheme might, for example, consider a depressive subtype of PTSD rather than comorbid PTSD and MDD. On the other hand, true comorbidities may be

present because trauma has been shown to induce depression without PTSD as well as other non-PTSD Axis I disorders. Resolution of this important question may have to await identification of specific neurobiological factors associated with one disorder or another. It will be possible to address this question only when we have a better understanding of the pathophysiology of PTSD so that we can determine how much it is unique and how much it overlaps with depression and other psychiatric disorders.
5. Although there are culture-specific posttraumatic idioms of distress, PTSD appears to characterize a universal human response to trauma that may be influenced by cultural factors.
6. Our understanding of PTSD is based mostly on evidence obtained with young and middle-aged adults. There are developmental issues at either end of the life span that should inform diagnostic assessment.
7. The growing body of evidence from neuroimaging, neurochemical, and psychophysiological studies should pave the way for a better refinement of our diagnostic measures.

References

Acierno R, Ruggiero KJ, Kilpatrick DG, et al: Risk and protective factors for psychopathology among older versus younger adults after the 2004 Florida hurricanes. Am J Geriatr Psychiatry 14:1051–1059, 2006

American Psychiatric Association: Diagnostic and Statistical Manual: Mental Disorders. Washington, DC, American Psychiatric Association, 1952

American Psychiatric Association: Diagnostic and Statistical Manual of Mental Disorders, 3rd Edition. Washington, DC, American Psychiatric Association, 1980

American Psychiatric Association: Diagnostic and Statistical Manual of Mental Disorders, 3rd Edition, Revised. Washington, DC, American Psychiatric Association, 1987

American Psychiatric Association: Diagnostic and Statistical Manual of Mental Disorders, 4th Edition. Washington, DC, American Psychiatric Association, 1994

American Psychiatric Association: Diagnostic and Statistical Manual of Mental Disorders, 4th Edition, Text Revision. Washington, DC, American Psychiatric Association, 2000

Amir M, Ramati A: Post-traumatic symptoms, emotional distress and quality of life in long-term survivors of breast cancer: a preliminary research. J Anxiety Disord 16:195–206, 2002

Anthony JL, Lonigan CJ, Hecht SA: Dimensionality of posttraumatic stress disorder symptoms in children exposed to disaster: results from confirmatory factory analysis. J Abnorm Psychol 108:326–336, 1999

Asmundson GJG, Frombach I, McQuaid JR, et al: Dimensionality of posttraumatic stress symptoms: a confirmatory factor analysis of DSM-IV symptom clusters and other symptom models. Behav Res Ther 38:203–214, 2000

Blanchard EB, Kolb LC, Pallmeyer, et al: A psychophysiological study of post traumatic stress disorder in Vietnam veterans. Psychiatr Q 54:220–229, 1982

Bracha HS, Williams AE, Haynes SN, et al: The STRS (shortness of breath, tremulousness, racing heart, and sweating): a brief checklist for acute distress, with panic-like sympathetic indicators; development and factor structure. Ann Gen Hosp Psychiatry 3(1):8, 2004

Bremner JD, Innis RB, Ng CK, et al: PET measurement of central metabolic correlates of yohimbine administration in posttraumatic stress disorder. Arch Gen Psychiatry 54:146–156, 1997

Breslau N, Kessler RC: The stressor criterion in DSM-IV posttraumatic stress disorder: an empirical investigation. Biol Psychiatry 50:699–704, 2001

Breslau N, Lucia VC, Davis GC: Partial PTSD versus full PTSD: an empirical examination of associated impairment. Psychol Med 34:1205–1214, 2004

Brewin CR, Andrews B, Rose S: Fear, helplessness, and horror in posttraumatic stress disorder: investigating DSM-IV criterion A2 in victims of violent crime. J Trauma Stress 13:499–509, 2000

Bryant RA, Harvey AG: Delayed-onset posttraumatic stress disorder: a prospective evaluation. Aust N Z J Psychiatry 36:205–209, 2002

Buckley TC, Blanchard EB, Hickling EJ: A confirmatory factor analysis of posttraumatic stress symptoms. Behav Res Ther 36:1091–1099, 1998

Carlier IV, Gersons BP: Partial posttraumatic stress disorder (PTSD): the issue of psychological scars and the occurrence of PTSD symptoms. J Nerv Ment Dis 183:107–109, 1995

Caspi A, Sugden K, Moffitt TE, et al: Influence of life stress on depression: moderation by a polymorphism in the 5HTT gene. Science 301:386–389, 2003

Charney DS: Psychobiological mechanisms of resilience and vulnerability: implications for the successful adaptation to extreme stress. Am J Psychiatry 161:195–216, 2004

Charney DS, Deutch AY, Krystal JH, et al: Psychobiologic mechanisms of posttraumatic stress disorder. Arch Gen Psychiatry 50:295–305, 1993

Chrousos GP, Gold PW: The concepts of stress and stress system disorders: overview of physical and behavioral homeostasis. JAMA 267:1244–1252, 1992

Cook JM, Niederehe G: Trauma in older adults, in Handbook of PTSD: Science and Practice. Edited by Friedman MJ, Keane TM, Resick PA. New York, Guilford, 2007, pp 252–276

Creamer M, Bell R, Failla S: Psychometric properties of the Impact of Event Scale–Revised. Behav Res Ther 41:1489–11496, 2003

Creamer M, McFarlane AC, Burgess P: Psychopathology following trauma: the role of subjective experience. J Affect Disord 86:175–182, 2005

Davidson JR, Foa EB: Diagnostic issues in posttraumatic stress disorder: considerations for the DSM-IV. J Abnorm Psychol 100:346–355, 1991

Davis M, Whalen PJ: The amygdala: vigilance and emotion. Mol Psychiatry 1:13–34, 2001

de Jong JT, Komproe IH, Van Ommeren M, et al: Lifetime events and posttraumatic stress disorder in 4 postconflict settings. JAMA 286:555–562, 2001

Demyttenaere K, Bruffaerts R, Posada-Villa J, et al: Prevalence, severity, and unmet need for treatment of mental disorders in the World Health Organization World Mental Health Surveys. JAMA 291:2581–2590, 2004

Foa EB, Kozak MJ: Emotional processing of fear: exposure to corrective information. Psychol Bull 99:20–35, 1986

Foy DW, Wood JL, King DW, et al: Los Angeles Symptom Checklist: psychometric evidence with an adolescent sample. Assessment 4:377–384, 1997

Friedman MJ: Future pharmacotherapy for PTSD: prevention and treatment. Psychiatr Clin North Am 25:427–441, 2002

Friedman MJ: Psychobiological laboratory assessment of PTSD, in Assessing Psychological Trauma and PTSD, 2nd Edition. Edited by Wilson JP, Keane TM. New York, Guilford, 2004, pp 419–438

Friedman MJ, McEwen BS: PTSD, allostatic load, and medical illness, in Trauma and Health: Physical Health Consequences of Exposure to Extreme Stress. Edited by Schnurr PP, Green BL. Washington, DC, American Psychological Association, 2004, pp 157–188

Friedman MJ, Yehuda R: Post-traumatic stress disorder and comorbidity: psychobiological approaches to differential diagnosis, in Neurobiological and Clinical Consequences of Stress: From Normal Adaptation to Post-traumatic Stress Disorder. Edited by Friedman MJ, Charney DS, Deutch AY. Philadelphia, PA, Lippincott-Raven, 1995, pp 429–445

Geffen DB, Blaustein A, Amir M, et al: Post-traumatic stress disorder and quality of life in long-term survivors of Hodgkin's disease and non-Hodgkin's lymphoma in Israel. Leuk Lymphoma 44:1925–1929, 2003

Gilbertson MW, Shenton ME, Ciszewski A, et al: Smaller hippocampal volume predicts pathologic vulnerability to psychological trauma. Nat Neurosci 5:1242–1247, 2002

Gold SD, Marx SP, Soler-Baillo JM, et al: Is life stress more traumatic than traumatic stress? J Anxiety Disord 19:687–698, 2005

Green BL, Friedman MJ, de Jong J, et al: Trauma Interventions in War and Peace: Prevention, Practice, and Policy. Amsterdam, The Netherlands, Kluwer Academic/Plenum, 2003

Guthrie R, Bryant R: Auditory startle response in firefighters before and after trauma exposure. Am J Psychiatry 162:283–290, 2005

Herman JL: Complex PTSD: a syndrome in survivors of prolonged and repeated trauma. J Trauma Stress 5:377–391, 1992

Karam EG: Comorbidity of posttraumatic stress disorder and depression, in Posttraumatic Stress Disorder: Acute and Long-Term Responses to Trauma and Disaster. Edited by Fullerton CS, Ursano RJ. Washington, American Psychiatric Press, 1997, pp 77–90

Karam EG, Noujeim JC, Saliba SE, et al: PTSD: how frequently should the symptoms occur? The effect of epidemiologic research. J Trauma Stress 9:899–905, 1996

Karam EG, Mneimneh Z, Karam AN, et al: Prevalence and treatment of mental disorders in Lebanon: a national epidemiological survey. Lancet 367:1000–1006, 2006

Karam EG, Mneimneh Z, Fayyad JA, et al: Lifetime prevalence of mental disorders in Lebanon: first onset, treatment, and exposure to war. PLoS Med 5:e61, 2008

Kaufman J, Aikins D, Krystal J: Neuroimaging studies in PTSD, in Assessing Psychological Trauma and PTSD, 2nd Edition. Edited by Wilson JP, Keane TM. New York, Guilford, 2004a, pp 389–418

Kaufman J, Yang BZ, Douglas-Palumberi H, et al: Social supports and serotonin transporter gene moderate depression in maltreated children. Proc Natl Acad Sci USA 101:17316–17321, 2004b

Keane TM, Zimering RT, Caddell JM: A behavioral formulation of posttraumatic stress disorder in Vietnam veterans. Behav Ther 8:9–12, 1985

Keane TM, Kolb LC, Kaloupek DG, et al: Utility of psychophysiological measurement in the diagnosis of posttraumatic stress disorder: results from a Department of Veterans Affairs Cooperative Study. J Consult Clin Psychol 66:914–923, 1998

Kessler RC, Sonnega A, Bromet E, et al: Posttraumatic stress disorder in the National Comorbidity Survey. Arch Gen Psychiatry 52:1048–1060, 1995

Kilpatrick DG, Resnick HS, Freedy JR, et al: Posttraumatic stress disorder field trial: evaluation of the PTSD construct—criteria A through E, in DSM-IV Sourcebook, Vol 4. Edited by Widiger TA, Frances AJ, Pincus HA, et al. Washington, DC, American Psychiatric Association, 1998, pp 803–844

King DW, Leskin GA, King LA, et al: Confirmatory factor analysis of the Clinician-Administered PTSD Scale: evidence for the dimensionality of posttraumatic stress disorder. Psychol Assess 10:90–96, 1998

Kirmayer LJ: Confusion of the senses: implications of ethnocultural variations in somatoform and dissociative disorders for PTSD, in Ethnocultural Aspects of Posttraumatic Stress Disorder: Issues, Research, and Clinical Applications. Edited by Marsella AJ, Friedman MJ, Gerrity ET, et al. Washington, DC, American Psychological Association, 1996, pp 131–163

Knight JA, Taft CT: Assessing neuropsychological concomitants of trauma and PTSD, in Assessing Psychological Trauma and PTSD, 2nd Edition. Edited by Wilson JP, Keane TM. New York, Guilford, 2004, pp 344–388

Koenen KC, Harley RM, Kyons MJ, et al: A twin registry study of familial and individual risk factors for trauma exposure and posttraumatic stress disorder. J Nerv Ment Dis 190:209–218, 2002

Koenen KC, Lyons MJ, Goldberg J, et al: A high risk twin study of combat-related PTSD comorbidity. Twin Res 6:218–226, 2003

Kolb LC: Heterogeneity of PTSD (letter). Am J Psychiatry 146:811–812, 1989

Lang PJ: Imagery in therapy: an information processing analysis of fear. Behav Ther 8:862–886, 1977

Linehan MM, Tutek DA, Heard HL, et al: Interpersonal outcome of cognitive behavioral treatment for chronically suicidal borderline patients. Am J Psychiatry 151:1771–1776, 1994

Lipschitz DS, Rasmusson AM, Anyan W, et al: Clinical and functional correlates of posttraumatic stress disorder in urban adolescent girls at a primary care clinic. J Am Acad Child Adolesc Psychiatry 39:1104–1111, 2000

Malloy PF, Fairbank JA, Keane TM: Validation of a multimethod assessment of posttraumatic stress disorders in Vietnam veterans. J Consult Clin Psychol 51:488–494, 1983

Marsella AJ, Friedman MJ, Gerrity ET, et al (eds): Ethnocultural Aspects of Post-traumatic Stress Disorder: Issues, Research and Clinical Applications. Washington, DC, American Psychological Association, 1996

Marshall GN: Posttraumatic stress disorder symptom checklist: factor structure and English-Spanish measurement invariance. J Trauma Stress 17:223–230, 2004

Martinez A, Israeliski D, Walker C, et al: Posttraumatic stress disorder in women attending human immunodeficiency virus outpatient clinics. AIDS Patient Care STDs 16: 283–291, 2002

McEwen BS: Protective and damaging effects of stress mediators. N Engl J Med 338:171–179, 1998

McEwen BS, Stellar E: Stress and the individual: mechanisms leading to disease. Arch Intern Med 153:2093–2101, 1993

McWilliams LA, Cox BJ, Asmundson GJG: Symptom structure of posttraumatic stress disorder in a nationally representative sample. J Anxiety Disord 19:626–641, 2005

Mol SSL, Arntz A, Metsemakers JFM, et al: Symptoms of post-traumatic stress disorder after non-traumatic events: evidence from an open population study. Br J Psychiatry 186:494–499, 2005

Morgan CA, Wang S, Southwick SM, et al: Plasma neuropeptide-Y concentrations in humans exposed to military survival training. Biol Psychiatry 47:902–909, 2000

Morgan CA, Wang S, Rasmusson A, et al: Relationship among plasma cortisol, catecholamines, neuropeptide Y, and human performance during exposure to uncontrollable stress. Psychosom Med 63:412–422, 2001

Mylle J, Maes M: Partial posttraumatic stress disorder revisited. J Affect Disord 78:37–48, 2004

Norris FH, Friedman MJ, Watson PJ: 60,000 disaster victims speak, part I: an empirical review of the empirical literature, 1981–2001. Psychiatry 65:207–239, 2002a

Norris FH, Friedman MJ, Watson PJ: 60,000 disaster victims speak, part II: summary and implications of the disaster mental health research. Psychiatry 65:240–260, 2002b

Norris FH, Murphy AD, Baker CK, et al: Severity, timing, and duration of reactions to trauma in the population: an example from Mexico. Biol Psychiatry 53:769–778, 2003

North CS, Westerhaus ET: Applications from previous disaster research to guide mental health interventions after the September 11 attacks, in Terrorism and Disaster: Individual and Community Mental Health Interventions. Edited by Ursano RJ, Fullerton CS, Norwood AE. Cambridge, UK, Cambridge University Press, 2003, pp 93–106

North CS, Pfefferbaum B, Narayanan P, et al: Comparison of post-disaster psychiatric disorders after terrorist bombings in Nairobi and Oklahoma City. Br J Psychiatry 186:487–493, 2005

O'Brien LS: What constitutes a stressor? in Traumatic Mental Health. Edited by O'Brien LS. Cambridge, UK, Cambridge University Press, 1998, pp 119–143

Orr SP, Metzger LJ, Lasko NB: De novo conditioning in trauma-exposed individuals with and without posttraumatic stress disorder. J Abnorm Psychol 109:290–298, 2000

Orr SP, Metzger LJ, Miller MW, et al: Psychophysiological assessment of PTSD, in Assessing Psychological Trauma and PTSD, 2nd Edition. Edited by Wilson JP, Keane TM. New York, Guilford, 2004, pp 289–343

Osterman JE, de Jong JE: Cultural issues in trauma, in Handbook of PTSD: Science and Practice. Edited by Friedman MJ, Keane TM, Resick PA. New York, Guilford, 2007, pp 425–446

Peters L, Slade T, Andrews G: A comparison of ICD-10 and DSM-IV criteria for posttraumatic stress disorder. J Trauma Stress 12:335–343, 1999

Pitman RK, Orr SP, Forgue DF, et al: Psychophysiologic assessment of posttraumatic stress disorder imagery in Vietnam combat veterans. Arch Gen Psychiatry 44:970–975, 1987

Redd WH, DuHamel KN, Vickberg SMJ, et al: Long-term adjustment in cancer survivors: integration of classical-conditioning and cognitive-processing models, in Psychosocial Interventions for Cancer. Edited by Baum AS, Andersen BL. Washington, DC, American Psychological Association, 2001, pp 77–97

Roemer L, Orsillo SM, Borkovec TD, et al: Emotional response at the time of a potentially traumatizing event and PTSD symptomatology: a preliminary retrospective analysis of the DSM-IV criterion A-2. J Behav Ther Exp Psychiatry 29:123–130, 1998

Saxe GN, MacDonald HZ, Ellis H: Psychosocial approaches for children with posttraumatic stress disorder, in Handbook of PTSD: Science and Practice. Edited by Friedman MJ, Keane TM, Resick PA. New York, Guilford, 2007, pp 359–375

Schnurr PP, Green BL (eds): Trauma and Health: Physical Health Consequences of Exposure to Extreme Stress. Washington, DC, American Psychological Association, 2004

Schnurr PP, Ford JD, Friedman MJ, et al: Predictors and outcomes of posttraumatic stress disorder in World War II veterans exposed to mustard gas. J Consult Clin Psychol 68:258–268, 2000

Schnurr PP, Spiro A, Vielhauer MJ, et al: Trauma in the lives of older men: findings from the Normative Aging Study. Journal of Clinical Geropsychology 8:175–187, 2002

Selye H: The general adaptation syndrome and the diseases of adaptation. J Clin Endocrinol 6:117–230, 1946

Simms LJ, Watson D, Doebbeling BN: Confirmatory factor analysis of posttraumatic stress symptoms in deployed and nondeployed veterans of the Gulf War. J Abnorm Psychol 111:637–647, 2002

Southwick SM, Krystal JH, Morgan CA, et al: Abnormal noradrenergic function in posttraumatic stress disorder. Arch Gen Psychiatry 50:266–274, 1993

Southwick SM, Davis LL, Aikins DE, et al: Neurobiological alterations associated with PTSD, in Handbook of PTSD: Science and Practice. Edited by Friedman MJ, Keane TM, Resick PA. New York, Guilford, 2007, pp 166–189

Stein MB, Walker JR, Hazen AL, et al: Full and partial posttraumatic stress disorder: findings from a community survey. Am J Psychiatry 154:1114–1119, 1997

Summerfield DA: Cross-cultural perspectives on the medicalization of human suffering, in Posttraumatic Stress Disorder: Issues and Controversies. Edited by Rosen GM. Chichester, UK, Wiley, 2004, pp 233–245

Tarquinio C, Tarquinio P, Costantini ML: Sentiment d'effroi. ESPT et altération du Soi chez des victimes de hold-up (Fright reaction, PTSD and self concept among victims of a hold-up). Rev Francoph Stress Trauma 3:99–109, 2003

Taylor S, Koch WJ: Anxiety disorders due to motor vehicle accidents: nature and treatment. Clin Psychol Rev 15:721–738, 1995

Taylor S, Kuch K, Koch WJ, et al: The structure of posttraumatic stress symptoms. J Abnorm Psychol 107:154–160, 1998

Thorp SR, Stein MB: Posttraumatic stress disorder and functioning. PTSD Res Q 16:1–7, 2005

True WR, Rice J, Eisen SA, et al: A twin study of genetic and environmental contributions to liability for posttraumatic stress symptoms. Arch Gen Psychiatry 50:257–264, 1993

Vaiva G, Brunet A, Lebigot F: Fright (Effroi) and other peritraumatic responses after a serious motor vehicle accident: prospective influence on acute PTSD development. Can J Psychiatry 48:395–401, 2003

Vermetten E, Bremner JD: Circuits and systems in stress, II: applications to neurobiology and treatment in posttraumatic stress disorder. Depress Anxiety 16:14–38, 2002

Weiss DS, Marmar CR, Schlenger WE, et al: The prevalence of lifetime and partial posttraumatic stress disorder in Vietnam theater veterans. J Trauma Stress 5:365–376, 1992

Wolfe J, Erickson DJ, Sharkansky EJ, et al: Course and predictors of posttraumatic stress disorder among Gulf War veterans: a prospective analysis. J Consult Clin Psychol 67:520–528, 1999

Woodward SH, Kaloupek DG, Streeter CC, et al: Decreased anterior cingulate volume in combat-related PTSD. Biol Psychiatry 59:582–587, 2006

World Health Organization: The ICD-10 Classification of Mental and Behavioural Disorders: Clinical Descriptions and Diagnostic Guidelines. Geneva, World Health Organization, 1992

Yehuda R, Southwich SM, Krystal JH, et al: Enhanced suppression of cortisol following dexamethasone administration in posttraumatic stress disorder. Am J Psychiatry 150:83–86, 1993

Zlotnick C, Rodriguez BF, Weisberg RB, et al: Chronicity in posttraumatic stress disorder and predictors of the course of posttraumatic stress disorder among primary care patients. J Nerv Ment Dis 192:153–159, 2004

2

PANIC DISORDER

Carlo Faravelli, M.D.
Toshi A. Furukawa, M.D., Ph.D.
Elisabetta Truglia, M.D.

The existence of a syndrome characterized by recurrent paroxysmal anxiety within the more general diagnosis of anxiety neurosis/neurasthenia was recognized by most of the textbooks of psychiatry before 1980. The concept of panic disorder, however, began with Donald Klein's (1964) observation that paroxysmal anxiety was selectively responsive to imipramine. In 1980, with the publication of DSM-III (American Psychiatric Association 1980), the neuroses were abolished and panic disorder was formalized as an independent disorder. Seven years later, in DSM-III-R (American Psychiatric Association 1987), agoraphobia with panic attacks was inserted into the category of panic disorder. In DSM-IV (American Psychiatric Association 1994), there was a minor but important change in the conceptualization of agoraphobia, which was defined as avoidance in anticipation of panic.

The rationale for the creation of panic disorder in 1980 and for the subsequent modifications was largely based on Klein's original assumptions that 1) patients with panic attacks respond preferentially to antidepressants, whereas patients with generalized anxiety respond to anxiolytics; 2) the first panic attack occurs abruptly and unexpectedly in people with no evidence of temperamental or prodromic features; and 3) agoraphobia not preceded by panic does not exist. From this perspective, panic attacks are seen as a pathological, primary phenomenon central to the origin of the disorder. Their association with agoraphobia is interpreted as a secondary or derived avoidance behavior phenomenon, both etiopathogenetically and chronologically (Klein 1981, 1987). The panic attack is seen as a predominantly biological event, qualitatively distinct from the other forms of anxiety. Because agoraphobia is only considered a consequence of panic, agoraphobia is not considered to occur in the absence of panic.

This position never received general agreement, despite being supported by a variety of findings, including clinical observations and findings from challenge studies (Bourin et al. 1995; Charney and Heninger 1986; Charney et al. 1984; Woods et al. 1988), electroencephalographic sleep studies (Arriaga et al. 1996), and brain imaging studies (Rauch et al. 2003). In particular, there was a debate during the years 1980–1990, when this position (usually referred to as "the American view") was challenged by several European authors who put forth a "European view" (Faravelli et al. 2001). This latter position contends that panic per se is neither specific nor pathological. Panic becomes pathological when its occurrence is combined with some specific premorbid vulnerability factors. The European position maintains that a phobic attitude precedes the development of panic and that specific temperamental features and vulnerability to environmental events are necessary in order for panic disorder to occur.

There are findings to support the European position. All community epidemiological studies report the presence of a consistent rate of subjects affected by agoraphobia without panic attacks (Andrews and Slade 2002; Andrews et al. 2001; Angst and Dobler-Mikola 1985; Bijl et al. 1998; Faravelli et al. 1989; Goodwin et al. 2005; Jacobi et al. 2004; Kringlen et al. 2001; Pirkola et al. 2005; Weissman et al. 1985; Wittchen 1986). Patients affected by panic disorder were reported to show prodromal symptoms before the onset of the disorder (Fava and Mangelli 1999; Fava et al. 1988, 1992; Garvey et al. 1988; Lelliott et al. 1989). The presence of personality and temperamental traits predisposing to agoraphobia is also supported by empirical verification (Cassano et al. 1997; Perugi et al. 1998; Roth and Argyle 1988; Shear et al. 2001, 2002).

As often happens, findings used to support either position lend themselves to different interpretations. On one hand, none of the findings supporting the American view could be unequivocally interpreted as supporting the biological origin of panic. The response to a challenge, for instance, could be seen as the intrapsychic dramatization of bodily sensations rather than as a specific substance response. On the other hand, the findings in favor of the European view could be equally biased: the absence of panic before agoraphobia, for instance, could simply result from inadequate interviewing or recall bias. Klein's three assumptions themselves may be wrong. The selective response to antidepressants is certainly not true (Ballenger et al. 1988; Pohl et al. 1994); the existence of agoraphobia not preceded by panic, although at lower rates than reported by previous studies, has been repeatedly confirmed; and the "out of the blue" onset of panic disorder has been strongly questioned (Fava and Mangelli 1999).

The Panic Attack

Panic attack is defined as a brief period of intense fear accompanied by some symptoms. DSM-III required 4 symptoms from a list of 13—a requirement that remained constant in DSM-III-R and DSM-IV. This definition is precise and allows recognition of the panic attack, but it is questionable with regard to some aspects.

CRITERION SYMPTOMS

The list of criterion symptoms is unsorted. However, the symptoms could be grouped into three categories: a) autonomic symptoms (basically due to sympathetic activation), b) psychic symptoms (fear of dying, losing control, going crazy), and c) a third group of symptoms of less clear interpretation (derealization/depersonalization, dizziness). Another possible categorization would be the division between objectively observable symptoms (e.g., tachycardia, trembling) and subjectively reported ones (e.g., choking, fainting, dizziness, fear). The range of symptoms seems to be largely in agreement. Only a few studies do not agree with the symptom list; according to some authors, some of the symptoms not included in the list—especially "urge to escape"—would be more prevalent than some of those symptoms that are included (Cox et al. 1996; Hollifield et al. 2003; Neerakal and Srinivasan 2003). ICD-10 (World Health Organization 1992) includes "dry mouth." We were unable to find any empirical study that addressed the differential validity of these 13 criterion symptoms.

NUMBER OF SYMPTOMS REQUIRED

The diagnostic criteria require that a minimum number of symptoms are present for a diagnosis to be made. This implies that a threshold must be attained. Patients who have sudden attacks of anxiety but who report fewer than four symptoms are generally considered "subthreshold." There is a fairly good literature concerning these subthreshold or "limited symptom panic attacks" (Katerndahl 1990, 1999; Katerndahl and Realini 1993, 1998; Krystal et al. 1991; Rosenbaum 1987; Shioiri et al. 1997). The number of symptoms required for an attack (4 of 13) is totally arbitrary. Whereas typical full-blown attacks usually involve more than four symptoms, there is agreement that the limited-symptom attack may be as disabling as the full-blown one in terms of severity, outcome, comorbidity, and risk factors (Klerman et al. 1991). Within the same individuals with panic disorder, limited-symptom attacks were less severe but were otherwise similar to full-blown panic attacks (Krystal et al. 1991). Work disability was primarily confined to panic disorder patients, however, thus providing partial support to the 4-of-13 threshold (Katerndahl and Realini 1998).

MODE OF ONSET

DSM-III-R and DSM-IV require an attack to reach its peak within 10 minutes of the beginning of the first symptom. Two studies question the validity of this requirement. Among German adolescents with panic attacks, only 65% reported that the attack got worse within the first 10 minutes (Essau et al. 1999). Of 864 respondents to a panic disorder questionnaire, 18% reported long onset, but these did not differ significantly from those with rapid-onset panic on any clinical characteristics (Scupi et al. 1997).

SUBTYPES OF PANIC ATTACK

The different types of panic attack described in DSM-III and DSM-IV have been compared in several studies: expected versus unexpected panic attacks (Craske et al. 1990; Rachman et al. 1987; Street et al. 1989), and situational versus spontaneous panic attacks (Krystal et al. 1991).

The distinction between unexpected, situationally predisposed, and situationally bound attacks seems difficult—and possibly unnecessary—to operationalize. The distinction between predictable and unpredictable attacks (i.e., when there is temporal discontinuity between the cue and the attack) is likely to be simpler and clinically more valid (Barlow et al. 1994; Fava and Mangelli 1999).

PANIC ATTACK IN THE ABSENCE OF PANIC DISORDER

Panic attacks occur in disorders other than panic disorder and can be an indicator of greater severity of that disorder (Furukawa et al. 1995). Moreover, in community-based longitudinal follow-up studies of cohorts of children and adolescents, preexisting panic attacks significantly increased the risk of onset of a range of anxiety and substance use disorders (Goodwin et al. 2004b). The panic attack may occasionally occur in otherwise healthy people without any particular pathological consequence (so-called sporadic or infrequent panic attacks). Sporadic panic has been reported to affect many people, exceeding all the other types of panic (Telch et al. 1989; Vollrath et al. 1990). Two possibilities can be suggested:

1. The panic attacks in themselves are not intrinsically pathological; in most cases they do not reoccur and do not result in consequences on social adaptation or quality of life; other factors are necessary in order for them to evolve into clearly pathological forms.
2. Sporadic panic attacks represent a weaker subpathological form of panic disorder; in this case an early recognition of this form would be essential in order to prevent their evolution into disorders of increased intensity.

From Panic Attack to Panic Disorder

According to DSM-III and DSM-III-R, a minimum number of panic attacks in a given time period was required for the diagnosis of panic disorder. However, several subsequent studies showed that there was no difference in clinical characteristics or levels of disability between frequent and infrequent panics (Katerndahl 1990; Katon et al. 1995). On the basis of these observations, DSM-IV now places less emphasis on the frequency of attacks. Instead, the criterion has changed into the presence of recurrent unexpected attacks and the requirement that at least one of the attacks be followed by 1 month (or more) of one (or more) of the following: persistent concern about having additional attacks; worry about the implications of the attack or its consequences; or a significant change in behavior related to the attacks. These criteria have shown improved sensitivity without loss of specificity (Fyer et al. 1996).

THE PRODROME

The following quotations summarize the disputed issue of the onset of panic disorder.

> Patients are often feeling quite well when they suddenly are struck by a panic attack. (Klein 1981)

> Even though the first attack of panic often develops 'out of the blue,' more detailed investigation will usually reveal that the disorder has not emerged out of an entirely clear sky and that the complex repertoire of avoidance behaviours and helpless dependence on others were not entirely without premorbid antecedents. (Roth 1984)

> The large majority of patients (90%) suffer from mild phobic or hypochondriacal symptoms before the onset of panic attacks. Anxiety and hypochondriacal fears and beliefs are also exceedingly common. (Fava et al. 1988)

Basically, these statements subsume the three positions debated during the 1980s, which were

1. Phobic symptoms are mere consequences of the repeated panic attacks (Katerndahl 2000; Klein 1981, 1987). The panic attack is the central and primitive feature, and anticipatory anxiety and agoraphobia are the comprehensible psychological consequences of the recurrent, unpredictable panics. Agoraphobia not preceded by panic cannot exist. The panic attack is also seen as a primarily biological phenomenon, the origin of which is in some brain dysfunction. Biochemical (Bell and Nutt 1998; Redmond and Huang 1979) and brain imaging studies (Rauch et al. 2003), the possibility of inducing panic chemically

(Bourin et al. 1995), and the specific response to some drugs (Klein 1964) are all in accordance with this interpretation.
2. Panic disorder is the exacerbation of a preexisting phobic attitude (Marks 1983; Roth 1984). This position contends that a phobic attitude (cognition, temperament, traits) precedes the first panic attack and that the disorder derives by the abnormal (phobic) psychological response to an otherwise nonspecific phenomenon such as the panic attack. The presence of agoraphobia without panic in epidemiological studies, the presence of "neurotic" traits before the onset of the first panic attack (Fava and Mangelli 1999; Fava et al. 1988; Marks 1969, 1983; Roth 1984), and the fact that the first unexpected attack generally occurs in public places (Faravelli et al. 1992; Lelliott et al. 1989) are used to support this interpretation.
3. Panic disorder derives from the association of panic attacks with a phobic attitude (Andrews and Slade 2002; Goisman et al. 1994, 1995b; Goodwin and Hamilton 2001; Goodwin et al. 2004b; Reed and Wittchen 1998; Shear et al. 2001, 2002; Wittchen et al. 1998b). Both the somatic predisposition (including autonomic vulnerability [Bystritsky et al. 2000; Coupland et al. 2003; Faravelli et al. 1997; McCraty et al. 2001; Perugi et al. 1998; Shioiri et al. 2004; Tanabe et al. 2004]) to panic symptoms and preexisting phobic attitudes are necessary for the complete, typical presentation of panic disorder. Panic disorder or agoraphobia may occur singly or together without presumption of any particular causal sequence.

Classification systems vary according to the relative prevalence of these positions at the time. In 1980 DSM-III considered three separate categories: panic disorder, agoraphobia with panic disorder, and agoraphobia without panic disorder. However, a number of investigators (Buller et al. 1986; Garvey and Tuason 1984; Klein 1981) began to argue that agoraphobia was not a separate entity but rather a secondary response to panic disorder. They reported that agoraphobia before the onset of panic attacks was uncommon and that panic disorder and agoraphobia were similar in their clinical presentation. Studies of familial transmission of panic disorder and agoraphobia further supported the concept of agoraphobia as a more severe variant of panic rather than a separate entity (Noyes et al. 1986). Thus, consistent with this body of research, DSM-III-R reclassified agoraphobia as mainly a sequel of panic disorder, which could itself present either with or without agoraphobia, and this classification is maintained in DSM-IV. Agoraphobia without panic remained in these classification systems because of the repeated reports that agoraphobia without panic, although rare in the clinical practice of psychiatry, was continuing to be reported in community surveys. DSM-III-R and DSM-IV therefore emphasize panic as the central feature, with agoraphobia as a complication. ICD-10, conversely, classifies the association of panic and agoraphobia among phobic disorders, thus accepting the position that the phobic attitude is the core aspect of this disorder.

PHOBIC COGNITIONS AND ATTITUDES

A panic attack is made up of autonomic symptoms and fear or feelings of losing control. The same symptoms may be found in a variety of conditions, and some people experience a panic attack without developing panic disorder. Some classifications require either a minimum number of attacks or, following an attack, "persistent concern about having another panic attack, worry about the possible implications or consequences of the panic attack, a significant change in behavior related to the panic attack" (American Psychiatric Association 1994, p. 402).

The risk of having another panic attack does not justify entirely the overconcern experienced by these subjects: people at risk of more unpredictable and more dangerous pathological attacks (e.g., epileptic seizures) do not develop such fears. One key factor may be anxiety sensitivity, which refers to fears of anxiety-related sensations. It has three factors: physical concerns ("It scares me when I am short of breath"), mental incapacitation concerns ("When I am nervous, I worry that I am mentally ill"), and social concerns ("It is important to me not to appear nervous") (McNally 2002). Anxiety sensitivity has been shown to be a risk factor for occurrence of spontaneous panic attacks in two cohort studies (Schmidt et al. 1997, 1999). Gardenswarts and Craske (2001) impressively demonstrated the etiological role of anxiety sensitivity in a randomized controlled trial in which 14% of those with high anxiety sensitivity developed panic disorder in contrast to 2% of those with low anxiety sensitivity. Conversely, experience of a panic attack or general distress increases anxiety sensitivity (Schmidt et al. 2000). Anxiety sensitivity along with good heartbeat perception predicted non-remission of panic disorder in a 1-year prospective study (Ehlers 1995).

Cognitive therapists posit that these fears of anxiety-related sensations are based on catastrophic misinterpretation of certain body sensations (Clark 1986). These cognitive interpretations appear to be more cogent in explaining the maintenance of panic disorder than in explaining its onset. Patients avoid feared consequences rather than feared situations, and they seek safety instead of anxiety reduction. Thus the person afraid of fainting sits down, and the person afraid of having a heart attack refrains from exercising. By engaging in these in-situation safety behaviors, the patient not only experiences immediate relief but also unwittingly protects his or her catastrophizing belief from facing its disconfirmation. Each panic attack will now be interpreted as another "near miss" in which a safety behavior prevented the feared catastrophe (Salkovskis et al. 1999). Phobic attitudes/cognitions (avoidant behaviors, excessive concerns about health, excessive anticipation, intrusive repetitions, need for control, and "what if" thoughts) are common among people, without being necessarily associated with mental disorders (Guidano 1987; Marks 1969). It is possible to surmise, therefore, that panic disorder requires the combination of somatic (autonomic) vulnerability (Bystritsky et al. 2000; Coupland et al. 2003; Faravelli et al. 1997; McCraty et al. 2001; Perugi et al. 1998; Shioiri et al. 2004; Tanabe et al. 2004) and phobic cognitions/attitudes (Fava and Mangelli 1999; Fava et al. 1988; Marks 1969; Perugi et al. 1998; Roth 1984; Shear et al. 2001, 2002).

SUBTYPES OF PANIC DISORDER

DSM-IV does not provide any subtypes for panic disorder except for the presence/absence of agoraphobia. Whether it will be clinically more useful to have different subtypes (as with schizophrenia) or specifiers (as with mood disorders) is an empirical question. Some classifications of panic attacks that have been suggested include

1. Type 1 (classic or respiratory), type 2 (anticipatory panic attack), and type 3 (cognitive) (Ley 1992)
2. Derealization, cardiac, and respiratory panic (Bovasso and Eaton 1999, based on predominant symptoms according to Epidemiological Catchment Area study)
3. Cardio-respiratory symptoms versus pseudoneurological symptoms (Massana et al. 2001, based on predominant symptoms of experimentally induced panic attacks)
4. Early and late-onset panic with and without fear/anticipatory anxiety at the first attack (Goodwin and Hamilton 2001, based on clinically derived panic subtypes according to National Comorbidity Survey)
5. Early onset, agoraphobia, and dyspnea (Goodwin et al. 2002, based on clinically derived panic subtypes according to National Comorbidity Survey)
6. Prototypic, cognitive, and non-fearful panic (Schmidt et al. 2002, based on the coupling or decoupling of verbal-cognitive and physiological symptoms)
7. With nocturnal attacks (Craske and Barlow 1989; Krystal et al. 1991; Norton et al. 1999)
8. Fearful versus nonfearful (Beitman et al. 1987, 1990, 1992, 1993; Fleet et al. 2000; Schmidt et al. 2002)

The clinical significance of these subtypes has yet to be established. Overall, the differences seem to be of minor importance, because these subtypes of panic attacks are substantially similar in terms of severity, outcome, comorbidity, and risk factors (Bovasso and Eaton 1999; Goodwin et al. 2002; Norton et al. 1999; Schmidt et al. 2002). One probable exception to this may be the nonfearful panic attack, because patients with such attacks tend not to seek psychiatric treatment and if they do, it is more difficult to recognize their signs and symptoms as panic.

For example, among cardiology patients with atypical or nonanginal chest pain, 37% had panic disorder, and of these, 32% had nonfearful panic attacks and were not very different from fearful panic attack subjects, except that they showed less anticipatory anxiety and agoraphobic avoidance (Beitman et al. 1987; Kushner and Beitman 1990).

In addition to chest pain and tachycardia, vomiting and paresthesia can be limited-symptom panic attacks (Rosenbaum 1987). Twenty-three percent of neurological patients with negative medical workup met criteria for nonfearful panic disorder. In addition, these patients all experienced panic upon lactate infusion and responded to antipanic medication (Russell et al. 1991). Inclusion of one word, *discomfort,* in DSM-III-R and DSM-IV in addition to *fear* in DSM-III may therefore not suffice. Establishing this group as having a clearly defined panic disorder subtype would aid in the accurate identification and treatment of their condition (Kushner and Beitman 1990).

Agoraphobia

DSM-IV defines *agoraphobia* as avoidance in the expectation (fear) of panic, whereas in DSM-III and DSM-III-R the fear was more general (fear of sudden incapacitation). This clearly reflects the acceptance of the position according to which agoraphobia is a direct consequence of panic. The definition of *agoraphobia* is therefore gradually shifting from "fear of open spaces" (Spitzer et al. 1978) to "fear of places from which escape is difficult" (DSM-III), to "panicophobia" (DSM-IV, DSM-IV-TR [American Psychiatric Association 2000]). Thus the problem of the existence of agoraphobia without panic is solved tautologically. But does agoraphobia without panic really exist?

EPIDEMIOLOGICAL STUDIES

In clinical studies, agoraphobia without panic is almost nonexistent, whereas it is common in epidemiological studies. Table 2–1 summarizes the rate of agoraphobics without panic in studies that adopted DSM-III or DSM-III-R criteria.

It is true that 62%–95% of individuals diagnosed with agoraphobia without panic on the basis of the Composite International Diagnostic Interview (CIDI), University of Michigan-CIDI, and Munich-CIDI or the Diagnostic Interview Schedule failed on reinterview to be rediagnosed as having agoraphobia (Andrews and Slade 2002; Horwath et al. 1993; Weissman and Merikangas 1986; Wittchen et al. 1998b). The fact remains, however, that there is a substantial proportion of subjects who avoid public places or open spaces without having ever experienced a panic attack. In the Sesto Fiorentino study, an epidemiological survey conducted by clinical interviewers (Faravelli et al. 2004a, 2004b), 75 subjects met the crite-

TABLE 2–1. Percentage of individuals with agoraphobia without panic in community and clinical samples

Study	Agoraphobia N	Agoraphobia without panic N	%
Epidemiological studies			
Angst and Dobler-Mikola 1985	22	15	68
Wittchen 1986	26	13	50
Joyce et al. 1989	76	35	46
Thompson et al. 1989	104	88	85
Horwath et al. 1993	961	656	68
Clinical studies			
Di Nardo et al. 1983	23	0	0
Torgersen 1983	26	8	31
Thyer et al. 1985	28	0	0
Argyle 1986	42	5	12
Breier et al. 1986	54	0	0
Noyes et al. 1986	67	0	0
Barlow 1988	42	1	2
Pollard et al. 1989	993	61	6

rion of "marked fear and avoidance of being in places or situations from which escape might be difficult or help not promptly available in case of occurrence of any of symptoms of panic." Of these 75 subjects, 56 had panic attacks (always preceding agoraphobia) and 19 had no lifetime history of unexpected attacks. These subjects were reinterviewed by clinical psychiatrists with research experience in the field of anxiety disorders. There were no significant differences between the two groups regarding age at onset of the agoraphobia, the family concentration, the types of situations avoided, or the severity of agoraphobia (measured by the total score of the Mobility Inventory for Agoraphobia [Chambless et al. 1985]). The only significant difference was found in the answer to the question "Why do you avoid?," for which the answer "because of the fear of panic" was given by 50% of respondents with agoraphobia and panic attacks compared with less than 20% of those without attacks.

Therefore, the question of whether agoraphobia can occur in the absence of panic remains relevant to the definition of agoraphobia. If we accept a broader definition of agoraphobia, focusing on the avoidance rather than on the reported reason for avoidance, it seems that the relationship of agoraphobia to panic is less simple than usually thought.

PANIC–AGORAPHOBIC SPECTRUM

The concept of "spectrum" is conceptually different from that of "subthreshold." In this case, the nearness to the core of the disorder is viewed as qualitative rather than quantitative (*subthreshold* is "a bit less" than the typical disorder, whereas *spectrum* is "similar" to the typical disorder). The term *spectrum* is presently used in psychopathology with various meanings, but it generally indicates a group of manifestations having something in common. The *panic-agoraphobic spectrum* (Cassano et al. 1997; Shear et al. 2001, 2002) is defined as a combination of symptoms and signs correlated to the disorder as defined by the current diagnostic manuals: nuclear and accessory symptoms of panic disorder, atypical symptoms, isolated symptoms and signs, and temperamental and personality traits.

The panic-agoraphobic spectrum has been reported to be able to identify subjects who show clinically significant features without meeting DSM-IV criteria for any diagnosis (Cassano et al. 1997; Frank et al. 2005; Grunhaus and Birmaher 1985; Shear et al. 2001, 2002) and to predict the possible evolution in panic disorder (Perugi et al. 1998).

Comorbidity of Panic Disorder

The comorbidity of anxiety disorders with one another and with other disorders is common both in clinical (Brawman-Mintzer et al. 1993; Cassano et al. 1999; Garyfallos et al. 1999; Goisman et al. 1995a; Lecrubier and Weiller 1997; Maser 1998; Segui et al. 1995) and in community samples (Andrews et al. 1990, 2001, 2002; Angst 1992, 1993; Aoki et al. 1994; Degonda and Angst 1993; Merikangas and Angst 1995; Regier et al. 1998; Wittchen et al. 1998a). Panic disorder shows extremely high comorbidity rates with social phobia (Eaton et al. 1994; Goisman et al. 1995a; Jacobi et al. 2004; Starcevic et al. 1992; Weissman et al. 1997), generalized anxiety disorder (Ball et al. 1995; Eaton et al. 1994; Goisman et al. 1995a; Jacobi et al. 2004; Maser 1998; Noyes 2001; Starcevic et al. 1992; Weissman et al. 1997), specific phobias (Eaton et al. 1994; Goisman et al. 1995a, 1998; Jacobi et al. 2004; Starcevic and Bogojevic 1997; Starcevic et al. 1992; Weissman et al. 1997), and major depression (Ball et al. 1995; Breier et al. 1985; Eaton et al. 1994; Goodwin et al. 2004a; Jacobi et al. 2004; Kaufman and Charney 2000; Reich et al. 1993; Starcevic et al. 1992; Stein et al. 1990; Vollrath et al. 1990; Weissman et al. 1997).

The level of comorbidity of anxiety disorders prompted Andrews et al. (1990) and more recently Tyrer et al. (2003) to propose once again the concept of the general neurotic syndrome. Andrews et al. (2002) and Andrews and Slade (2002) analyzed the current comorbidity from the Australian National Survey of Mental Health and Well Being. They found that the panic/agoraphobic syndrome (combining panic disorder, panic disorder with agoraphobia, and agoraphobia) had a significant association with social phobia, generalized anxiety disorder, and Cluster A personality disorders. In this general population survey, the concurrent comorbidity was common (40% of the sample with any current disorder), especially within groups (i.e., affective disorders, anxiety disorders, substance use disorders, and personality disorders). Middeldorp et al. (2005) reviewed 22 twin studies and concluded that anxiety disorders and depression are distinct entities and not alternative phases of one disease. Their frequent co-occurrence can be explained by the shared genetic vulnerability between panic disorder and other anxiety disorders and between anxiety disorders and depressive disorders. Neuroticism may be the shared risk factor for anxiety and depression.

A more intriguing comorbidity is represented by the more-than-chance probability of the association of panic with bipolar disorder: the "panic-manic" comorbidity has been repeatedly reported (Birmaher et al. 2002; Bowen et al. 1994; Chen and Dilsaver 1995; Doughty et al. 2004; Goodwin and Hoven 2002; MacKinnon et al. 1997, 2002, 2003; Perugi et al. 1999; Savino et al. 1993) but scarcely studied. It would be interesting to explore the possibility of the existence of two kinds of panic: neurotic panic (with comorbidity with other anxiety disorder and depression), and bipolar panic (with comorbidity with bipolar disorder and possibility of panic-manic switch).

A caveat is necessary, however, regarding questions of comorbidity within the frame of operational criteria, especially with DSM-IV. DSM contains recognized problems of 1) overlapping criteria (e.g., same item in different categories, items inclusive of others, uncertain discrimination between criteria); 2) explicit exclusion criteria (e.g., general medical condition, substance related conditions); and 3) subtle hierarchy (e.g., "not better accounted for by..."). These characteristics of the diagnostic system are questionable and might create arbitrary boundaries between different disorders.

Etiological Factors

THE AMYGDALA CIRCUIT

Numerous investigations have searched for a neuroanatomical basis of panic disorder (Bechara et al. 1995; Charney 2003; Gorman et al. 2000). Preclinical animal studies from basic and behavioral neuroscience showed that some neuroanatomical pathways are involved in conditioned fear in animals (Gorman et al. 2000). This "fear network" is centered in the amygdala and involves interaction with the hippocampus and medial prefrontal cortex. The amygdala receives sensory information by two major pathways: downstream, from brainstem structures and sensory thalamus, and upstream, from the sensory cortex and via corticothalamic relays, allowing for higher level neurocognitive processing and modulation of sensory information. Contextual information is stored in memory in the hippocampus and conveyed directly to the amygdala. Major efferent pathways of the amygdala relevant to anxiety include the locus coeruleus (increases noradrenaline release, which contributes to physiological and behavioral arousal); the periaqueductal gray region (results in defensive behaviors and postural freezing); the hypothalamic paraventricular nucleus (activates the hypothalamic-pituitary-adrenal [HPA] axis, releasing adrenocorticoids); the hypothalamic lateral nucleus (activates the sympathetic nervous system); and the parabrachial nucleus (influences respiratory rate).

A similar fear network exists in humans, as shown by neuroimaging studies in human fear conditioning (Canli et al. 2000; Critchley at al. 2002; Fredrikson et al. 1995; Furmark et al. 1997; LaBar et al. 1998). Gorman et al. (2000) observed that physiological and behavioral consequences of response to a conditioned-fear stimulus is similar to a panic attack, and they postulated that panic originates in an abnormally sensitive fear network. More recent evidence seems to give support to this theory.

Neuroimaging Studies

A volumetric magnetic resonance imaging (MRI) study conducted with 13 patients with panic disorder and 14 healthy subjects showed smaller temporal lobe volume in panic disorder patients (Vythilingam et al. 2000). An MRI study conducted in 12 drug-free symptomatic panic disorder patients and 12 case-matched healthy comparison subjects found that panic disorder patients had smaller left-sided and right-sided amygdala volumes than control subjects (Massana et al. 2003). This is the first study using quantitative structural neuroimaging techniques to examine amygdala anatomy in panic disorder. In a recent study, F-fluorodeoxyglucose positron emission tomography (PET) was used to compare regional brain glucose utilization in 12 nonmedicated panic disorder patients—without their experiencing panic attacks during PET acquisition—and 22 healthy control subjects. Panic disorder patients exhibited significantly higher levels of glucose uptake in the bilateral amygdala, hippocampus, and thalamus, and in the midbrain, caudal pons, medulla, and cerebellum, compared with control subjects (Sakai et al. 2005). These results provided the first functional neuroimaging support in human patients for the neuroanatomical hypothesis of panic disorder focusing on the amygdala-based fear network.

Molecular Studies

A PET study conducted on 16 unmedicated symptomatic outpatients with panic disorder and 15 matched healthy control subjects showed reduced serotonin type 1A (5-HT$_{1A}$) receptor binding in panic disorder patients (Neumeister et al. 2004). Serotonin has an important regulatory role in the fear network (Gorman et al. 2000). A functional MRI (fMRI) study showed that individuals with one or two copies of the short allele of the serotonin transporter (5-HTT) promoter polymorphism, which has been associated with reduced 5-HTT expression and function and increased fear and anxiety-related behaviors, exhibit greater amygdala neuronal activity in response to fearful stimuli compared with individuals homozygous for the long allele (Hariri et al. 2002). Another fMRI study showed that activity in the amygdala is independently predicted by the personality style and the serotonin transporter genotype (Bertolino et al. 2005).

Animal Studies

Macaque monkeys who received bilateral amygdala lesions at 2 weeks of age showed an impaired ability to perceive potential danger in comparison with control monkeys (Bauman et al. 2004a). Rhesus monkeys who received bilateral lesions of the amygdala at 2 weeks of age produced more fear behaviors during social encounters than did control monkeys (Bauman et al. 2004b). These results are consistent with the view that the amygdala is related to the detection, evaluation, and avoidance of environmental dangers. 5-HT$_{1A}$ receptor knockout mice exhibit an anxiety-related phenotype characterized by an inappropriate generalization of fearful behavior to a context containing both fearful and neutral stimuli, a phenomenon that occurs in a subset of human anxiety disorders such as panic disorder (Klemenhagen et al. 2006). Serotonin has an important regulatory role in the fear network (Gorman et al. 2000).

THE STRESS HYPOTHESIS

The relationship between panic disorder and life stress has been an object of ample study. On one hand, the HPA axis has been thoroughly investigated, with controversial results. On the other hand, the role of early and recent life events has been an object of research.

HPA Axis in Panic Disorder

According to the fear network hypothesis (Gorman et al. 2000), there is an activation of the HPA axis, at least during the panic attack. In panic disorder subjects some studies have found normal physiological measurements: normal basal plasma levels of cortisol (Brambilla et al. 1992, 1995; Cameron et al. 1987; Gurguis et al. 1991; Liebowitz et al. 1985; Stein and Uhde 1988; Villacres et al. 1987;

Woods et al. 1988), normal urinary free cortisol levels (Uhde et al. 1988), normal adrenocorticotropic hormone (ACTH) levels (Rapaport et al. 1989), and normal cerebrospinal fluid/corticotropin-releasing hormone (CRH) levels (Jolkonen et al. 1987). Other studies found various abnormal measurements: elevated basal plasma levels of cortisol (Abelson and Curtis 1996; Goldstein et al. 1987; Nesse et al. 1984; Roy-Byrne et al. 1986b; Wedekind et al. 2000); elevated basal levels of free cortisol in the plasma (Wedekind et al. 2000), the urine (Bandelow et al. 1997; Lopez et al. 1990), and the saliva (Bandelow et al. 2000; Wedekind et al. 2000); increased basal ACTH levels (Brambilla et al. 1992); increased ACTH levels after CRH stimulation (Brambilla et al. 1992; Holsboer et al. 1987; Roy-Byrne et al. 1986b); dexamethasone nonsuppression (Avery et al. 1985; Coryell and Noyes 1988; Judd et al. 1987; Westberg et al. 1991); and dexamethasone/CRH nonsuppression (Schreiber et al. 1996). Similar alterations have been found in other psychiatric disorders, in particular posttraumatic stress disorder (PTSD) (Kellner and Yehuda 1999).

Life Events and Panic Disorder

The researchers that have investigated the life events in panic disorder have basically achieved sounder results. An excess of childhood trauma and adversity has been reported in prospective studies (Hubbard et al. 1995; Swanston et al. 1997; von Knorring et al. 1982) as well as in a consistent set of retrospective studies (Bandelow et al. 2002; Faravelli et al. 1985; Felitti 2002; Horesh et al. 1997; Kessler et al. 1997; Manfro et al. 1996; Moisan and Engels 1995; Safren et al. 2002; Servant and Parquet 1994; Tweed et al. 1989; Young et al. 1997). A perception of low maternal care has also been consistently shown (Faravelli et al. 1991; Hojat 1998; Nilzon and Palmerus 1997; Parker 1979, 1981). The matter is more controversial regarding recent life events prior to the onset of panic (life events as precipitating factors): according to some studies there is an excess of recent stressful life events before the onset of panic disorder (De Loof et al. 1989; Faravelli 1985; Faravelli and Pallanti 1989; Manfro et al. 1996; Roy-Byrne et al. 1986a; Wade et al. 1993); other studies, however, failed to confirm these findings (Rapee et al. 1990; Savoia and Bernik 2004). Panic might itself become a stressor. Like typical stressors that produce PTSD, panic attacks are sudden, unpredictable, and often perceived as life threatening. Structured interviews with 30 subjects with panic disorder revealed that 5 (17%) and 2 (7%) met lifetime and current DSM-III-R PTSD criteria, respectively, following their most terrifying panic attack (Burstein 1993; Lundy 1993; McNally and Lukach 1992).

Newer animal research, however, furnishes a solid basis for interpreting the role of life stress for anxiety. In animals, the augmented production of corticosteroids caused by the stress induces a hyperactivation of corticosteroid receptors. This receptor hyperactivation, via second messengers, leads to an inhibition of the transcription factor CREB (cyclic adenosine monophosphate [cAMP] response element binding). Inhibition of CREB causes a reduced expression of brain derived neurotrophic factor mRNA in the hippocampus and gyrus dentatus, with consequent atrophy of these structures (Gross and Hen 2004a, 2004b; Mirescu and Gould 2004; Mirescu et al. 2004; Santarelli et al. 2003; Vogel 2003).

We can also hypothesize that there is a parallelism between general adaptation syndrome findings (Selye 1956) from neurobiological studies and stress-related disorders. In the general adaptation syndrome there is an alarm, followed by a reaction of resistance characterized by a process of allostasis. If the alarm persists, there is an exhaustion of the responses of the organism. Neurobiological findings show that the stress causes an activation involving, first, monoamines and a fear circuitry (centered on amygdala) and, then, the HPA axis and other neural networks (with prominent role of the hippocampus); if stress persists, neural atrophy occurs. Stress-related disorders might include anxiety at a first level, depression at a second level, and finally death (exhaustion of the stress response).

Proposals for Future Research

For future research it would be useful to evaluate panic attacks, phobic cognition, and agoraphobia independent of panic disorder. We need to prepare operational definitions for these phenomena that are independent of each other (e.g., avoid defining agoraphobia as the fear of panic), with description, association with overt symptoms and other disorders, and long-term outcome. It would also be useful to describe the natural aggregations of panic attacks, agoraphobia, and phobic cognition with one another and with other disorders and to explore the most promising etiological hypotheses within this frame. Whereas during the past few decades the large majority of the studies have been directed at distinguishing among disorders, investigation into shared features of the disorders would be welcome.

We will learn most if we can plan two types of studies: one clinical cohort study and one general population study. The former should focus on a relatively narrow group of patients, directed at exploring single issues/pathogens (e.g., treatment, imaging, cognitions). In such a study it is important to focus on an inception cohort—that is, a cohort of patients at about the same stage of the clinical course of the disease; otherwise we would be mixing green oranges with ripe oranges with rotten oranges. The population studies should aim at a broad spectrum, preferably using a representative developmental twin population. In these epidemiological surveys, it is vital to examine a random subsample of those who screened negative to probe questions, otherwise we would not be able to know the true sensitivity/specificity of any characteristic for any target disorder.

References

Abelson JL, Curtis GC: Hypothalamic-pituitary-adrenal axis activity in panic disorder: 24-hour secretion of corticotropin and cortisol. Arch Gen Psychiatry 53:323–331, 1996

American Psychiatric Association: Diagnostic and Statistical Manual of Mental Disorders, 3rd Edition. Washington, DC, American Psychiatric Association, 1980

American Psychiatric Association: Diagnostic and Statistical Manual of Mental Disorders, 3rd Edition, Revised. Washington, DC, American Psychiatric Association, 1987

American Psychiatric Association: Diagnostic and Statistical Manual of Mental Disorders, 4th Edition. Washington, DC, American Psychiatric Association, 1994

American Psychiatric Association: Diagnostic and Statistical Manual of Mental Disorders, 4th Edition, Text Revision. Washington, DC, American Psychiatric Association, 2000

Andrews G, Slade T: Agoraphobia without a history of panic disorder may be part of the panic disorder syndrome. J Nerv Ment Dis 190:624–630, 2002

Andrews G, Stewart G, Morris-Yates A, et al: Evidence for a general neurotic syndrome. Br J Psychiatry 157:6–12, 1990

Andrews G, Henderson S, Hall W: Prevalence, comorbidity, disability and service utilization: overview of the Australian National Mental Health Survey. Br J Psychiatry 178:145–153, 2001

Andrews G, Slade T, Issakidis C: Deconstructing the current comorbidity: data from the Australian National Survey of Mental Health and Well Being. Br J Psychiatry 181:306–314, 2002

Angst J: Comorbidity of panic disorder in a community sample. Clin Neuropharmacol 1(suppl) 1:176A–177A, 1992

Angst J: Comorbidity of anxiety, phobia, compulsion and depression. Int Clin Psychopharmacol 15(suppl 1):21–25, 1993

Angst J, Dobler-Mikola A: The Zurich Study: anxiety and phobia in young adults. Eur Arch Psychiatr Neurol Sci 235:171–178, 1985

Aoki Y, Fujihara S, Kitamura T: Panic attacks and panic disorder in Japanese non-patient population: epidemiology and psychosocial correlates. J Affect Disord 32:51–59, 1994

Argyle N: Anxiety and panic disorders. Practitioner 230:453–459, 1986

Arriaga F, Paiva T, Matos-Pires A, et al: The sleep of non-depressed patients with panic disorder: a comparison with normal controls. Acta Psychiatr Scand 93:191–194, 1996

Avery DH, Osgood TB, Ishiki DM, et al: The DST in psychiatric outpatients with generalized anxiety disorder, panic disorder, or primary affective disorder. Am J Psychiatry 142:844–848, 1985

Ball SG, Buchwald AM, Waddell MT, et al: Depression and generalized anxiety symptoms in panic disorder: implications for comorbidity. J Nerv Ment Dis 183:304–308, 1995

Ballenger JC, Burrows GD, DuPont RL Jr, et al: Alprazolam in panic disorder and agoraphobia: results from a multicenter trial, I: efficacy in short-term treatment. Arch Gen Psychiatry 45:413–422, 1988

Bandelow B, Sengos G, Wedekind D, et al: Urinary excretion of cortisol, norepinephrine, testosterone, and melatonin in panic disorder. Pharmacopsychiatry 30:113–117, 1997

Bandelow B, Wedekind D, Pauls J, et al: Salivary cortisol in panic attacks. Am J Psychiatry 157:454–456, 2000

Bandelow B, Spath C, Tichauer GA, et al: Early traumatic life events, parental attitudes, family history, and birth risk factors in patients with panic disorder. Compr Psychiatry 43:269–278, 2002

Barlow DH: Anxiety and Its Disorders: The Nature and Treatment of Anxiety and Panic. New York, Guilford, 1988

Barlow DH, Brown TA, Craske MG: Definitions of panic attacks and panic disorder in the DSM-IV: implications for research. J Abnorm Psychol 103:553–564, 1994

Bauman MD, Lavenex P, Mason WA, et al: The development of mother–infant interactions after neonatal amygdala lesions in rhesus monkeys. J Neurosci 24:711–721, 2004a

Bauman MD, Lavenex P, Mason WA, et al: The development of social behavior following neonatal amygdala lesions in rhesus monkeys. J Cogn Neurosci 16:1388–1411, 2004b

Bechara A, Tranel D, Damasio H, et al: Double dissociation of conditioning and declarative knowledge relative to the amygdala and hippocampus in humans. Science 269:1115–1118, 1995

Beitman BD, Basha I, Flaker G, et al: Non-fearful panic disorder: panic attacks without fear. Behav Res Ther 25:487–492, 1987

Beitman BD, Kushner M, Lamberti JW, et al: Panic disorder without fear in patients with angiographically normal coronary arteries. J Nerv Ment Dis 178:307–312, 1990

Beitman BD, Thomas AM, Kushner MG: Panic disorder in the families of patients with normal coronary arteries and non-fear panic disorder. Behav Res Ther 30:403–406, 1992

Beitman BD, Mukerji V, Russell JL, et al: Panic disorder in cardiology patients: a review of the Missouri Panic/Cardiology Project. J Psychiatr Res Suppl 27:35–46, 1993

Bell CJ, Nutt DJ: Serotonin and panic. Br J Psychiatry 172:465–471, 1998

Bertolino A, Arciero G, Rubino V, et al: Variation of human amygdala response during threatening stimuli as a function of 5-HTTLPR genotype and personality style. Biol Psychiatry 57:1517–1525, 2005

Bijl RV, Ravelli A, van Zessen G: Prevalence of psychiatric disorders in the general population: results from the Netherlands Mental Health Survey and Incidence Study (NEMESIS). Soc Psychiatry Psychiatr Epidemiol 33:587–595, 1998

Birmaher B, Kennah A, Brent D, et al: Is bipolar disorder specifically associated with panic disorder in youths? Clin Psychiatry 63:414–419, 2002

Bourin M, Malinge M, Guitton B: Provocative agents in panic disorder. Therapie 50:301–306, 1995

Bovasso G, Eaton W: Types of panic attacks and their association with psychiatric disorder and physical illness. Compr Psychiatry 40:469–477, 1999

Bowen R, South M, Hawkes J: Mood swings in patients with panic disorder. Can J Psychiatry 39:91–94, 1994

Brambilla F, Bellodi L, Perna G, et al: Psychoimmunoendocrine aspects of panic disorder. Neuropsychobiology 26:12–22, 1992

Brambilla F, Bellodi L, Arancio C, et al: Alpha 2-adrenergic receptor sensitivity in panic disorder, II: cortisol response to clonidine stimulation in panic disorder. Psychoneuroendocrinology 20:11–19, 1995

Brawman-Mintzer O, Lydiard RB, Emmanuel N, et al: Psychiatric comorbidity in patients with generalized anxiety disorder. Am J Psychiatry 150:1216–1218, 1993

Breier A, Charney DS, Heninger GR: The diagnostic validity of anxiety disorders and their relationship to depressive illness. Am J Psychiatry 142:787–797, 1985

Breier A, Charney DS, Heninger GR: Agoraphobia with panic attacks: development, diagnostic stability, and course of illness. Arch Gen Psychiatry 43:1029–1036, 1986

Buller R, Maier W, Benkert O: Clinical subtypes in panic disorder: their descriptive and prospective validity. J Affect Disord 11:105–114, 1986

Burstein A: Panic as a posttraumatic stressor. Am J Psychiatry 150:842, 1993

Bystritsky A, Craske M, Maidenberg E, et al: Autonomic reactivity of panic patients during a CO_2 inhalation procedure. Depress Anxiety 11:15–26, 2000

Cameron OG, Lee MA, Curtis GC, et al: Endocrine and physiological changes during "spontaneous" panic attacks. Psychoneuroendocrinology 12:321–331, 1987

Canli T, Zhao Z, Brewer J, et al: Event-related activation in the human amygdala associates with later memory for individual emotional experience. J Neurosci 20:RC99, 2000

Cassano GB, Michelini S, Shear MK, et al: The panic-agoraphobic spectrum: a descriptive approach to the assessment and treatment of subtle symptoms. Am J Psychiatry 154(suppl):27–38, 1997

Cassano GB, Pini S, Saettoni M, et al: Multiple anxiety disorder comorbidity in patients with mood spectrum disorders with psychotic features. Am J Psychiatry 156:474–476, 1999

Chambless DL, Caputo GC, Jasin SE, et al: The Mobility Inventory for Agoraphobia. Behav Res Ther 23:35–44, 1985

Charney DS: Neuroanatomical circuits modulating fear and anxiety behaviors. Acta Psychiatr Scand 417(suppl):38–50, 2003

Charney DS, Heninger GR: Abnormal regulation of noradrenergic function in panic disorders: effects of clonidine in healthy subjects and patients with agoraphobia and panic disorder. Arch Gen Psychiatry 43:1042–1054, 1986

Charney DS, Heninger GR, Breier A: Noradrenergic function in panic anxiety: effects of yohimbine in healthy subjects and patients with agoraphobia and panic disorder. Arch Gen Psychiatry 41:751–763, 1984

Chen YW, Dilsaver SC: Comorbidity of panic disorder in bipolar illness: evidence from the Epidemiologic Catchment Area Survey. Am J Psychiatry 152:280–282, 1995

Clark DM: A cognitive approach to panic. Behav Res Ther 24:461–470, 1986

Coryell W, Noyes R: HPA axis disturbance and treatment outcome in panic disorder. Biol Psychiatry 24:762–766, 1988

Coupland NJ, Wilson SJ, Potokar JP, et al: Increased sympathetic response to standing in panic disorder. Psychiatry Res 118:69–79, 2003

Cox BJ, Cohen E, Direnfeld DM, et al: Does the Beck Anxiety Inventory measure anything beyond panic attack symptoms? Behav Res Ther 34:949–954, 1996

Craske MG, Barlow DH: Nocturnal panic. J Nerv Ment Dis 177:160–167, 1989

Craske MG, Miller PP, Rotunda R, et al: A descriptive report of features of initial unexpected panic attacks in minimal and extensive avoiders. Behav Res Ther 28:395–400, 1990

Critchley HD, Mathias CJ, Dolan RJ: Fear conditioning in humans: the influence of awareness and autonomic arousal on functional neuroanatomy. Neuron 33:653–663, 2002

De Loof C, Zandbergen J, Lousberg H, et al: The role of life events in the onset of panic disorder. Behav Res Ther 27:461–463, 1989

Degonda M, Angst J: The Zurich study, XX: social phobia and agoraphobia. Eur Arch Psychiatry Clin Neurosci 243:95–102, 1993

Di Nardo PA, O'Brien GT, Barlow DH, et al: Reliability of DSM-III anxiety disorder categories using a new structured interview. Arch Gen Psychiatry 40:1070–1074, 1983

Doughty CJ, Wells JE, Joyce PR, et al: Bipolar-panic disorder comorbidity within bipolar disorder families: a study of siblings. Bipolar Disord 6:245–252, 2004

Eaton WW, Kessler RC, Wittchen HU, et al: Panic and panic disorder in the United States. Am J Psychiatry 151:413–420, 1994

Ehlers A: A 1-year prospective study of panic attacks: clinical course and factors associated with maintenance. J Abnorm Psychol 104:164–172, 1995

Essau CA, Conradt J, Petermann F: Frequency of panic attacks and panic disorder in adolescents. Depress Anxiety 9:19–26, 1999

Faravelli C: Life events preceding the onset of panic disorder. J Affect Disord 9:103–105, 1985

Faravelli C, Pallanti S: Recent life events and panic disorder. Am J Psychiatry 146:622–626, 1989

Faravelli C, Webb T, Ambonetti A, et al: Prevalence of traumatic early life events in 31 agoraphobic patients with panic attacks. Am J Psychiatry 142:1493–1494, 1985

Faravelli C, Guerrini Degl'Innocenti B, Giardinelli L: Epidemiology of anxiety disorders in Florence. Acta Psychiatr Scand 79:308–312, 1989

Faravelli C, Panichi C, Pallanti S, et al: Perception of early parenting in panic and agoraphobia. Acta Psychiatr Scand 84:6–8, 1991

Faravelli C, Pallanti S, Biondi F, et al: Onset of panic disorder. Am J Psychiatry 149:827–828, 1992

Faravelli C, Marinoni M, Spiti R, et al: Abnormal brain hemodynamic responses during passive orthostatic challenge in panic disorder. Am J Psychiatry 154:378–383, 1997

Faravelli C, Ricca V, Truglia E: Panic disorder: pathogenesis and treatment, in Anxiety Disorders: An Introduction to Clinical Management and Research. Edited by Griez E, Faravelli C, Nutt D, et al. West Sussex, United Kingdom, Wiley and Sons, 2001, pp 81–103

Faravelli C, Abrardi L, Bartolozzi D, et al: The Sesto Fiorentino Study: background, methods and preliminary results: lifetime prevalence of psychiatric disorders in an Italian community sample using clinical interviewers. Psychother Psychosom 73:216–225, 2004a

Faravelli C, Abrardi L, Bartolozzi D, et al: The Sesto Fiorentino Study: point and one year prevalences of psychiatric disorders in an Italian community sample using clinical interviewers. Psychother Psychosom 73:226–234, 2004b

Fava GA, Mangelli L: Subclinical symptoms of panic disorder: new insights into pathophysiology and treatment. Psychother Psychosom 68:281–289, 1999

Fava GA, Grandi S, Canestrari R: Prodromal symptoms in panic disorder with agoraphobia. Am J Psychiatry 145:1546–1547, 1988

Fava GA, Grandi S, Rafanelli C, et al: Prodromal symptoms in panic disorder with agoraphobia: a reduplication study. J Affect Disord 26:85–88, 1992

Felitti VJ: The relationship of adverse childhood experiences to adult health: turning gold into lead. Z Psychosom Med Psychother 48:359–369, 2002

Fleet RP, Martel JP, Lavoie KL, et al: Non-fearful panic disorder: a variant of panic in medical patients? Psychosomatics 41:311–320, 2000

Frank E, Shear MK, Rucci P, et al: Cross-cultural validity of the Structured Clinical Interview for Panic-Agoraphobic Spectrum. Soc Psychiatry Psychiatr Epidemiol 40:283–290, 2005

Fredrikson M, Wik G, Fischer H, et al: Affective and attentive neural networks in humans: a PET study of Pavlovian conditioning. Neuroreport 7:97–101, 1995

Furmark T, Fisher H, Wik G, et al: The amygdala and individual differences in human fear conditioning. Neuroreport 6:3957–3960, 1997

Furukawa T, Awaji R, Nakazato H, et al: Persistence of chronic mood disorders: a 2 year follow-up. Psychiatry Clin Neurosci 49:19–24, 1995

Fyer AJ, Katon W, Hollifield M, et al: The DSM-IV panic disorder field trial: panic attack frequency and functional disability. Anxiety 2:157–166, 1996

Gardenswarts CA, Craske MG: Prevention of panic disorder. Behav Ther 32:725–738, 2001

Garvey MJ, Tuason VB: The relationship of panic disorder to agoraphobia. Compr Psychiatry 25:529–531, 1984

Garvey MJ, Cook B, Noyes R Jr: The occurrence of a prodrome of generalized anxiety in panic disorder. Compr Psychiatry 29:445–449, 1988

Garyfallos G, Adamopoulou A, Karastergiou A, et al: Psychiatric comorbidity in Greek patients with generalized anxiety disorder. Psychopathology 32:308–318, 1999

Goisman RM, Warshaw MG, Peterson LG, et al: Panic, agoraphobia, and panic disorder with agoraphobia: data from a multicenter anxiety disorder study. J Nerv Ment Dis 182:72–79, 1994

Goisman RM, Goldenberg I, Vasile RG, et al: Comorbidity of anxiety disorders in a multicenter anxiety study. Compr Psychiatry 36:303–311, 1995a

Goisman RM, Warshaw MJ, Steketee GS, et al: DSM-IV and the disappearance of agoraphobia without a history of panic disorder: new data on a controversial diagnosis. Am J Psychiatry 152:1438–1443, 1995b

Goisman RM, Allsworth J, Rogers MP, et al: Simple phobia as a comorbid anxiety disorder. Depress Anxiety 7:105–112, 1998

Goldstein S, Halbreich U, Asnis G, et al: The hypothalamic-pituitary-adrenal system in panic disorder. Am J Psychiatry 144:1320–1323, 1987

Goodwin RD, Hamilton SP: Panic attack as a marker of core psychopathological processes. Psychopathology 34:278–288, 2001

Goodwin RD, Hoven CW: Bipolar-panic comorbidity in the general population: prevalence and associated morbidity. J Affect Disord 70:27–33, 2002

Goodwin RD, Hamilton SP, Milne BJ, et al: Generalizability and correlates of clinically derived panic subtypes in the population. Depress Anxiety 15:69–74, 2002

Goodwin RD, Fergusson DM, Horwood LJ: Panic attacks and the risk of depression among young adults in the community. Psychother Psychosom 73:158–165, 2004a

Goodwin RD, Lieb R, Höfler M, et al: Panic attack as a risk factor for severe psychopathology. Am J Psychiatry 161:2207–2214, 2004b

Goodwin RD, Faravelli C, Rosi S, et al: The epidemiology of panic disorder and agoraphobia in Europe. Eur Neuropsychopharmacol 15:435–443, 2005

Gorman JM, Kent JM, Sullivan GM, et al: Neuroanatomical hypothesis of panic disorder, revised. Am J Psychiatry 157:493–505, 2000

Gross C, Hen R: The developmental origins of anxiety. Nat Rev Neurosci 5:545–552, 2004a

Gross C, Hen R: Genetic and environmental factors interact to influence anxiety. Neurotox Res 6:493–501, 2004b

Grunhaus L, Birmaher B: The clinical spectrum of panic attacks. J Clin Psychopharmacol 5:93–99, 1985

Guidano V: Complexity of the Self: A Developmental Approach to Psychopathology and Therapy. New York, Guilford, 1987

Gurguis GN, Mefford IN, Uhde TW: Hypothalamic-pituitary-adrenocortical activity in panic disorder: relationship to plasma catecholamine metabolites. Biol Psychiatry 30:502–506, 1991

Hariri AR, Mattay VS, Tessitore A, et al: Serotonin transporter genetic variation and the response of the human amygdala. Science 297:400–403, 2002

Hojat M: Satisfaction with early relationships with parents and psychosocial attributes in adulthood: which parent contributes more? J Genet Psychol 159:203–220, 1998

Hollifield M, Finley MR, Skipper B: Panic disorder phenomenology in urban self-identified Caucasian-Non-Hispanics and Caucasian-Hispanics. Depress Anxiety 18:7–17, 2003

Holsboer F, von Bardeleben U, Buller R, et al: Stimulation response to corticotropin-releasing hormone (CRH) in patients with depression, alcoholism and panic disorder. Horm Metab Res 16(suppl):80–88, 1987

Horesh N, Amir M, Kedem P, et al: Life events in childhood, adolescence and adulthood and the relationship to panic disorder. Acta Psychiatr Scand 96:373–378, 1997

Horwath E, Lish JD, Johnson J, et al: Agoraphobia without panic: clinical reappraisal of an epidemiologic finding. Am J Psychiatry 150:1496–1501, 1993

Hubbard J, Realmuto GM, Northwood AK, et al: Comorbidity of psychiatric diagnosis with post-traumatic stress disorder in survivors of childhood trauma. J Am Child Adolesc Psychiatry 34:1167–1173, 1995

Jacobi F, Wittchen HU, Holting C, et al: Prevalence, co-morbidity and correlates of mental disorders in the general population: results from the German Health Interview and Examination Survey (GHS). Psychol Med 34:597–611, 2004

Jolkonen J, Lepola U, Bissett G: CSF corticotropin-releasing factor is not affected in panic disorder. Biol Psychiatry 33:136–138, 1987

Joyce PR, Bushnell JA, Oakley-Browne MA, et al: The epidemiology of panic symptomatology and agoraphobic avoidance. Compr Psychiatry 30:303–312, 1989

Judd FK, Norman TR, Burrows GD, et al: The dexamethasone suppression test in panic disorder. Pharmacopsychiatry 20:99–101, 1987

Katerndahl DA: Infrequent and limited-symptom panic attacks. J Nerv Ment Dis 178:313–317, 1990

Katerndahl DA: Progression of limited symptom attacks. Depress Anxiety 9:138–140, 1999
Katerndahl DA: Predictors of the development of phobic avoidance. J Clin Psychiatry 61:618–623, 2000
Katerndahl DA, Realini JP: Lifetime prevalence of panic states. Am J Psychiatry 150:246–249, 1993
Katerndahl DA, Realini JP: Associations with subsyndromal panic and the validity of DSM-IV criteria. Depress Anxiety 8:33–38, 1998
Katon W, Hollifield M, Chapman T, et al: Infrequent panic attacks: psychiatric comorbidity, personality characteristics and functional disability. J Psychiatr Res 29:121–131, 1995
Kaufman J, Charney D: Comorbidity of mood and anxiety disorders. Depress Anxiety 12(suppl):69–76, 2000
Kellner M, Yehuda R: Do panic disorder and post traumatic stress disorder share a common psychoneuroendocrinology? Psychoneuroendocrinology 24:485–504, 1999
Kessler RC, Davis CG, Kendler KS: Childhood adversity and adult psychiatric disorders in the US National Comorbidity Survey. Psychol Med 27:1001–1019, 1997
Klein DF: Delineation of two drug-responsive anxiety syndromes. Psychopharmacology 5:397–408, 1964
Klein DF: Anxiety reconceptualized, in Anxiety: New Research and Changing Concepts. Edited by Klein DF, Raskin J. New York, Raven Press, 1981, pp 235–236
Klein DF: Anxiety reconceptualized, in Anxiety. Edited by Klein DF. Basel, Switzerland, Karger, 1987, pp 1–35
Klemenhagen KC, Gordon JA, David DJ, et al: Increased fear response to contextual cues in mice lacking the 5-HT1A receptor. Neuropsychopharmacology 31:101–111, 2006
Klerman GL, Weissman MM, Ouellette R, et al: Panic attacks in the community: social morbidity and health care utilization. JAMA 265:742–746, 1991
Kringlen E, Torgersen S, Cramer V: A Norwegian psychiatric epidemiological study. Am J Psychiatry 158:1091–1098, 2001
Krystal JH, Woods SW, Hill CL, et al: Characteristics of panic attack subtypes: assessment of spontaneous panic, situational panic, sleep panic, and limited symptom attacks. Compr Psychiatry 32:474–480, 1991
Kushner MG, Beitman BD: Panic attacks without fear: an overview. Behav Res Ther 28:469–479, 1990
LaBar KS, Gatenby JC, Gore JC, et al: Human amygdala activation during conditioned fear acquisition and extinction: a mixed-trial fMRI study. Neuron 20:283–289, 1998
Lecrubier Y, Weiller E: Comorbidities in social phobia. Int Clin Psychopharmacol 6(suppl):S17–S21, 1997
Lelliott P, Marks I, McNamee G, et al: Onset of panic disorder with agoraphobia: toward an integrated model. Arch Gen Psychiatry 46:1000–1004, 1989
Ley R: The many faces of Pan: psychological and physiological differences among three types of panic attacks. Behav Res Ther 30:347–357, 1992
Liebowitz MR, Gorman JM, Fyer AJ, et al: Lactate provocation of panic attacks, II: biochemical and physiological findings. Arch Gen Psychiatry 42:709–719, 1985

Lopez AL, Kathol RG, Noyes R Jr: Reduction in urinary free cortisol during benzodiazepine treatment of panic disorder. Psychoneuroendocrinology 15:23–28, 1990

Lundy MS: Panic as a posttraumatic stressor. Am J Psychiatry 150:841–842, 1993

MacKinnon DF, McMahon FJ, Simpson SG, et al: Panic disorder with familial bipolar disorder. Biol Psychiatry 42:90–95, 1997

MacKinnon DF, Zandi PP, Cooper J, et al: Comorbid bipolar disorder and panic disorder in families with a high prevalence of bipolar disorder. Am J Psychiatry 159:30–35, 2002

MacKinnon DF, Zandi PP, Gershon ES, et al: Association of rapid mood switching with panic disorder and familial panic risk in familial bipolar disorder. Am J Psychiatry 160:1696–1698, 2003

Manfro GG, Otto MW, McArdle ET, et al: Relationship of antecedent stressful life events to childhood and family history of anxiety and the course of panic disorder. J Affect Disord 41:135–139, 1996

Marks I: Fears and Phobias. London, England, Heinemann, 1969

Marks I: Panic disorder. Br Med J (Clin Res Ed) 287:290, 1983

Maser JD: Generalized anxiety disorder and its comorbidities: disputes at the boundaries. Acta Psychiatr Scand Suppl 393:12–22, 1998

Massana J, Lopez Risueno JA, Masana G, et al: Subtyping of panic disorder patients with bradycardia. Eur Psychiatry 16:109–114, 2001

Massana G, Serra-Grabulosa JM, Salgado-Pineda P, et al: Amygdalar atrophy in panic disorder patients detected by volumetric magnetic resonance imaging. Neuroimage 19:80–90, 2003

McCraty R, Atkinson M, Tomasino D, et al: Analysis of twenty-four hour heart rate variability in patients with panic disorder. Biol Psychol 56:131–150, 2001

McNally RJ: Anxiety sensitivity and panic disorder. Biol Psychiatry 52:938–946, 2002

McNally RJ, Lukach BM: Are panic attacks traumatic stressors? Am J Psychiatry 149:824–826, 1992

Merikangas KR, Angst J: Comorbidity and social phobia: evidence from clinical, epidemiologic, and genetic studies. Eur Arch Psychiatry Clin Neurosci 244:297–303, 1995

Middeldorp CM, Cath DC, Van Dyck R, et al: The co-morbidity of anxiety and depression in the perspective of genetic epidemiology; a review of twin and family studies. Psychol Med 35:611–624, 2005

Mirescu C, Gould E: From neurotoxin to neurotrophin. Nat Neurosci 7:899–900, 2004

Mirescu C, Peters JD, Gould E: Early life experience alters response of adult neurogenesis to stress. Nat Neurosci 7:841–846, 2004

Moisan D, Engels ML: Childhood trauma and personality disorder in 43 women with panic disorder. Psychol Rep 76:1133–1134, 1995

Neerakal I, Srinivasan K: A study of the phenomenology of panic attacks in patients from India. Psychopathology 36:92–97, 2003

Nesse RM, Cameron OG, Curtis GC, et al: Adrenergic function in patients with panic anxiety. Arch Gen Psychiatry 41:771–776, 1984

Neumeister A, Bain E, Nugent AC, et al: Reduced serotonin type 1A receptor binding in panic disorder. J Neurosci 24:589–591, 2004

Nilzon KR, Palmerus K: The influence of familial factors on anxiety and depression in childhood and early adolescence. Adolescence 32:935–943, 1997

Norton GR, Norton PJ, Walker JR, et al: A comparison of people with and without nocturnal panic attacks. J Behav Ther Exp Psychiatry 30:37–44, 1999

Noyes R Jr: Comorbidity in generalized anxiety disorder. Psychiatr Clin North Am 24:41–55, 2001

Noyes R Jr, Crowe RR, Harris EL, et al: Relationship between panic disorder and agoraphobia: a family study. Arch Gen Psychiatry 43:227–232, 1986

Parker G: Parental representations of patients with anxiety neurosis. Acta Psychiatr Scand 63:33–36, 1979

Parker G: Reported parental characteristic of agoraphobics and social phobics. Br J Psychiatry 135:555–560, 1981

Perugi G, Toni C, Benedetti A, et al: Delineating a putative phobic–anxious temperament in 126 panic-agoraphobic patients: toward a rapprochement of European and US views. J Affect Disord 47:11–23, 1998

Perugi G, Akiskal HS, Ramacciotti S, et al: Depressive comorbidity of panic, social phobic, and obsessive-compulsive disorders re-examined: is there a bipolar II connection? J Psychiatr Res 33:53–61, 1999

Pirkola S, Isometsä E, Suvisaari J, et al: DSM-IV mood-, anxiety and alcohol use disorders and their comorbidity in the Finish general population: result from the Health 2000 Study. Soc Psychiatry Psychiatr Epidemiol 40:1–10, 2005

Pohl R, Balon R, Berchou R, et al: Lactate-induced anxiety after imipramine and diazepam treatment. Anxiety 1:54–63, 1994

Pollard CA, Bronson SS, Kenney MR: Prevalence of agoraphobia without panic in clinical settings. Am J Psychiatry 146:559, 1989

Rachman S, Levitt K, Lopatka C: A simple method for distinguishing between expected and unexpected panics. Behav Res Ther 25:149–154, 1987

Rapaport MH, Risch SC, Golshan S: Neuroendocrine effects of ovine corticotropin-releasing hormone in panic disorder patients. Biol Psychiatry 26:344–348, 1989

Rapee RM, Litwin EM, Barlow DH: Impact of life events on subjects with panic disorder and on comparison subjects. Am J Psychiatry 147:640–644, 1990

Rauch SL, Shin LM, Wright CI: Neuroimaging studies of amygdala function in anxiety disorders. Ann N Y Acad Sci 985:389–410, 2003

Redmond DE, Huang YH: Current concepts II: new evidence for a locus coeruleus norepinephrine connection with anxiety. Life Sci 25:2149–2162, 1979

Reed V, Wittchen HU: DSM-IV panic attacks and panic disorder in a community sample of adolescents and young adults: how specific are panic attacks? J Psychiatr Res 32:335–345, 1998

Regier DA, Rae DS, Narrow WE, et al: Prevalence of anxiety disorders and their comorbidity with mood and addictive disorders. Br J Psychiatry Suppl (34):24–28, 1998

Reich J, Warshaw M, Peterson LG, et al: Comorbidity of panic and major depressive disorder. J Psychiatr Res 27(suppl):23–33, 1993

Rosenbaum JF: Limited-symptom panic attacks. Psychosomatics 28:407–408, 411–412, 1987

Roth M: Agoraphobia, panic disorder and generalized anxiety disorder. Psychiatr Dev 2:31–52, 1984

Roth M, Argyle N: Anxiety, panic and phobic disorders: an overview. J Psychiatr Res Suppl 22:33–54, 1988

Roy-Byrne P, Geraci M, Uhde T: Life events and the course of illness in patients with panic disorder. Am J Psychiatry 143:1033–1035, 1986a

Roy-Byrne PP, Uhde TW, Post RM, et al: The corticotropin-releasing hormone stimulation test in patients with panic disorder. Am J Psychiatry 143:896–899, 1986b

Russell JL, Kushner MG, Beitman BD, et al: Nonfearful panic disorder in neurology patients validated by lactate challenge. Am J Psychiatry 148:361–364, 1991

Safren SA, Gershuny BS, Marzol P, et al: History of childhood abuse in panic disorder, social phobia, and generalized anxiety disorder. J Nerv Ment Dis 190:453–456, 2002

Sakai Y, Kumano H, Nishikawa M, et al: Cerebral glucose metabolism associated with a fear network in panic disorder. Neuroreport 16:927–931, 2005

Salkovskis PM, Clark DM, Hackmann A, et al: An experimental investigation of the role of safety-seeking behaviours in the maintenance of panic disorder with agoraphobia. Behav Res Ther 37:559–574, 1999

Santarelli L, Saxe M, Gross C, et al: Requirement of hippocampal neurogenesis for the behavioral effects of antidepressants. Science 301:805–809, 2003

Savino M, Perugi G, Simonini E, et al: Affective comorbidity in panic disorder: is there a bipolar connection? J Affect Disord 28:155–163, 1993

Savoia MG, Bernik M: Adverse life events and coping skills in panic disorder. Rev Hosp Clin Fac Med Sao Paulo 59:337–340, 2004

Schmidt NB, Lerew DR, Jackson RJ: The role of anxiety sensitivity in the pathogenesis of panic: prospective evaluation of spontaneous panic attacks during acute stress. J Abnorm Psychol 106:355–364, 1997

Schmidt NB, Lerew DR, Jackson RJ: Prospective evaluation of anxiety sensitivity in the pathogenesis of panic: replication and extension. J Abnorm Psychol 108:532–537, 1999

Schmidt NB, Lerew DR, Joiner TE Jr: Prospective evaluation of the etiology of anxiety sensitivity: test of a scar model. Behav Res Ther 38:1083–1095, 2000

Schmidt NB, Forsyth JP, Santiago HT, et al: Classification of panic attack subtypes in patients and normal controls in response to biological challenge: implications for assessment and treatment. J Anxiety Disord 16:625–638, 2002

Schreiber W, Lauer CJ, Krumrey K, et al: Dysregulation of the hypothalamic-pituitary-adrenocortical system in panic disorder. Neuropsychopharmacology 15:7–15, 1996

Scupi BS, Benson BE, Brown LB, et al: Rapid onset: a valid panic disorder criterion? Depress Anxiety 5:121–126, 1997

Segui J, Salvador L, Canet J, et al: Comorbidity of panic disorder and social phobia. Actas Luso Esp Neurol Psiquiatr Cienc Afines 23:43–47, 1995

Selye H: Stress and psychiatry. Am J Psychiatry 113:423–427, 1956

Servant D, Parquet PJ: Life events and anxiety. Encephale 20:333–337, 1994

Shear MK, Frank E, Rucci P, et al: Panic-agoraphobic spectrum: reliability and validity of assessment instruments. J Psychiatr Res 35:59–66, 2001

Shear MK, Cassano GB, Frank E, et al: The panic-agoraphobic spectrum: development, description, and clinical significance. Psychiatr Clin North Am 25:739–756, 2002

Shioiri T, Someya T, Fujii K, et al: Differences in symptom structure between panic attack and limited symptom panic attack: a study using cluster analysis. Psychiatry Clin Neurosci 51:47–51, 1997

Shioiri T, Kojima M, Hosoki T, et al: Momentary changes in the cardiovascular autonomic system during mental loading in patients with panic disorder: a new physiological index "rho(max)." J Affect Disord 82:395–401, 2004

Spitzer RL, Endicott J, Robins E: Research Diagnostic Criteria: rationale and reliability. Arch Gen Psychiatry 35:773–779, 1978

Starcevic V, Bogojevic G: Comorbidity of panic disorder with agoraphobia and specific phobia: relationship with the subtypes of specific phobia. Compr Psychiatry 38:315–320, 1997

Starcevic V, Uhlenhuth EH, Kellner R, et al: Patterns of comorbidity in panic disorder and agoraphobia. Psychiatry Res 42:171–183, 1992

Stein MB, Uhde TW: Cortisol response to clonidine in panic disorder: comparison with depressed patients and normal controls. Biol Psychiatry 24:322–330, 1988

Stein MB, Tancer ME, Uhde TW: Major depression in patients with panic disorder: factors associated with course and recourrence. J Affect Disord 19:287–296, 1990

Street LL, Craske MG, Barlow DH: Sensations, cognitions and the perception of cues associated with expected and unexpected panic attacks. Behav Res Ther 27:189–198, 1989

Swanston HV, Tebbutt JS, O'Toole BJ, et al: Sexually abused children 5 years after presentation: a case-control study. Pediatrics 100:600–608, 1997

Tanabe Y, Harada H, Sugihara S, et al: 123I-Metaiodobenzylguanidine myocardial scintigraphy in panic disorder. J Nucl Med 45:1305–1308, 2004

Telch MJ, Lucas JA, Nelson P: Nonclinical panic in college students: an investigation of prevalence and symptomatology. J Abnorm Psychol 98:300–306, 1989

Thompson AH, Bland RC, Orn HT: Relationship and chronology of depression, agoraphobia, and panic disorder in the general population. J Nerv Ment Dis 177:456–463, 1989

Thyer BA, Himle J, Curtis GC, et al: A comparison of panic disorder and agoraphobia with panic attacks. Compr Psychiatry 26:208–214, 1985

Torgersen S: Genetic factors in anxiety disorders. Arch Gen Psychiatry 40:1085–1089, 1983

Tweed JL, Schoenbach VJ, George LK, et al: The effects of childhood parental death and divorce on six-month history of anxiety disorders. Br J Psychiatry 154:823–828, 1989

Tyrer P, Seivewright H, Johnson T: The core elements of neurosis: mixed anxiety-depression (cothymia) and personality disorder. J Personal Disord 17:129–138, 2003

Uhde TW, Joffe RT, Jimerson DC, et al: Normal urinary free cortisol and plasma MHPG in panic disorder: clinical and theoretical implications. Biol Psychiatry 23:575–585, 1988

Villacres EC, Hollifield M, Katon WJ, et al: Sympathetic nervous system activity in panic disorder. Psychiatry Res 21:313–321, 1987

Vogel G: Neuroscience: depression drugs' powers may rest on new neurons. Science 301:757, 2003

Vollrath M, Koch R, Angst J: The Zurich Study, IX: panic disorder and sporadic panic: symptoms, diagnosis, prevalence, and overlap with depression. Eur Arch Psychiatry Neurol Sci 239:221–230, 1990

von Knorring AL, Bohman M, Sigvardsson S: Early life experiences and psychiatric disorders: an adoptee study. Acta Psychiatr Scand 65:283–291, 1982

Vythilingam M, Anderson ER, Goddard A, et al: Temporal lobe volume in panic disorder: a quantitative magnetic resonance imaging study. Psychiatry Res 99:75–82, 2000

Wade SL, Monroe SM, Michelson LK: Chronic life stress and treatment outcome in agoraphobia with panic attacks. Am J Psychiatry 150:1491–1495, 1993

Wedekind D, Bandelow B, Broocks A, et al: Salivary, total plasma and plasma free cortisol in panic disorder. J Neural Transm 107:831–837, 2000

Weissman MM, Merikangas KR: The epidemiology of anxiety and panic disorder: an update. J Clin Psychiatry 47(suppl):11–17, 1986

Weissman MM, Loof PJ, Holzer CE: The epidemiology of anxiety disorders: a highlight of recent evidence. Psychopharmacol Bull 21:538–541, 1985

Weissman MM, Bland RC, Canino GJ, et al: The cross-national epidemiology of panic disorder. Arch Gen Psychiatry 54:305–309, 1997

Westberg P, Modigh K, Lisjo P, et al: Higher postdexamethasone serum cortisol levels in agoraphobic than in nonagoraphobic panic disorder patients. Biol Psychiatry 30:247–256, 1991

Wittchen HU: Epidemiology of panic attacks and panic disorders, in Panic and Phobias: Empirical Evidences of Theoretical Models and Long-Term Effects of Behavioral Treatments. Edited by Hand I, Wittchen HU. Berlin, Germany, Springer–Verlag, 1986, pp 18–28

Wittchen HU, Nelson CB, Lachner G: Prevalence of mental disorders and psychosocial impairment in adolescents and young adults. Psychol Med 28:109–126, 1998a

Wittchen HU, Reed V, Kessler R: The relationship of agoraphobia and panic in a community sample of adolescent and young adults. Arch Gen Psychiatry 55:1017–1024, 1998b

Woods SW, Charney DS, Goodman WK, et al: Carbon dioxide-induced anxiety: behavioral, physiologic, and biochemical effects of carbon dioxide in patients with panic disorders and healthy subjects. Arch Gen Psychiatry 45:43–52, 1988

World Health Organization: The ICD-10 Classification of Mental and Behavioural Disorders: Clinical Descriptions and Diagnostic Guidelines. Geneva, Switzerland, World Health Organization, 1992

Young EA, Abelson JL, Curtis JC: Childhood adversity and vulnerability to mood and anxiety disorders. Depress Anxiety 5:66–72, 1997

3

SOCIAL PHOBIA

Susan Bögels, Ph.D.
Murray B. Stein, M.D., FRCPC, M.P.H.

Social phobia (also known as social anxiety disorder [SocAD]) has at its core the fear of being negatively evaluated by other people. In community samples, social phobia is the most prevalent anxiety disorder; in Western society, lifetime prevalence estimates range from 4% to 13% among adults (Grant et al. 2005; Kessler et al. 2005; Narrow et al. 2002) and adolescents (Essau et al. 1999; Romano et al. 2001). In children from community samples, it is the second most prevalent disorder after simple phobia (Costello et al. 2003; Gau et al. 2005). In clinical samples, social phobia is the most prevalent anxiety disorder among adults and children (Barrett et al. 1996; Nauta et al. 2003). Mean age of onset is between 10 and 17 years, and new cases are rarely seen after the age of 25 (Grant et al. 2005; Wittchen and Fehm 2003). Social phobia seriously affects quality of life (Simon et al. 2002), and the economic costs of the disorder are huge (Lipsitz and Schneider 2000). Social phobia is a chronic illness; duration of 10–25 years is retrospectively reported in epidemiological and clinical studies (Davidson et al. 1993; DeWit et al. 1999; Kessler et al. 1998; Perugi et al. 1999). A prospective study found complete remission in an 8-year period to occur only in one-third of the cases (Yonkers et al. 2001).

Although social phobia is the most prevalent anxiety disorder, little is known about its etiology. Family studies suggest that social phobia is familial; in one study, an odds ratio of 4.7 was found between parental and offspring social phobia (Lieb et al. 2000). Moreover, specific familial transmission for social phobia (rather than anxiety disorders in general) has been found, suggesting that the disorder "breeds true" (Cooper et al. 2006; Feyer et al. 1995; Reich and Yates 1988), although there is also evidence that social phobia is part of an affective spectrum

(Hudson et al. 2003). Behavior genetic studies suggest that genetic factors influence susceptibility to social phobia and that the underlying structure of the genetic and environmental risk factors for social phobia is similar between men and women (Hettema et al. 2005). Underlying traits thought to predispose to social phobia include personality characteristics such as behavioral inhibition and fear of negative evaluation (e.g., Biederman et al. 2001; Robinson et al. 1992; M.B. Stein et al. 2002). With regard to behavioral inhibition, new data suggest possible links between this childhood trait and variation in genes that encode for corticotropin-releasing factor (Smoller et al. 2003, 2005).

Little is known about specific individual and shared environmental factors that might promote or protect against social phobia. There is hardly any evidence of a causative role for specific life events, and the existing evidence is nonspecific—that is, it concerns life events that form a risk for psychopathology in general. For example, Tiet et al. (2001) found that of 26 life events assessed in youth, only having a family member with an alcohol or drug problem predicted social phobia, but this life event also predicted most other forms of psychopathology. Models that have been tested with respect to shared environment or rearing merely concern general rearing factors, such as overprotection and rejection, that are thought to predispose to many forms of psychopathology (Rapee and Spence 2004). More recently, Hirshfeld-Becker et al. (2004) failed to find significant associations between behavioral inhibition and any of the following psychosocial factors: socioeconomic status; an index of adversity factors found in previous studies to be additively associated with child psychopathology; family intactness, conflict, expressiveness, and cohesiveness; exposure to parental psychopathology; sibship size; birth order; and gender.

Our goal in this chapter is to review the DSM criteria of the social phobia disorder in order to stimulate research on the pathways toward development of this severe and common disorder. Increased knowledge of the etiology of social phobia will eventually inform prevention and treatment. We start with a brief overview of the history of the DSM definition of social phobia and its consequences for prevalence ratings. Then we critically review the criteria, with a specific focus on the subtype definitions of this heterogeneous disorder. Finally, we propose promising hypotheses to be tested concerning etiology and pathophysiology, based on the proposed dimensions of social phobia.

History of Social Phobia Diagnosis in Adults and Children

SOCIAL PHOBIA FROM DSM-III TO DSM-IV

The diagnosis of social phobia has been subject to substantial changes from its first appearance in DSM-III (American Psychiatric Association 1980) to DSM-IV

(American Psychiatric Association 1994). In DSM-III, phobic disorders and anxiety states were regarded as two types of anxiety disorders, and social phobia was placed with the phobic disorders. The idea that social anxiety generalizes to many different social situations did not exist at the time, as is illustrated by the remark in DSM-III that "[g]enerally an individual has only one social phobia" (American Psychiatric Association 1980, p. 227). The examples given in DSM-III concerned social phobias that were later considered simple social phobias: "speaking or performing in public, using public lavatories, eating and writing in public" (p. 227). A generalized type had not yet been defined. With respect to the boundaries between social phobia and avoidant personality disorder, DSM-III criterion C specified that symptoms must not be due to avoidant personality disorder. Children with social anxiety could, in DSM-III, also be diagnosed under avoidant disorder in children and adolescents, defined as a persistent and excessive shrinking from contact with strangers sufficiently severe as to interfere with social functioning in peer relationships. In addition, the diagnosis of overanxious disorder in childhood and adolescence, which most resembled generalized anxiety disorder, was also considered for children with social fears, because of the criteria: preoccupation with appropriateness of behavior in the past; excessive concern with competence in various areas, including social; and marked self-consciousness and susceptibility to embarrassment and humiliation.

In DSM-III-R (American Psychiatric Association 1987), examples of social phobic fears were extended to include the reason why individuals would fear rejection: "*being unable to continue talking* while speaking in public, *choking on food* when eating in front of others, *being unable to urinate* in a public lavatory, *hand-trembling* when writing in the presence of others, and *saying foolish things or not being able to answer questions* in social situations" (p. 243, emphasis added). In DSM-III-R a generalized type was defined, and social phobia and avoidant personality disorder were no longer mutually exclusive; in fact, the diagnostic criteria recommended that the clinician "also consider the *additional* diagnosis of Avoidant Personality Disorder" (p. 243, emphasis added).

In DSM-IV and its text revision, DSM-IV-TR (American Psychiatric Association 2000), a new name, "social anxiety disorder," was introduced for the disorder, put between brackets after "social phobia." This new synonym is presumed to serve as a reminder that this condition is, indeed, an anxiety disorder. The reason why individuals would fear rejection was further elaborated and extended: "individuals with social phobia…are afraid that others will judge them to be anxious, weak, 'crazy,' stupid or that they will appear inarticulate" (pp. 450–451). Furthermore, fear of showing anxiety symptoms was specifically addressed; in fact, in criterion A it was added as the primary source of fear: "The individual fears that he or she will act in a way *(or show anxiety symptoms)* that will be humiliating or embarrassing" (p. 456, emphasis added). Under diagnostic features the anxiety symptoms are more clearly described:

> Individuals with social phobia almost always experience symptoms of anxiety (e.g., palpitations, tremors, sweating, gastrointestinal discomfort, diarrhea, muscle tension, blushing, confusion) and in severe cases these symptoms might meet the criteria for a Panic Attack. Blushing may be more typical of Social Phobia. (p. 451)

Other associated features include "observable signs of anxiety (e.g., cold clammy hands, tremors, shaky voice)" (p. 452).

With respect to the overlap with avoidant personality disorder, common associated features previously used to characterize avoidant personality disorder, such as low self-esteem, feelings of inferiority, and hypersensitivity to criticism, are added to the social phobia diagnostic feature description in DSM-IV, and avoidant personality disorder is in fact incorporated in the social phobia diagnosis: "Avoidant Personality Disorder may be a more severe variant of Social Phobia, Generalized, that is not qualitatively different" (p. 455). Test anxiety is indirectly included in the diagnosis of social phobia: "Individuals with social phobia also often fear indirect evaluation, such as taking a test…often underachieve in school due to test anxiety" (p. 452).

Concerning the diagnosis of social phobia in childhood, major changes were made in DSM-IV. Both avoidant disorder and overanxious disorder in childhood and adolescence were removed from the childhood section, the former because of its high overlap with social phobia (65%–100% comorbidity; Francis et al. 1992). Instead, for the first three criteria, specific child notes were added as in the previous avoidant disorder criteria: children have to be capable of age-appropriate social relations with familiar people, the anxiety must occur in peer settings and not just in interaction with adults, and the anxiety can be expressed by crying, tantrums, freezing, or shrinking from unfamiliar people. Finally, children, unlike adults, do not have to be able to recognize their fear is excessive or unreasonable.

Finally, DSM-IV introduced *Taijin Kyofusho* (TK), a culture-bound syndrome (e.g., Japan and Korea) referring to an individual's "intense fear that his or her body, its parts or its functions, displease, embarrass, or are offensive to other people in appearance, odor, facial expression, or movement" (p. 849).

In summary, the diagnosis of social phobia has evolved in the following ways: social phobia 1) was once conceptualized as a circumscribed phobia but is now thought to be an anxiety state, with addition of a generalized type; 2) was once discriminated from avoidant disorder in childhood and avoidant personality disorder in adulthood, but now has both of these disorders subsumed under its diagnosis; 3) now takes into account that anxiety symptoms are a primary source of fear of rejection and includes test anxiety; and 4) recognizes cultural differences in the expression of the disorder.

Prevalence of Social Phobia as a Function of Changing Criteria

As DSM-defined social phobia has evolved from a narrowly defined phobia to a broader anxiety state, prevalence ratings have increased. For adults, early (pre-1990) studies based on DSM-III revealed low lifetime prevalence estimates ranging between 1% and 4%. Subsequent studies, relying on the thoroughly revised DSM-III-R criteria, revealed lifetime rates ranging between 4.1% and 16%. Finally, in line with the only minor differences between DSM-III-R and DSM-IV, studies relying on DSM-IV criteria reported lifetime prevalence rates between 3.9% and 13.7%, comparable to the DSM-III-R studies (Bourdon et al. 1988; Kessler et al. 1994, 2005; see Fehm et al. 2005 for an overview of European community studies). Studies that have focused on social phobia with clear evidence of impairment (not merely distress) have tended to report lifetime prevalence rates of 4%–5% (Grant et al. 2005; Narrow et al. 2002).

For children, prevalence estimates of social phobia in New Zealand and the United States, based on DSM-III and DSM-III-R, were only 1% at various ages (Anderson et al. 1987; Kashani et al. 1991; McGee et al. 1990). Higher prevalence ratings for childhood social phobia could be expected based on DSM-IV criteria. Indeed, a recent epidemiological study in Taiwan based on DSM-IV reported a much higher prevalence of childhood social phobia: a 3-month prevalence of 3.4% in seventh-grade children (Gau et al. 2005).

Strengths and Weaknesses of Current Criteria for Social Phobia

SOCIAL PHOBIA OR SOCIAL ANXIETY DISORDER

The name "social phobia" might be misleading, because it suggests that *avoidance* of a *circumscribed* object, activity, or situation is an essential element of the disorder. However, many persons meeting criteria of social phobia do not overtly avoid social situations, because there is societal pressure to execute social roles despite discomfort or fear, and social interaction is hard to avoid because it is everywhere. Moreover, the stimuli that persons with social phobia fear can often not be narrowly circumscribed, because rejection may be feared in many different social situations (e.g., job interview, dating), in relation to many different types of people (e.g., authority figures, romantic figures), and on the basis of different concerns (e.g., blushing, making mistakes, being boring). As a result of the suggestion that social phobia concerns avoidance of a circumscribed situation, the condition might not be recognized by clinicians in patients with more generalized social phobia if they do not use a structured diagnostic interview. Therefore, we advise the preferential use of the name "social anxiety disorder" in DSM-V. In line with this, we only use the name social anxiety disorder for the remainder of this chapter. We do not use "SAD," because this acronym is also used to describe separation anxiety disorder and seasonal affective disorder.

GENERALIZED SOCIAL ANXIETY DISORDER

The main problem with the generalized subtype in contrast to the nongeneralized is that it is defined as a quantitative (or severity) rather than a qualitative difference. Research so far on the difference between the two subtypes has, consistent with the quantitative distinction, simply shown that generalized SocAD cases are more severe—that is, they have earlier onset and longer duration; report more anxiety, more avoidance, more skill deficits (reported and objective); have greater impairment and more problems with work, family, friends, and daily activities; have more suicidal behavior; and have a poorer response to psychological and psychopharmacological treatment (Furmark et al. 2000; M.B. Stein et al. 2000; see also Hook and Valentiner 2002 for a summary).

It has been argued that the different subtypes of SocAD, as defined in DSM, can be conceptualized as lying on a continuous spectrum, with nongeneralized SocAD as the least severe, generalized SocAD in the middle, and generalized SocAD plus avoidant personality disorder as the most severe form (e.g., M.B. Stein et al. 2000). There is little evidence that generalized and nongeneralized SocAD are characterized by qualitatively different treatment response (D.J. Stein et al. 2001), although this is an area in which additional research is required. It is unclear whether the current subtypes add to our understanding of the etiology, maintenance, and treatment response of social phobia, as long as we cannot define the subtypes in a more qualitative way. Based on the empirical literature, one may argue for a new qualitative description of subtypes, if any.

Hook and Valentiner (2002) also argued for a qualitative description of the former generalized subtype—that is, to view it as interpersonal social anxiety, rooted in beliefs of the self being unlovable that were probably developed in early childhood, given the early onset of generalized SocAD. In support of possible qualitative distinctions, individuals with generalized SocAD reported higher childhood shyness, higher neuroticism, and lower extraversion than individuals with nongeneralized SocAD (Stemberger et al. 1995). Moreover, Norton et al. (1997) found that anxiety sensitivity and neuroticism are two different traits underlying SocAD, of which anxiety sensitivity was the stronger predictor of nonclinical nongeneralized SocAD, and neuroticism the stronger predictor of nonclinical generalized SocAD. This research suggests that there is a form of SocAD that originates from a certain personality development.

Chartier et al. (2001) investigated potential childhood risk factors for social phobia and found that lack of a close relationship with an adult, especially for severe (probably generalized) SocAD cases, was a strong risk factor. It could be speculated that lack of a close relationship in early childhood may cause self schemas of being unlovable, which may lead to interpersonal behaviors of avoiding intimacy and being distant, submissive, or even aggressive in interpersonal relationships (Alden and Taylor 2004). More recently, in a Japanese clinical sample of SocAD patients, a relationship subtype emerged from a cluster analysis, which supports cross-cultural validity for an interpersonal subtype (Sakurai et al. 2005).

Taken together, there seems to exist a form of SocAD that may be called the interpersonal subtype, rooted in early schema of the self being unlovable, boring, or weak and characterized by a more neurotic, shy, and less extroverted early personality development, which may have resulted from lack of closeness with an adult. This subtype hypothesis should be tested in the future, preferentially in prospective longitudinal studies.

NONGENERALIZED, SIMPLE, OR CIRCUMSCRIBED SOCIAL ANXIETY DISORDER

The nongeneralized "subtype" is, as DSM-IV-TR acknowledges, a heterogeneous group "that includes persons who fear a single performance situation as well as those who fear several, but not most, social situations" (p. 452). Within nongeneralized SocAD, there seems to be a "performance" subtype that appears to be different from other types of SocAD in a number of ways. *Performance* refers to situations in which a person has to perform for a real or imagined audience (e.g., music, drama, dance, sports, speech) as well as a testing situation. A performance requires an active role of the performer and little or no interaction with the public; the person is the object of others' attention and evaluation.

Research on psychophysiological differences between generalized and nongeneralized SocAD consistently shows that individuals with SocAD of the nongeneralized type have stronger heart rate acceleration during a speech task than individuals with generalized SocAD (Boone et al. 1999; Heimberg et al. 1990; Hofmann et al. 1995; Levin et al. 1993), a difference not found in a social interaction task (Boone et al. 1999). Because most of the people in the nongeneralized group in the referred studies had speech phobia, the finding that they have a higher heart rate response only in a speech task supports a performance subtype. Individuals with nongeneralized SocAD—mostly people with performance anxiety—respond to beta-blockers, unlike people with generalized SocAD (Liebowitz et al. 1992; Turner et al. 1994). Furthermore, those with performance anxiety report more traumatic experiences related to their social phobia than other individuals with social phobia (Stemberger et al. 1995), and this suggests a stronger conditioning history in performance anxiety. Further support for a performance subtype comes from social anxiety questionnaire research in which performance anxiety appears a separate factor from interaction anxiety (Mattick and Clarke 1998). On the basis of these differences, it could even be argued that performance anxiety bears more resemblance to other specific phobias than to more generalized SocAD and might be better placed within that category. Nonetheless, for the time being, the comparable nature of the cognitions (i.e., concern about embarrassment) in nongeneralized and generalized SocAD could argue for their retention within the single SocAD diagnostic category. In any case, there seems to be substantial evidence to suggest a performance subtype of social phobia.

What other social anxieties have been included under the simple or nongeneralized social phobia? Fears of eating or writing in public have been classified as simple social phobias. Such fears are, in most cases, directly related to fear of trembling, just as is fear of drinking, lighting a cigarette, or singing. Fears of eating and writing have also been called "performance fears," suggesting that eating or writing—daily activities in human life—are a performance. Many patients with SocAD have bodily symptoms such as blushing, trembling, or sweating, and for almost half of the patients in a Dutch clinical sample this was the primary source of fear (Bögels and Reith 1999). These bodily reactions have in common that they are observable by others and therefore can attract attention to the person and become a fear themselves. What they also have in common is that they are bodily reactions that are not readily inhibited. Like panic attacks, they can play both stimulus and response roles in the conditioning of social fears (Evans 1972; McNally 1990). Fear of blushing is most common in Dutch referred patients with SocAD, followed by fear of trembling and fear of sweating (Bögels 2006). A similar order was found in Japanese SocAD patients: most frequent was fear of blushing; second, fear of feeling tense; third, fear of emitting body odor (Matsunaga et al. 2001). However, fear of showing bodily symptoms such as blushing cannot be regarded as a nongeneralized fear according to a quantitative definition (although it has been categorized under nongeneralized [Scholing and Emmelkamp 1993]) because visible bodily reactions occur in many different social situations and therefore have the power to condition the social fear to many different social situations of the performance and the interaction type.

Research from various areas suggests that fear of showing bodily symptoms is indeed a distinct social fear. Several studies investigating ratings of objective social behavior of SocAD patients found that social skills ratings comprised two factors: a visible anxiety factor and a social behavior factor (Voncken and Bögels 2008). Even more convincing, the same visible anxiety and social behavior factors were found in children with SocAD while they performed social tasks (Cartwright-Hatton et al. 2003). Patients with fear of blushing as the primary source of fear had indeed higher blushing responses, as measured by a photo-plethysmograph, than SocAD patients without this primary fear in two studies (Gerlach et al. 2001; Voncken and Bögels 2008), and they were also identified by independent observers as blushing more often and more intensively (Voncken and Bögels 2006). Interestingly, they did not show higher skin conductance response, which is an indication of general fear. Another argument for distinguishing a fear of showing bodily symptoms subtype is that this problem seems highly common in Asiatic cultures (Kleinknecht et al. 1997) and is the predominant fear in SocAD patients with TK (Matsunaga et al. 2001). With respect to the learning history of a fear of blushing, Mulkens and Bögels (1999) found that people with subclinical, as well as clinical, SocAD with fear of blushing as the primary complaint reported more traumatic experiences preceding the fear, suggesting that, just as in performance anxiety, conditioning may play an important role in the learning history.

A last form of more circumscribed SocAD, not mentioned in any DSM, is social appearance anxiety or social physique anxiety (Hart et al. 1989). Some individuals with SocAD, when their physiques are observed by others, become anxious and are concerned about being negatively evaluated because of their physical appearance. For example, their concerns may focus on aspects of their bodily appearance, hair growth on their body, clothes, or way of walking. With respect to the learning history of social physique anxiety, Cash et al. (1986) found that being teased about one's appearance as a child is a risk factor, but so is actual appearance (e.g., body fat [Hart et al. 1989]). In line with this, D.J. Stein et al. (2004) included body-focused concerns as one of the dimensions in their social anxiety disorder spectrum approach. It is unknown to what extent these types of pathological social concerns about body image overlap with the DSM-IV diagnostic category of body dysmorphic disorder; however, based on the frequent comorbidity between that and SocAD (Coles et al. 2006), the possibility of a social physique "subtype" of SocAD overlapping with current conceptualizations of body dysmorphic disorder should be strongly considered.

RECOGNITION OF IRRATIONALITY OF FEAR

Criterion C states that adults—but not necessarily children—should recognize that their fear is irrational or exaggerated. It is our clinical impression that some adult SocAD patients do not recognize the "irrationality" of their fears. This criterion was formulated to distinguish SocAD from psychotic disorders but is not included in some other anxiety disorders, such as panic disorder. In other anxiety disorders the criterion is less stringent; for example, in obsessive-compulsive disorder, *at some point during the course of the disorder,* the person has recognized that the obsessions or compulsions are excessive or unreasonable. It might not be necessary to mutually exclude social phobia and psychotic disorders, because psychotic patients with a comorbid diagnosis of SocAD might benefit from treatment for SocAD. In fact, there are indications that treating social phobia might prevent psychotic relapse (Bögels and Tarrier 2004). Another reason to reevaluate criterion C is that some SocAD patients with TK lose insight into their symptoms (Matsunaga et al. 2001). Poor insight tended to be more frequent in nonresponders to (pharmacological) treatment. Matsunaga et al. (2001) argue for a "poor insight" specifier in SocAD just as DSM-IV has recognized in some other anxiety disorders (e.g., obsessive-compulsive disorder). It might be sufficient that the interviewer recognizes the fear as exaggerated, that is, that the fear of being rejected because of X is larger than necessary, given X.

SUBTHRESHOLD SOCIAL ANXIETY DISORDER

Criterion E concerns the interference as a result of social anxiety: the SocAD should interfere with social or professional (school) functioning. In clinical samples, the failure to discern demonstrable psychosocial impairment (as opposed to distress about having the illness) is a prime reason for failing to meet full diagnostic criteria for DSM-IV social phobia (Zimmerman et al. 2004). Subthreshold SocAD concerns social fears that might bother the person and lead to suffering but do not clearly interfere with functioning. Structured diagnostic interviews such as the Anxiety Disorder Interview Schedule (Albano and Silverman 1996; DiNardo et al. 1994) allow for such subthreshold diagnoses by assigning interference scores below 4. Including subthreshold social phobia in DSM-V would have certain advantages in the light of research findings. First, the diagnosis of SocAD is more stable over the life course when subthreshold levels of SocAD are included. Second, because social phobia is the precursor of many other severe types of psychopathology, such as depression (D.J. Stein et al. 2001), conduct disorder, psychotic disorder, and addictions (Bögels and Tarrier 2004), preventing SocAD by intervening in subthreshold stages might preclude such severe outcomes. On the other hand, there is merit to excluding from diagnostic status a set of symptoms that merely serve as a risk factor for other disorders. As such, it might be better to educate clinicians about subthreshold social anxiety symptoms without codifying them as a diagnostic entity.

SOCIAL ANXIETY DISORDER AS A COMORBID STATE IMPORTANT FOR TREATMENT

Criterion G states that pervasive developmental disorder (PDD) and social phobia are mutually exclusive, that is, the social anxiety should not be attributed to PDD. As was already argued in the context of psychotic disorder, persons with PDD and excessive social anxiety might benefit from SocAD treatment (Sverd 2003; Tantam 2000). These individuals also present a different clinical picture from those with PDD with conduct problems or depression. Therefore, it could be considered to change this statement to "Consider also a diagnosis of PDD if the social fears are related to symptoms of PDD."

Overlap Between Social Phobia and Avoidant Personality Disorder

The overlap between avoidant personality disorder and social phobia, especially of the generalized subtype, is enormous (i.e., up to 89%; Schneier et al. 1991, 1992). The distinction, as described in DSM-III, is that in both disorders humiliation is a concern, but a specific situation, such as public speaking, is avoided rather than personal relationships. Note that in DSM-III, SocAD was still regarded as a phobia rather than an anxiety state. In DSM-III-R, there was one criterion of avoidant personality disorder that clearly differentiated SocAD from avoidant personality disorder, concerning avoidance of situations because of fear of physical vulnerability; in DSM-IV, however, this criterion was removed. This makes it questionable whether the current distinction between (generalized) SocAD and avoidant personality disorder is still valid. The pattern of family aggregation of SocAD and avoidant personality disorder also suggests that the latter and social phobia represent a dimension of severity of social anxiety rather than separate disorders, because the relatives of both avoidant personality disorder and SocAD patients are at risk for having social phobia (Tillfors et al. 2001), and both avoidant personality disorder and generalized SocAD are seen at markedly elevated rates among first-degree relatives of patients with generalized SocAD (M.B. Stein et al. 1998).

Emerging Hypotheses That Can Be Tested in the Not Too Distant Future

Generalized social phobia is characterized by altered amygdala reactivity to salient social cues (e.g., emotional faces) (Phan et al. 2005; M.B. Stein et al. 2002). Moreover, it is likely that greater amygdala activation in this context is associated with higher levels of social anxiety and may not be restricted to persons with SocAD. As such, heightened amygdala activation to certain types of emotional processing demands may characterize an endophenotype for SocAD and related disorders, such as enduring childhood behavioral inhibition (Schwartz et al. 2003). When technological advances enable the conduct of multicenter neuroimaging studies, it will be possible to study enough individuals to test this hypothesis.

As noted earlier, there exist compelling data for genetic and environmental contributors to SocAD, but with the exception of twin studies, these two areas of research have not been well integrated. It seems likely that gene–environment interactions might explain the propensity for some individuals with high familial risk to develop SocAD, whereas others do not. Testing for gene–environment interactions is impossible with certain study designs and, even when possible, requires large sample sizes. Once specific candidate genes for SocAD are identified, testing for such interactions will be possible (see Caspi et al. 2003 for an example in major depression) although large samples will still be required.

Another interesting research area concerning the etiology of SocAD concerns the specific psychophysiological responses that may underlie social phobia. Already in 1983, the landmark study of Amies, Gelder and Shaw revealed that the only bodily symptom that is more pronounced in social phobia, compared with agoraphobia, is blushing (Amies et al. 1983). The study relied on self-report, but now that blushing is being assessed with a cheek photo-plethysmograph (e.g., Bogels et al. 2002; Mulkens et al. 2001), it can be tested whether a more intense blushing response is a pathway toward either SocAD in general or a certain subtype of SocAD: social anxiety due to fear of showing bodily symptoms. Because such a blushing response can be assessed very early in childhood, it can be used as a potential early marker for a socially anxious development.

Conclusion

Social anxiety disorder has, in recent decades, emerged from a phobic reaction to a circumscribed social situation to an anxiety state with large variety in severity, content of fears, and insight in irrationality of fears. Despite the progress that has been made in understanding maintenance factors and developing effective treatments, the etiology of SocAD is largely unknown. The subtype classification as defined in DSM concerns a quantitative (severity) rather than a qualitative differentiation, and one can argue that such subtyping does not add to our understanding of the etiology. On the basis of the empirical literature, we argue for qualitative subtypes or dimensions, if any. SocAD can be conceptualized in four dimensions: 1) performance fear, 2) fear of showing bodily symptoms, 3) social physical fear, and 4) interpersonal anxiety. Different etiological routes in terms of predisposition (e.g., psychophysiology), rearing, and life events may underlie these dimensions and can be tested, preferably with experimental and longitudinal designs, starting from early childhood. Perhaps most progress in this field may come from testing gene (or predisposition)-environment interactions. Finally, testing the stability of etiological routes and SocAD subtypes across cultures may enhance our understanding of the essential characteristics of SocAD.

References

Albano AM, Silverman AM: Anxiety Disorders Interview Schedule for DSM-IV Child Version, Clinical Manual. San Antonio, TX, Psychological Corporation, 1996

Alden LE, Taylor CT: Interpersonal processes in social phobia. Clin Psychol Rev 24:857–882, 2004

American Psychiatric Association: Diagnostic and Statistical Manual of Mental Disorders, 3rd Edition. Washington, DC, American Psychiatric Association, 1980

American Psychiatric Association: Diagnostic and Statistical Manual of Mental Disorders, 3rd Edition, Revised. Washington, DC, American Psychiatric Association, 1987

American Psychiatric Association: Diagnostic and Statistical Manual of Mental Disorders, 4th Edition. Washington, DC, American Psychiatric Association, 1994

American Psychiatric Association: Diagnostic and Statistical Manual of Mental Disorders, 4th Edition, Text Revision. Washington, DC, American Psychiatric Association, 2000

Amies PL, Gelder MG, Shaw PM: Social phobia: a comparative clinical study. Br J Psychiatry 142:174–179, 1983

Anderson JC, Williams SM, McGee R, et al: DSM-III disorders in pre-adolescent children: prevalence in a large sample from the general population. Arch Gen Psychiatry 44:69–76, 1987

Barrett PM, Dadds MR, Rapee RM: Family treatment of childhood anxiety: a controlled trial. J Consult Clin Psychol 20:459–468, 1996

Biederman JDR, Hirshfeld-Becker JF, Rosenbaum C, et al: Further evidence of association between behavioral inhibition and social anxiety in children. Am J Psychiatry 158:1673–1679, 2001

Bögels SM: Task concentration training versus applied relaxation, in combination with cognitive therapy, for social phobia patients with fear of blushing, trembling, and sweating. Behav Res Ther 44:1119–1210, 2006

Bögels SM, Reith W: Validity of two questionnaires to assess social fears: the Dutch Social Phobia and Anxiety Inventory and the Blushing, Trembling and Sweating Questionnaire. J Psychopathol Behav Assess 21:51–66, 1999

Bögels SM, Tarrier N: Unexplored issues and future direction in social phobia research. Clin Psychol Rev 24:731–736, 2004

Bögels SM, Rijsemus W, De Jong PJ: Self-focused attention and social anxiety: the effects of experimentally heightened self-awareness on fear, blushing, cognitions, and social skills. Cognit Ther Res 26:461–472, 2002

Boone ML, McNeil DW, Masia CL, et al: Multimodal comparisons of social phobia subtypes and avoidant personality disorder. J Anxiety Disord 13:271–292, 1999

Bourdon KH, Boyd JH, Rae DS, et al: Gender differences in phobias: results of the ECA community survey. J Anxiety Disord 2:227–241, 1988

Cartwright-Hatton S, Hodges L, Porter J: Social anxiety in childhood: the relationship between self and observer rated social skills. J Child Psychol Psychiatry 44:1–6, 2003

Cash TF, Winstead BA, Janda LH: Body image survey report: the great American shape-up. Psychol Today 20:30–37, 1986

Caspi A, Sugden K, Moffitt TE, et al: Influence of life stress on depression: moderation by a polymorphism in the 5-HTT gene. Science 301:386–389, 2003

Chartier MJ, Walker JR, Stein MB: Social phobia and potential childhood risk factors in a community sample. Psychol Med 31:307–315, 2001

Coles ME, Phillips KA, Menard W et al: Body dysmorphic disorder and social phobia: cross-sectional and prospective data. Depress Anxiety 23:26–33, 2006

Cooper PJ, Fearn V, Willets L, et al: Affective disorders in the parents of a clinical sample of children with anxiety disorders. J Affect Disord 93:205–212, 2006

Costello EJ, Mustillo S, Erkanli A, et al: Prevalence and development of psychiatric disorders in childhood and adolescence. Arch Gen Psychiatry 60:837–844, 2003

Davidson JRT, Hughes DL, George LK, et al: The epidemiology of social phobia: findings from the Duke epidemiological catchment area study. Psychol Med 23:709–718, 1993

DiNardo PA, Brown TA, Barlow DH: Anxiety Disorders Interview Schedule for DSM-IV: Lifetime Version (ADIS-IV-L). San Antonio, TX, Psychological Corporation, 1994

DeWit DJ, Ogborne A, Offord DR, et al: Antecedents of the risk of recovery from DSM-III-R social phobia. Psychol Med 29:569–582, 1999

Essau CA, Conradt J, Petermann F: Frequency and comorbidity of social phobia and social fears in adolescents. Behav Res Ther 37:831–843, 1999

Evans IM: A conditioning model of a common neurotic pattern—fear of fear. Psychotherapy: Theory, Research, and Practice 9:238–242, 1972

Fehm L, Pelisso A, Furmark T, et al: Size and burden of social phobia in Europe. Eur Neuropsychopharmacol 15:453–462, 2005

Feyer A, Mannuzza S, Chapman T, et al: Specificity in familial aggregation of phobic disorders. Arch Gen Psychiatry 52:564–573, 1995

Francis G, Last CG, Strauss CC: Avoidant disorder and social phobia in children and adolescents. J Am Acad Child Adolesc Psychiatry 31:1086–1089, 1992

Furmark T, Tillfors M, Stattin H, et al: Social phobia subtypes in the general population revealed by cluster analysis. Psychol Med 30:1335–1344, 2000

Gau SFS, Chong MY, Chen THH, et al: A 3-year panel study of mental disorders among adolescents in Taiwan. Am J Psychiatry 162:1344–1350, 2005

Gerlach AL, Wilhelm FH, Gruber K, et al: Blushing and physiological arousability in social phobia. J Abnorm Psychol 110:247–258, 2001

Grant BF, Hasin DS, Blanco C, et al: The epidemiology of social anxiety disorder in the United States: results from the National Epidemiologic Survey on Alcohol and Related Conditions. J Clin Psychiatry 66:1351–1361, 2005

Hart EA, Leary MR, Rejeski WJ: The measurement of social physique anxiety. J Sport Exerc Psychol 11:94–104, 1989

Heimberg RG, Hope DA, Dodge CS, et al: DSM-III-R subtypes of social phobia: comparison of generalized social phobics and public speaking phobics. J Nerv Ment Dis 178:172–179, 1990

Hettema JM, Prescott CA, Myers JM, et al: The structure of genetic and environmental risk factors for anxiety disorders in men and women. Arch Gen Psychiatry 62:182–189, 2005

Hirshfeld-Becker DH, Biederman J, Faraone SV, et al: Lack of association between behavioral inhibition and psychosocial adversity factors in children at risk for anxiety disorders. Am J Psychiatry 161:547–555, 2004

Hofmann SG, Newman MG, Ehlers A, et al: Psychophysiological differences between subgroups of social phobia. J Abnorm Psychol 104:224–231, 1995

Hook JN, Valentiner DP: Are specific and generalized social phobias qualitatively distinct? Clin Psychol Sci Pract 9:379–395, 2002

Hudson JI, Mangweth B, Pope HG, et al: Family study of affective spectrum disorder. Arch Gen Psychiatry 60:170–177, 2003

Kashani JH, Dandoy AC, Orvaschel H: Current perspectives on anxiety disorders in children and adolescents: an overview. Compr Psychiatry 32:481–495, 1991

Kessler RC, McGonagle KA, Zhao S, et al: Lifetime and 12-month prevalence of DSM-III-R psychiatric disorders in the United States. Results from the National Comorbidity Survey. Arch Gen Psychiatry 51:8–19, 1994

Kessler RC, Stein MB, Berglund P: Social phobia subtypes in the National Comorbidity Survey. Am J Psychiatry 155:613–619, 1998

Kessler RC, Berglund P, Demler O, et al: Lifetime prevalence and age-of-onset distributions of DSM-IV disorders in the National Comorbidity Survey Replication. Arch Gen Psychiatry 62:593–602, 2005

Kleinknecht RA, Dinnel DL, Kleinknecht EE, et al: Cultural factors in social anxiety: a comparison of social phobia symptoms and Taijin Kyofusho. J Anxiety Disord 11:157–177, 1997

Levin AP, Saoud JB, Strauman T, et al: Responses of "generalized" and "discrete" social phobics during public speaking. J Anxiety Disord 7:207–221, 1993

Lieb R, Wittchen H, Höfler M, et al: Parental psychopathology, parenting styles, and the risk of social phobia in offspring. Arch Gen Psychiatry 57:859–865, 2000

Liebowitz MR, Schneier F, Campeas R, et al: Phenelzine vs atenolol in social phobia: a placebo-controlled comparison. Arch Gen Psychiatry 49:290–300, 1992

Lipsitz JD, Schneider FR: Social phobia: epidemiology and costs of illness. Pharmacoeconomics 18:23–32, 2000

Matsunaga H, Kiriike N, Matsui T, et al: Taijin kyofusho: a form of social anxiety that responds to serotonin reuptake inhibitors? Int J Neuropsychopharmacol 4:231–237, 2001

Mattick RP, Clarke JC: Development and validation of measures of social phobia scrutiny fear and social interaction anxiety. Behav Res Ther 36:455–470, 1998

McGee R, Feehan M, Williams S, et al: DSM-III disorders in a large sample of adolescents. J Am Acad Child Adolesc Psychiatry 29:611–619, 1990

McNally RJ: Psychological approaches to panic disorder: a review. Psychol Bull 108:3–20, 1990

Mulkens S, Bögels SM: Learning history in fear of blushing. Behav Res Ther 37:1159–1167, 1999

Mulkens S, Bogels SM, de Jong PJ, et al: Fear of blushing: effects of task concentration training versus exposure in vivo on fear and physiology. J Anxiety Disord 15:413–432, 2001

Narrow WE, Rae DS, Robins LN, et al: Revised prevalence estimates of mental disorders in the United States: using a clinical significance criterion to reconcile 2 surveys' estimates. Arch Gen Psychiatry 59:115–123, 2002

Nauta M, Scholing A, Emmelkamp P, et al: Cognitive-behavior therapy for children with anxiety disorders in a clinical setting: no additional effect of a cognitive parent training. J Am Acad Child Adolesc Psychiatry 42:1270–1278, 2003

Norton GR, Cox BJ, Hewitt PL, et al: Personality factors associated with generalized and non-generalized social anxiety. Pers Individ Dif 22:655–660, 1997

Perugi G, Nassani S, Socci C et al: Avoidant personality in social phobia and panic-agoraphobia disorder: a comparison. J Affect Disord 54:277–282, 1999

Phan KL, Fitzgerald DA, Nathan PJ et al: Association between amygdala hyperactivity to harsh faces and severity of social anxiety in generalized social phobia. Biol Psychiatry 59:424–429, 2005

Rapee RM, Spence SH: The etiology of social phobia: empirical evidence and an initial model. Clin Psychol Rev 24:737–767, 2004

Reich J, Yates W: Family history of psychiatric disorders in social phobia. Compr Psychiatry 29:72–75, 1988

Robinson JAL, Kagan J, Reznick JS, et al: The heritability of inhibited and uninhibited behavior: a twin study. Dev Psychol, 28:1030–1037, 1992

Romano E, Tremblay RE, Vitaro F: Prevalence of psychiatric diagnoses and the role of perceived impairment: findings from an adolescent community sample. J Child Psychol Psychiatry 42:451–461, 2001

Sakurai A, Nagata T, Harai H, et al: Is "relationship fear" unique to Japan? symptom factors and patient clusters of social anxiety disorder among the Japanese clinical population. J Affect Disord 87:131–137, 2005

Scholing A, Emmelkamp PM: Cognitive and behavioural treatments of fear of blushing, sweating or trembling. Behav Res Ther 31:155–170, 1993

Schneier FR, Spitzer RL, Gibbon M, et al: The relationship of social phobia subtypes and avoidant personality disorders. Compr Psychiatry 6:496–502, 1991

Schneier FR, Johnsons J, Hornig CD, et al: Social phobia: comorbidity and morbidity in an epidemiologic sample. Arch Gen Psychiatry 49:282–288, 1992

Schwartz CE, Wright CI, Shin LM, et al: Inhibited and uninhibited infants "grown up": adult amygdalar response to novelty. Science 300:1952–1953, 2003

Simon NM, Otto MW, Korlby NB, et al: Quality of life in social anxiety disorder compared with panic disorder and the general population. Psychiatr Serv 53:714–718, 2002

Smoller JW, Rosenbaum JF, Biederman J, et al: Association of a genetic marker at the corticotropin-releasing hormone locus with behavioral inhibition. Biol Psychiatry 54:1376–1381, 2003

Smoller JW, Yamaki LH, Fagerness JA, et al: The corticotropin-releasing hormone gene and behavioral inhibition in children at risk for panic disorder. Biol Psychiatry 57:1485–1492, 2005

Stein DJ, Stein MB, Goodwin W, et al: The selective serotonin reuptake inhibitor paroxetine is effective in more generalized and less generalized social anxiety disorder. Psychopharmacology 158:267–272, 2001

Stein DJ, Ono Y, Tajima O, et al: The social anxiety disorder spectrum. J Clin Psychiatry 65:27–33, 2004

Stein MB, Chartier MJ, Hazen AZ, et al: A direct-interview family study of generalized social phobia. Am J Psychiatry 155:90–97, 1998

Stein MB, Torgrud LJ, Walker JR: Social phobia symptoms, subtypes, and severity: findings from a community survey. Arch Gen Psychiatry 57:1046–1052, 2000

Stein MB, Jang KL, Livesley J: Heritability of social anxiety-related concerns and personality characteristics: a twin study. J Nerv Ment Dis 190:219–224, 2002

Stemberger R, Turner SM, Beidel DC, et al: Social phobia: an analysis of possible developmental factors. J Abnorm Psychol 104:526–531, 1995

Sverd J: Psychiatric disorders in individuals with pervasive developmental disorder. J Psychiatr Pract 9:111–127, 2003

Tantam D: Psychological disorder in adolescents and adults with Asperger syndrome. Autism 4:47–62, 2000

Tiet QQ, Bird HR, Hoven CW: Relationship between specific aversive life events and psychiatric disorders. J Abnorm Child Psychol 29:153–164, 2001

Tillfors M, Furmark T, Ekselius L, et al: Social phobia and avoidant personality disorder as related to parental history of social anxiety: a general population study. Behav Res Ther 39:289–298, 2001

Turner SM, Beidel DC, Jacob RG: Social phobia: a comparison of behaviour therapy and atenolol. J Consult Clin Psychol 62:350–358, 1994

Voncken MJ, Bögels SM: Physiological responses, anxious appearance, and social skills in social phobia, in Afraid of Being Disliked: From Distorted Cognitions to Interpersonal Problems in Social Phobia. Doctoral thesis, Voncken MJ. Maastricht, The Netherlands, University Press, 2006, pp 47–77

Voncken MJ, Bögels SM: Social performance deficits in social anxiety disorder: reality during conversation and biased perception during speech. J Anxiety Disord February 9, 2008 [Epub ahead of print]

Wittchen HU, Fehm L: Epidemiology and natural course of social fears and social phobia. Acta Psychiatr Scand 108:4–18, 2003

Yonkers KA, Dijck IR, Keller MB: An eight-year longitudinal comparison of clinical course and characteristics of social phobia among men and women. Psychiatr Serv 52:637–643, 2001

Zimmerman M, Chelminski I, Young D: On the threshold of disorder: a study of the impact of the DSM-IV clinical significance criterion on diagnosing depressive and anxiety disorders in clinical practice. J Clin Psychiatry 65:1400–1405, 2004

4

SPECIFIC PHOBIAS

Paul M.G. Emmelkamp, Ph.D.
Hans-Ulrich Wittchen, Ph.D.

Our purpose in this chapter is to discuss the current status of research on the epidemiology, clinical features, course and prognosis, and familial and genetic patterns of specific phobias and to provide some directions for future research. We examine evidence for separating subtypes of specific phobia and for delineating specific phobias from other anxiety disorders.

Description of the Disorder

According to almost all epidemiological surveys in the community, specific phobia (formerly simple phobia in DSM-III-R [American Psychiatric Association 1987]) is the most widespread of all anxiety disorders. Specific phobias are focused upon, and restricted to, specific objects and situations, such as animals, heights, storm, closed spaces, or darkness, and it is well known that specific phobias can develop in response to almost any type of object (Marks 1987). According to the diagnostic criteria of DSM-IV (American Psychiatric Association 1994) and DSM-IV-TR (American Psychiatric Association 2000), specific phobia should be diagnosed in the case of a marked and persistent, excessive, and/or irrational fear that occurs in response to a real or anticipated circumscribed stimulus, such as an object or situation (criterion A), and that is accompanied by all of the following features: the confrontation provokes almost invariably an immediate anxiety reaction that might reach the severity threshold of a situational bound panic attack (criterion B); the person recognizes that the anxiety is excessive or unreasonable (criterion C); the person avoids or endures the situation or object with intense anxiety (criterion D); and the fear, associated anticipatory anxiety, or avoidance behavior interferes significantly with the person's normal life or is associated with clinically significant suffering (criterion E). The situationally bound fear reaction, panic, or avoidance should not be better explained by other mental disorders, such as from the content of the obsessions of obsessive-compulsive disorder (OCD), trauma of posttraumatic stress disorder (PTSD), separation anxiety, social phobia, or panic disorder/agoraphobia trigger stimuli. For specific phobias that frequently occur as early as childhood, the DSM-IV-TR criteria also highlight at least three modified criteria—namely, that panic-like features (criterion B) might be manifest with different emotional responses, that children are not required to consider their fear as irrational or excessive, and that the duration in children must be of at least 6 months to warrant a diagnosis.

The diagnostic criteria for specific phobia in ICD-10 (World Health Organization 1992) are very similar to those in DSM-IV-TR; however, ICD-10 does not require that the fear is recognized as unreasonable. Debates about this difference seem to have come to the conclusion that the DSM-IV-TR version is preferable, because exaggerated anxiety responses to stressors alone are not considered to be clinically sufficient; also, the unreasonable component enhances the clinical utility because persons who seek treatment typically do so when they recognize that their anxiety is unreasonable (Tyrer 1989).

DSM-IV-TR—unlike ICD-10, which uses fewer distinctions—distinguishes five types of specific phobias: animal (e.g., spiders, dogs, cats, snakes, and birds), natural environment (e.g., storms, heights, or water), blood-injection-injury (e.g., injections, dental phobia), situational (e.g., tunnels, bridges, elevators, flying, driving, or enclosed places), and a residual category (e.g., choking, vomiting, loud sounds, costumed characters). The decision to distinguish different types of phobia arises from research suggesting that each type has sufficiently distinct features with regard to age at onset, physiological response (e.g., fainting, panic), fear of physiological response, and patterns of comorbidity (e.g., Antony et al. 1997; Lipsitz et al. 2002). However, there is debate about how useful and meaningful these distinctions are.

Epidemiology

PREVALENCE

Despite considerable methodological differences, convergent evidence from many studies around the world suggests a lifetime prevalence of specific phobias in the community of greater than 10% (Bijl et al. 1997; Bland et al. 1988; Burnam et al. 1987; Karno et al. 1987; Kessler et al. 1994; Magee et al. 1996; Myers et al. 1984; Robins et al. 1984; Wittchen 1988; Wittchen and Jacobi 2005; Wittchen et al.

1998) and reveals that specific phobia is the most common of all mental disorders. There are some—albeit minor—indications that rates might vary by culture, although it is not clear whether this is simply due to instruments that are not culturally adapted and the fact that some studies restrict the diagnostic assessment to only certain forms of specific phobias. Brown et al. (1990) suggested that fears and phobias are more prevalent in African Americans and Mexican Americans born in the United States (Karno et al. 1989). Higher rates have also been reported from Brazil (Da Motta et al. 2000). The recent European-wide Size and Burden of Disorders of the Brain Project (Wittchen and Jacobi 2005) reported little evidence for substantial cross-national variation in Europe. In all these studies, depressive disorders and specific phobias rank as the most common mental disorders, both over the lifetime and in the past 12 months. Lower figures for 12-month prevalence were reported in Japan, but the rank order was similar (Kawakami et al. 2005): major depression (2.9%), specific phobia (2.7%), and alcohol abuse/dependence (2.0%) were the most prevalent.

Few studies have examined the prevalence of various subtypes of specific phobia, which is remarkable. Wittchen et al. (1998, 1999) reported the following rank order by frequency for a community sample of adolescents: The cumulative incidence up to age 19 years was as follows: animal (7%), blood-injection-injury (6%), situational (4%), and natural-environmental type (3.4%). However, later in life the highest rates were for phobias of the situational and natural environment type.

The prevalence of fears that do not meet DSM-IV-TR criteria is considerably higher, especially in children. For example, in a sample of 4- to 12-year-olds, 75% of children reported fears of circumscribed objects or situations (Muris et al. 2000). In children, specific fears are common and are often "passing episodes in a normal developmental process" (Emmelkamp 1982) and developmentally appropriate, and disappear within a few months. DSM-IV-TR requires that, for young persons, a specific phobia must last at least 6 months before a formal diagnosis can be made. Specific phobias can also be differentiated from such normal developmental fears in that the phobic reaction is excessive.

Age Differences

The prevalence of specific phobias varies considerably across the lifespan (Kessler et al. 1994; Wittchen and Jacobi 2005). Because specific phobias are typically persistent disorders, the reason for this variation is not yet well explained. Studies in childhood, adolescent, and young adult samples usually report the highest prevalence (lifetime rates, 11%–15%; 12-month, 6%–8%), whereas prevalence rates among older adults (after age of 50) seem to be substantially lower (lifetime rates, 6%–9%; 12-month, 4%–6%). The age-at-onset distribution appears to be fairly similar, indicating that at least two-thirds of specific phobias have their first onset in childhood or adolescence. Whereas community surveys covering the whole age range usually report mean onset in the mid-teens (Kessler et al. 2005a), there is some evidence that recall bias shifts the age onset reports in older subjects to higher ages of onset. Also, studies that date the onset of the first fear, as opposed to the full criteria of phobia, typically state lower ages of onset. Prospective-longitudinal studies with incidence estimates in adolescent cohorts (Wittchen et al. 1999) suggest that most specific phobias started up to the early teens; after age of 16, the assumed mean age of onset in adult studies, only few incident cases are observed for any of the five subtypes. This is consistent with earlier clinical studies suggesting that animal and blood-injection-injury phobia tend to have an earlier onset in childhood (Öst 1987), whereas situational and height phobias tend to start later in adolescence. In clinical samples, the mean onset age is estimated to be about 8 years for animal phobia and blood-injury phobia (Öst and Hellström 1997), 12 years for dental phobia, and 20 years for claustrophobia (Öst 1987).

Gender Differences

Research has consistently found that certain specific phobias according to the DSM criteria (animals, lightning, enclosed spaces, and darkness) are more common in women, compared with men (Curtis et al. 1998; Frederikson et al. 1996; Goisman et al. 1998), whereas smaller gender differences are observed for phobias of heights, flying, injections, and dentists. The reason for the overall substantial two-to-one preponderance of women remains a matter of debate. The hypothesis of underreporting of men (Pierce and Kirkpatrick 1992) is indirectly supported by the finding that the gender difference is less pronounced before age 10 years and increases with age (Craske 2003).

IMPAIRMENT

The impairment criterion is the most problematic of all DSM-IV-TR criteria because there are no uniform measurements for determining social-role impairment that are applicable in an identical way to children, adolescents, adults, and the elderly. Furthermore, in the early stages of specific phobia, failure to reach expected normative role transitions might be more easily detectable than in lifelong cases, where individual adaptations and well-established avoidance behaviors might have led to stable social integration, although at a low level. A further complication is that avoidance of the feared situations—if successful—leads to prolonged periods of relative freedom from more severe anxiety reactions, acute suffering, and impairment. The diagnosis is less problematic when specific phobia can lead to intense panic and extreme immediate avoidance of the specific situations. In some cases, this might have immediate severe consequences such as when a blood phobic avoids medical treatment or a claustrophobic refuses to undergo a scan. As reviewed later, however, even strong fears do not seem to motivate many individuals to refer themselves for treatment. It is not clear to what degree the potential lack of awareness about having a mental disorder in early childhood and adolescence contributes to this finding. When people with specific phobias do seek treatment, it is often because they anticipate that circumstances will force confrontation with a dreaded cue stimulus, or probably more commonly, when secondary psychopathological complications have emerged, such as depressive demoralization or depression. This might explain why it usually takes decades before subjects with specific phobias ultimately receive professional attention (Kessler et al. 2005b).

Few studies have addressed specifically the issue of impairment approaches to specific phobias. Wittchen and Jacobi (2005) raised the question to what degree the DSM-IV-TR impairment and distress criteria and the way they are assessed in diagnostic instruments are sufficiently adapted to the diagnosis-specific and age-group–related social role and social functioning pattern. Zimmerman et al. (2004) found that adding the criterion of clinically significant impairment reduced the number of specific phobia diagnoses substantially, more so than in major depression, generalized anxiety disorder (GAD), and PTSD. In a recent study in Europe (conducted in Belgium, France, Germany, Italy, the Netherlands, and Spain), mental disorders were found to be important determinants of work-role disability and quality of life (Alonso et al. 2004). However, specific phobia had lower independent impact on work loss days than panic disorder, agoraphobia, PTSD, major depressive episode, and dysthymia. However, this study did not control for differences in age-group composition of subjects with specific phobia and other mental disorders that occur more frequently in later life. The National Comorbidity Survey investigated whether individuals with an anxiety disorder were also impaired in terms of a physical disorder (Sareen et al. 2005). Anxiety disorders were positively associated with physical disorders even after adjusting for other mental disorders. However, PTSD and panic disorder with or without agoraphobia were more likely to be associated with physical disorders than were GAD, social phobia, or specific phobia. Interestingly, specific phobias were strongly linked with respiratory disease, which corroborates findings from a study by Goodwin et al. (2003) that found an association between specific phobia and a diagnosis of asthma.

There have also been only a few studies that have directly compared impairment among different anxiety disorders. In a study using the Work and Social Adjustment Scale, specific-phobic patients were clearly less impaired than patients with agoraphobia and social phobia, especially in the areas of work and relationships (Mataix-Cols et al. 2005). As to quality of life, Cramer et al. (2005) found, in a study with more than 2,000 individuals, that in contrast to social phobia, panic disorder, and GAD, specific phobias had only a small effect on quality of life. Furthermore, in contrast to other anxiety disorders, such as panic disorder, social phobia, and OCD, patients with specific phobias were not found to be neuropsychologically impaired in terms of episodic memory and executive functioning.

COMORBIDITY

All anxiety disorders, phobias, and specific phobias are frequently comorbid with one another. In a cross-tabulation of lifetime prevalence findings in 14- to 24-year-olds, including specific phobia subtypes, Wittchen et al. (2003) showed that all anxiety disorders are substantially associated with one another, with most odds ratios being 2 or greater. For example, specific phobia, animal type was significantly associated with specific phobia, environmental type (OR=3.5) and with specific phobia, situational type (OR=2.4). The blood-injury type was associated with the environmental (OR=4.8) and the situational type (OR=3.5). Specific phobias were particularly highly associated also with all other anxiety disorders except PTSD and OCD; in most of these comorbid patterns, the onset of specific phobias clearly preceded the onset of the other types of anxiety disorders. Comorbid patterns of specific phobias with a wide range of other disorders, including depression, somatoform, bipolar disorders, substance use, and eating disorders have also been extensively documented (Kessler et al. 2005b). The combined finding that specific phobias are early-onset disorders and are significantly associated with many forms of subsequent psychopathology has recently created more interest in exploring whether specific phobias are risk factors for subsequent psychopathology.

An interesting prospective study over the first decades of life was reported by Bittner et al. (2004), who used the Early Developmental Stages of Psychopathology sample and found that the proportion of pure (i.e., not comorbid) specific phobias and other anxiety disorders was low only among young adolescents, whereas by each progressive follow-up investigation, the proportion of comorbid and multi-comorbid other mental disorders increased steadily. This study investigated whether specific anxiety disorders and impairment associated with anxiety disorders predicted major depression 4 years later. After other disorders were controlled for, specific phobia predicted subsequent major depression, but the odds ratio was modest (1.9). Other anxiety disorders in early adolescence were better able to predict the first onset of major depression: GAD at baseline was the best predictor (OR=4.5), followed by panic disorder (OR=3.4), agoraphobia (OR=3.1), and social phobia (OR=2.9). Furthermore, severe impairment in one or more social roles was also found to be associated with a significantly greater risk of major depressive disorder.

High comorbidity among anxiety and depressive disorders is a consistent finding in both clinical and community studies. The causes of the comorbidity, however, are not yet well understood, and few studies have investigated whether normal personality traits mediate this comorbidity. A notable exception is a study by Andrews et al. (1990) that found that higher levels of neuroticism were associated with more anxiety and depressive disorders in the same person. In a more recent study (Bienvenu and Stein 2003; Bienvenu et al. 2001), comorbidity among phobic, panic, and major depressive disorders was found to be related to a five-factor model of personality traits. In a subset of subjects ($N=320$) in the Baltimore Epidemiologic Catchment Area Follow-up Study, the Revised NEO Personality Inventory was completed, and neuroticism was found to be significantly associated with the prevalence of specific phobias as well as with other anxiety disorders and major depression. Neither agreeableness, nor conscientiousness, nor openness had statistically significant relationships with the prevalence of any of these disorders. Results of this study indicate that the associations among phobic, panic, and major depressive disorders are substantially reduced when personality correlates in common (i.e., neuroticism and introversion) are taken into account.

In summary, there is some evidence that specific phobia in adolescence is a risk factor for subsequent depression and, possibly, also for other disorders such as illicit substance–abuse disorders (Bittner et al. 2004; Wittchen et al. 2000). This association seems to be mainly due to the severity of anxiety reactions, avoidance behavior, and degree of associated avoidance. As discussed later, there is little evidence for specific phobia being a specific marker for subsequent major depression or substance abuse independent from other anxiety disorders. Furthermore, prospective studies are needed to investigate whether specific phobia additionally contributes to the other anxiety/mood disorders in predicting subsequent major depression.

STRUCTURE OF FEAR

The high degree of comorbidity within anxiety and between anxiety and depression has generated interest in higher-order factors. Many factor-analysis studies of fear and phobia surveys have been conducted, but the results are sometimes difficult to interpret because of the non-representative samples used (e.g., students rather than community) as well as methodological problems. More recently, investigators used the National Comorbidity Survey dataset to investigate the structure of fears in terms of DSM phobias. In a study investigating the structure of the specific phobias listed in DSM, some evidence was found in latent-class analyses that two types of specific phobias could be distinguished: fear of heights, and blood and animal phobias (Curtis et al. 1998). A more recent study investigated the structure of all phobias in the National Comorbidity Survey (Cox et al. 2003). Explorative- and confirmatory-factor analysis revealed the following structure:

- Agoraphobia: Public places, crowd, away from home, cars/trains/buses
- Speaking: Public speaking, speaking to a group, talking to others
- Heights/water: Flying, heights, crossing a bridge, water/lake/pool
- Being observed: Public eating, public toilet use, writing
- Threat: Blood/needles, storm/thunder, snakes/animals, being alone, closed spaces

Thus, the original split between two types of specific phobias (Curtis et al. 1998) was supported in these subsequent analyses. Furthermore, two types of social fears—speaking and being observed—could be distinguished. Higher-order factor analyses revealed two second-order fear factors: social fears and specific fears. At the third-order level one general fear factor was identified.

By performing factor analysis of data obtained from 5,491 young adult students from 11 countries, Arrindell et al. (2003) found evidence for separate diagnostic constructs for the blood-injection-injury type and for the animal type. However, the natural-environment and situational types represented one single common factor. Similar findings were obtained by Muris et al. (1999) in a sample of 996 Dutch 7- to 19-year-old school children, and by Fredrikson et al. (1996) in 704 Swedish 18- to 70-year-olds from the general population. This latter study used only 10 items to measure fears, which implies that, of all possible fears, only a very limited number were assessed. Hence, the lack of evidence from this study for a difference between natural environments versus situational fears may have been due to the use of an insufficient number of representative items. In contrast, Muris et al. (1999) and Arrindell et al. (2003) used a larger number of representative items. They found support for a factor model in which the natural-environment type and the situational type would be indistinguishable.

A different way of testing if diagnostic categories represent different phenomena is to test if they differ with respect to comorbidity. Positive findings would indicate that they might have different etiological mechanisms, with different long-term consequences, or might require subtype-specific treatment. Several studies have assessed comorbidity rates in cases of specific phobia (Dhossche et al. 2002; Essau et al. 2000; Last et al. 1987; Ollendick et al. 2002; Silverman et al. 1999). These studies found high rates of comorbidity with other anxiety disorders, but also with affective and somatoform disorders and, to a lesser extent, with behavior and substance-use disorders. Unfortunately, these studies did not investigate comorbidity patterns according to phobia subtype.

Some studies have assessed differences between phobia subtypes with respect to comorbidity with panic disorder (Antony et al. 1997; Lipsitz et al. 2002; Starcevic and Bogojevic 1997). For example, Lipsitz et al. (2002) found that situational specific phobia was differentiated from other subtypes by the presence of panic attacks. Starcevic and Bogojevic (1997) found that both the situational subtype and the natural-environment subtype were associated with panic disorder, whereas other subtypes were not. Antony et al. (1997) found an association of agoraphobia with the natural environment subtype but not with the other subtypes. Hence, results of these studies that tried to delineate subtypes of specific phobia are inconsistent. Furthermore, they merely considered comorbidity with panic disorder, whereas comorbidity with other problems, such as other anxiety problems, affective problems, somatoform symptoms, and behavior disorders, may be important as well (Dhossche et al. 2002; Essau et al. 2000; Last et al. 1987; Ollendick et al. 2002; Silverman et al. 1999).

In summary, these explorations remain inconclusive, especially with regard to the justification of subtypes.

CONDITIONAL STIMULUS AND UNCONDITIONAL STIMULUS

Learning

Originally, behavior theorists held that specific phobias are acquired through a process of conditioning, in which conditional stimulus and unconditioned stimulus are paired, but the conditioning models of fear acquisition do not seem to be tenable in their original forms (e.g., Emmelkamp 1982) and need broader reconceptualization within broader vulnerability stress models. Recollection of traumatic experiences linked with the first phobic reactions have been reported in many specific phobias, but—unfortunately for the conditioning theory—nonphobic individuals also report having experienced traumatic events in these situations. Research to date suggests that apart from conditioning experiences, modeling and negative information transmission are also important factors in the etiology of specific phobias (Muris and Merckelbach 2001). Furthermore, many factors other than the experienced pairings of conditional stimulus and unconditioned stimulus can affect the strength of the association between these events, including beliefs and expectancies about possible danger associated with a particular conditional stimulus, and culturally transmitted information about the conditional stimulus–unconditioned stimulus contingency (Davey 1997).

Information Processing

Theories propose that attentional, as well as pre-attentive, biases for threatening information are either contributing to or maintaining anxiety disorders. One common method used in experimental studies into attentional bias is the *emotional Stroop paradigm* (Williams et al. 1997). In the emotional Stroop task, the participant is required to report the color of a word as fast as possible while ignoring the meaning of the word. Words with threatening content have been shown to increase color-naming latencies in anxious individuals, and this so-called Stroop interference is presumed to reflect an automatic tendency to attend to threatening information. *Nonmasked* Stroop interference has been shown in spider-phobic adults (Kindt and Brosschot 1997, 1998; Thorpe and Salkovskis 1997; Wikström et al. 2004). In children with spider phobia, however, Stroop interference failed to differentiate between phobic and nonphobic control subjects (Kindt and Brosschot 1999; Kindt et al. 1997). Although pre-attentive Stroop interference involving *masked* words has been shown in clinical anxiety patients (e.g., Lundh et al. 1999; Mogg et al. 1995; Williams et al. 1997), results with regard to specific phobias are inconclusive. Only one study found Stroop interference for masked threat words (van den Hout et al. 1997), whereas negative results were reported in two other studies involving subjects with specific phobias (Thorpe and Salkovskis 1997; Wikström et al. 2004). The van den Hout et al. (1997) study has been criticized for lack of a control group, no reporting of awareness check, and a very small masked Stroop effect, actually much smaller than in the unmasked condition (Wikström et al. 2004). The difference in results with respect to masked stimuli between specific phobia, on the one hand, and other anxiety disorders, on the other, suggests that a broader construct of "negative affect" may be associated with the masked Stroop interference for threat words in anxiety disorders other than specific phobia (Wikström et al. 2004).

Preparedness

It is remarkable that there exists a selection of objects or situations that persons with specific phobias fear. Surprisingly, some phobias never occur, such as gun phobia, mixer phobia, car phobia, mower phobia, or hammer phobia. The preparedness theory attempts to explain this phenomenon. According to this perspective, most phobias are based on a genetic disposition or preparedness to develop fear of those objects and situations (e.g., snakes, spiders, enclosed places, angry faces) that were threatening to our prehistoric ancestors. This preconscious fear response is thought of as genetically "prepared" through evolution in order to facilitate fear conditioning for aversive stimuli that may threaten survival. According to this model of Öhman (1997a, 1997b, 1997c), only a limited range of threatening stimuli may be physiologically arousing when exposed at a level below conscious awareness. In a series of studies, threatening pictorial stimuli that were shown at a pre-attentive level of awareness were shown to elicit skin conductance responses in spider- and snake-fearful subjects. In a study by Hettema et al. (2003), some evidence was provided for a genetic factor accounting for acquisition of fear and extinction of fear for evolutionary relevant stimuli.

Temperament

There is some evidence that temperament may be involved in the etiology of anxiety disorders, including specific phobias. Research so far has focused on two related constructs: neuroticism/emotional lability and behavioral inhibition. In recent years, a number of studies have provided evidence for both emotional lability and behavioral inhibition being risk factors for developing anxiety disorders. Measures of negative affectivity at 3 years of age predict anxiety disorders in adolescence (Craske et al. 2001), but this was not specifically related to specific phobias. Similarly, two studies in adolescence found negative affectivity to predict internalizing symptoms 3–4 years later (Hayward et al. 2000; Krueger et al. 1996). Although there is some evidence that measures of negative affectivity at one point in time predict anxiety disorders at a later point in time, there is no evidence yet that there is a specific link between predisposing vulnerability and the development of specific phobias. Rather, the relationship between the predisposing influence of emotional lability is presumably much broader, including not only anxiety disorders in general but also depressed mood (Roberts and Kendler 1999).

Another temperamental vulnerability candidate for the development of specific phobias is behavioral inhibition. Behavioral inhibition can be regarded as a temperamental trait characterized by the tendency of children and adolescents to react with fear and withdrawal in novel and/or unfamiliar situations (Kagan 1997). A number of studies have shown that children who are behaviorally inhibited are at increased risk for developing anxiety disorders (e.g., Emmelkamp and Scholing 1997; Turner et al. 1996). For example, in a longitudinal study by Biederman et al. (1993), children initially identified as behaviorally inhibited were subsequently more likely to develop anxiety disorders compared with control children. Multiple anxiety disorders were significantly more prevalent in the subsample of children with behavioral inhibition. Here, again, the question remains whether behavioral inhibition in children is specifically linked to specific phobias, anxiety disorders in general, or broader psychopathology, such as depression (Reznick et al. 1992).

From the results of the prospective studies into temperament as vulnerability for phobias, it seems plausible that temperamental factors such as behavioral inhibition and emotional lability/negative affectivity not only are antecedents for specific phobias and other anxiety disorders but also serve as vulnerability factors for the development of subsequent depression. There is some evidence that these temperamental factors may lead to non-specific anxiety, which in turn results in subsequent depression. For example, high levels of anxiety at one point in time predicted high levels of depression at a subsequent point in time, even after prior levels of depression were controlled for (Cole et al. 1998). In line with this, employing structural-equations modeling, Muris et al. (2001) found that a pathway of "behavioral inhibition–anxiety–depression" provided the best fit for their data.

Course and Prognosis

As indicated earlier, in young children, simple fears (mostly fears of animals) often improve "spontaneously" without any treatment. However, specific phobias that continue from childhood into adolescence seldom recover spontaneously. Evidence from prospective-longitudinal investigations in community samples of adolescents (Wittchen et al. 2003) from age 14 to the third decade of life suggests that there is a relatively high degree of homotypic and, even more so, heterotypic continuity.

Children and adolescents with a DSM-IV-TR specific phobia at baseline retained this diagnosis in 41% of all cases (homotypic continuity; Figure 4–1A). This rate increased to 73% when allowing for diagnostic changes to other anxiety disorders and depression (heterotypic continuity). Even more important, complete remission, in terms of having neither specific phobia nor any other DSM-IV-TR disorder, was extremely low (i.e., 10%). A closer examination by type of specific phobia revealed that spontaneous remission rates for none of the subtypes exceeded 25%, and lowest complete remission rates were found for animal phobias. Strict homotypic continuity (same specific phobia diagnosis at following waves was highest for blood injury [34%] and situational phobias [30%] and lowest for other specific phobias and phobias not otherwise specified [Figure 4–1B]). Thus, this study highlighted a considerable degree of continuity of specific phobias and that is much greater than that found for other anxiety disorders and depressive disorders, in particular.

COURSE IN TREATMENT STUDIES

Specific phobias are especially responsive to behavioral treatment; exposure therapy has proven successful in alleviating symptoms of specific phobia (Emmelkamp 2004). A number of controlled-outcome studies have demonstrated the effectiveness of exposure therapy delivered in a single-session format (Emmelkamp and Felten 1985; Hellström and Öst 1995; Öst 1989; Öst et al. 1992). One-session exposure treatment for specific phobias takes up to 3 hours and incorporates prolonged in vivo exposure and participant modeling to the feared stimulus. Öst's one-session exposure procedure involves cognitive and behavioral interventions to facilitate change; however, it is unclear what the additional benefit of cognitive interventions is (Emmelkamp and Felten 1985). In a recent study by Koch et al. (2004), the addition of cognitive methods to the one-session exposure treatment did not enhance outcomes in terms of behavioral, cognitive, or somatic phobic symptoms. Interestingly, both treatments were equally effective in promoting cognitive change. A recent development regarding treatment involves exposure to virtual environments rather than real environments. Such virtual reality exposure therapy has been found as effective as exposure in vivo in patients with specific phobia (Emmelkamp 2005; Emmelkamp et al. 2002). There is no evidence that pharmacotherapy is of lasting benefit to patients with specific phobia (Emmelkamp 2004).

BIOLOGICAL AND NEUROBIOLOGICAL FACTORS

Certain childhood fears are part of normal development. As cognitive development advances, children first become anxious when separated from their mothers or when facing strangers; later, children become fearful of animals and, finally, of social situations. In general, these fears are transitory and can be regarded as adaptive and protective responses of the developing organism; even among adults, certain stimuli are more likely to trigger phobias (Marks 1987). It is well established that some childhood fears are innate and might reflect past evolutionary dangers.

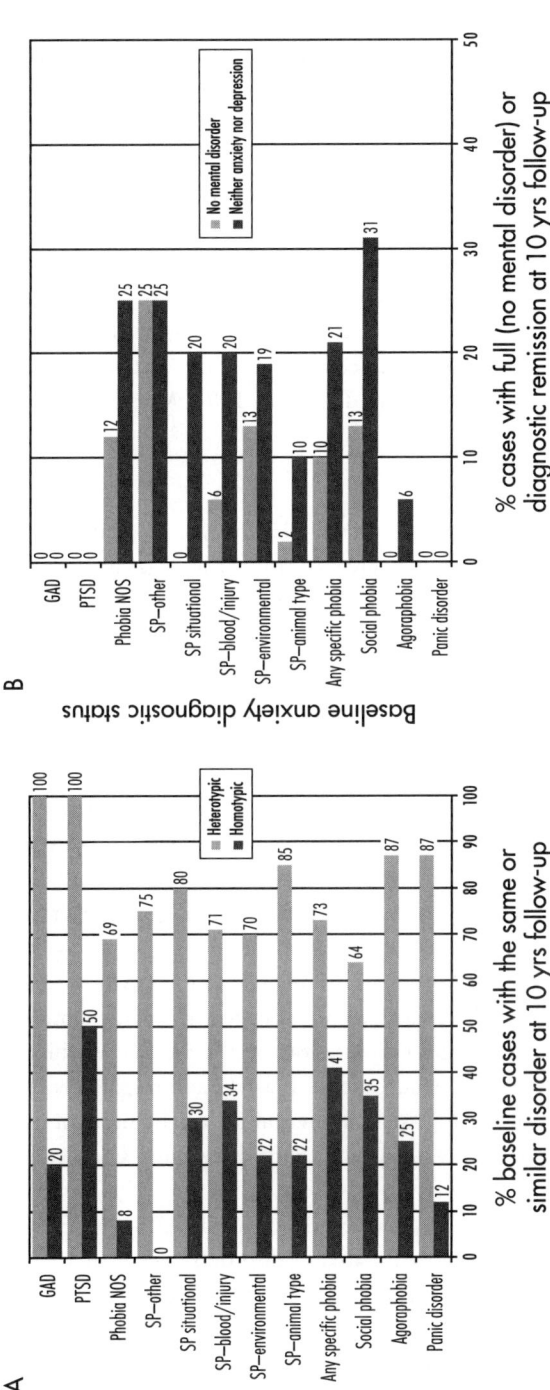

FIGURE 4–1. DSM-IV anxiety disorders from childhood to adulthood.

A. Proportion (%) of baseline cases with an anxiety disorder meeting criteria for exactly the same diagnosis 10 years later (black bar=strict homotypic continuity) compared to those exhibiting broader heterotypic continuity (meets criteria for either anxiety or depression, or both). B. Proportion (%) of baseline cases with an anxiety disorder NOT meeting criteria for any mental disorder 10 years later (gray bar=full remission), compared to those not meeting criteria for any anxiety or depression disorder.

N=3021; 10 years cumulative follow-up; diagnoses are based on DSM-IV Composite International Diagnostic Interview data. GAD=generalized anxiety disorder; NOS=not otherwise specified; PTSD=posttraumatic stress disorder; SP=specific phobia.

Source. Wittchen H-U, Gloster AT, Klotsche J, Hoefler M, Beesdo K, Lieb R: "The longitudinal prospective structure of common mental disorders during adolescence and early adulthood." Unpublished manuscript.

Seligman (1971) hypothesized that humans, like animals, are "prepared" to develop certain fears, as we discussed earlier. Such genetic predispositions are well known in animals. For instance, monkeys fear snakes even if they have never been exposed to them. Behaviorists originally believed that the mind is a tabula rasa and that, with appropriate intervention, any stimulus might become a trigger for anxiety (J.B. Watson and Morgan 1917). Several studies, however, strongly suggest that persons become conditioned more easily to certain stimuli—for instance, to snakes and spiders—than to other, more traumatic experiences such as air raids (Rachman 1977). The fact that humans are "hardwired" to respond to certain situations with fear may explain the prominence of certain phobias. One also has to consider that persons may become sensitized to certain stimuli by frequent environmental exposure, making them look "prepared" (Davey 1995; Marks 1987).

FAMILIAL AND GENETIC PATTERNS

Clearly there are familial influences on fears during childhood and adulthood. Family genetic studies have shown moderate degrees of familial aggregation of specific phobias. Positive correlations have been found routinely between the fears of children and their mothers (Emmelkamp and Scholing 1997). The influence of mothers' and siblings' fears on the fears of children is probably greater among younger than among older children. Familial influences might also be relatively stronger among children from lower socioeconomic strata. Although these data suggest that social learning factors are important in the development of specific phobias (Chapman 1997), other factors may also be involved. Like social learning factors (e.g., modeling), the experience of stressful life events (e.g., parental loss or separation, child abuse) may be related to the development of anxiety disorders, but its effects are largely nonspecific across disorders. In addition, genetic factors may account for the co-occurrence of specific phobias in families.

In a recent study by Bolton et al. (2006), patterns of genetic and environmental influences on early onset anxiety disorders were investigated. In a large sample of more than 4,500 twins, the heritability estimate for specific phobia was high (60%) for diagnostic status (symptom syndrome with associated impairment), with remaining variance attributed to non-shared environment. The heritability estimate suggests that the genetic effects on specific phobia are more significant than environmental effects.

In contrast, studies by Skre et al. (1993) and Kendler et al. (1992) suggest that although there is a common genetic variance for anxiety disorders in general, there is some evidence for a specific genetic vulnerability to specific phobia. For example, the concordances of blood-injury phobias and animal phobias were higher among monozygotic than among dizygotic twins (Torgersen 1979). In family studies, Fyer et al. (1990, 1995) presented evidence for a specific genetic contribution to specific phobias. Relatives of probands with specific phobias were at increased risk for specific phobias but not for other phobias. Finally, those with blood-injury phobia had more relatives with similar problems than did those with other phobias. Among blood-phobic subjects, about 60% had first-degree relatives who were also blood phobic; this is three to six times more frequent than for panic disorder, OCD, agoraphobia, and social, dental, or animal phobia (Marks 1987; Öst et al. 1992). In female twins, Neale et al. (1994) found that different factors are responsible for illness and blood-injection-injury phobias. Results of this study revealed that genetic factors were primarily responsible for the familial aggregation of blood-injection-injury fears but that aggregation of illness fears was better accounted for by shared environment.

Hettema et al. (2005) used multivariate structural equation modeling to investigate whether the comorbidity of anxiety disorders in a community sample (twin register) could be explained by underlying genetic and environmental risk factors. The results of this study suggest that etiologically, the anxiety disorders possess a relatively simple genetic architecture. In the best-fitting model, the genetic influences on anxiety were best explained by two additive genetic factors common across the disorders. The first loaded primarily in GAD, panic disorder, and agoraphobia, whereas the second loaded strongly in two specific phobias: situational and animal phobia. Risk across all of the anxiety disorders may be further increased by life experiences either shared or non-shared with family members. The finding that the specific phobias load primarily on a second genetic factor uncorrelated with the first suggests that their genetic etiology may be largely distinct from the other disorders. Additional analyses including blood-injury phobia revealed that blood-injury phobia is more related genetically to agoraphobia than to the specific phobias.

The same research group investigated the heritability of fear conditioning in same-sex twin pairs (Hettema et al. 2003). Results revealed that genetic factors play a significant role in the acquisition and extinction of fears. Interestingly, different results were found for evolutionary relevant stimuli (snakes, spiders) as compared with evolutionary irrelevant stimuli (triangles, circles), thus providing some support for the preparedness theory of phobia acquisition.

In summary, evidence is increasing that heritability plays an important role in the etiology of specific phobias. However, what remains unclear is what exactly is inherited. More theoretically driven research is needed to investigate which mechanisms are involved. Good candidates for further studies into the genetic basis for specific fears, apart from conditioning of fear (Hettema et al. 2005), are personality traits associated with fears, automatic threat processing, and looming maladaptive style.

NEUROIMAGING

In recent years brain-imaging techniques, such as positron emission tomography (PET), single-photon emission computed tomography (SPECT), and, more recently, functional magnetic resonance imaging (fMRI), have been used to investigate the neuroanatomical substrate of specific phobias, particularly animal phobias. These studies typically involve exposing subjects to phobic objects such as snakes or spiders, either pictures or live animals, during scanning. To date, these studies have yielded conflicting results (Charney 2003; Veltman et al. 2004). It is puzzling that, despite the use of specific-phobia–related challenges, little conclusive research has been done to establish specific phobias as a separate disorder.

Whereas Mountz et al. (1989), in an early PET study, reported negative results, subsequent studies such as those of Wik et al. (1993) found increased regional cerebral blood flow (rCBF) in secondary visual cortex but decreased rCBF in hippocampus and orbitofrontal, prefrontal, temporopolar, and posterior cingulate cortex with exposure to phobic stimuli. Johanson et al. (1998), using ^{133}Xe SPECT, reported decreased right lateral prefrontal flow during presentation of a spider video compared with a neutral video, particularly in near-panicking subjects. In contrast, Rauch et al. (1995), in their subjects with small-animal phobias, found increased rCBF in left posterior orbitofrontal, left insular, and left somatosensory cortex, as well as in the right anterior temporal and anterior cingulate cortex, but not in the amygdala complex during presentation of phobic objects, compared with baseline. Similar findings were reported by Reiman (1997). In a recent study by Straube et al. (2006b) using fMRI, subjects with spider phobia showed greater responses to spiders versus mushrooms in the left amygdala, left insula, left anterior cingulate gyrus, and left dorsomedial prefrontal cortex.

Inconsistencies in these findings may reflect methodological differences, such as imaging modality and data-analytic techniques (region of interest vs. voxel by voxel methods). In addition, few studies have controlled for decrements in subjects' responses in time due to habituation after repeated exposure to phobic stimuli. Given that a single session of exposure *in vivo* can result in significant improvement in specific phobia, Veltman et al. (2004) used PET to investigate neurophysiological changes (habituation) during repeated exposures to phobic stimuli in spider-phobic patients. To this end, a behavior therapy paradigm (prolonged visual stimulation) was adapted by also including a neutral control condition (pictures of butterflies). The imaging data showed a clear dissociation between main effects for condition and habituation effects. Main effects for spider-versus-butterfly pictures were found predominantly in the fusiform/parahippocampal gyrus, but also in the bilateral peri-rhinal cortex, right posterior lateral prefrontal cortex, and right medial amygdala region. Habituation effects (decreases over time) were found exclusively in so-called limbic structures involving the bilateral anterior medial temporal lobe, including the amygdala, as well as in the posterior insula and hypothalamus.

In another recent study, brain activation (fMRI) to spider videos was measured before and after cognitive-behavioral therapy in spider-phobic subjects. After treatment, a significant reduction of hyperactivity in the insula and anterior cingulate gyrus was found in patients who had received therapy as compared with a no-treatment control group (Straube et al. 2006a).

Phobic responses may be associated with implicit (without conscious awareness) memories linked to the amygdala (Mineka and Ohman 2002). Some investigators have suggested that the amygdala is central to conditioned fear of discrete objects, whereas the hippocampus is linked with conditioned anxiety to environmental context (for overview see Craske 2003).

Conclusion and Future Research

This review has highlighted a considerable paradox. Despite specific phobias being the most frequent of all mental disorders, despite their continuity and persistence, and despite the considerable—but less dramatically acute—suffering and impairment they cause, there has been surprisingly little systematic basic and clinical research that can guide us in designing improved diagnostic criteria for them. There is little doubt that specific phobias are almost prototypical disorders of the brain and that they belong to the family of "fear-circuitry disorders," but the specific evidence for subtypes and the systematic delineation from social phobia, agoraphobia, and other anxiety disorders is meager.

This paradox is also evident when we compare the well-established effectiveness of cognitive-behavioral therapy for specific phobias, on the one hand, with the fact that only a fraction of individuals with specific phobias ever receive established treatment, and if so, usually many years, if not decades, after onset. In absence of the explanations, we can only speculate that patients with specific phobia are rarely a core group in psychiatric specialty settings as a result of both little active help-seeking behavior on the side of patient and the fact that clinicians do not take specific phobias seriously. It is likely that this combination acts as a vicious circle.

Against this more general background, reviewed evidence seems to suggest various potentially helpful measures.

DIAGNOSTIC AND CLASSIFICATORY ISSUES

1. There are several indications from cross-sectional and longitudinal studies that the decision in DSM-IV/DSM-IV-TR to apply basically the same criteria of specific phobia to children and adults remains problematic. There is some evidence that childhood phobias are somehow different from late-adolescent and adult phobias: there are differences in reliability and stability of diagnoses, predictive value, complications, severity, and prognosis. Proof of these indicators has been established for specific phobias after age of 14, but not in the same way for younger age groups. It might be conceivable that different and more dimensional criteria for childhood phobias would improve the problem. In

contrast, in adolescence and adulthood, the delineation of normal variations in phobic liability and specific phobic disorders seems to be less of a problem if DSM-IV-TR criteria are rigidly applied.

2. Applying DSM-IV-TR criteria will certainly not remedy two other issues—namely, the more comprehensive validation and exploration of various subtypes of specific phobia in both childhood and higher ages. Clearly, blood-injury and situational phobias are different from specific phobias, but there is not enough systematic evidence to justify a more coherent and clinically useful subtyping. Latent-class and factor-analytic studies have failed so far to provide conclusive evidence of a higher-order grouping but at least suggest some empirical guidance about reducing the number of subtypes. Illness phobia appears to be highly prevalent in the general population (Edelmann 1992; Eifert and Forsyth 1996; Noyes et al. 2000) and is associated with significant distress and impairment. Persons with illness phobias have been observed both to require medical examination sooner than control subjects and to avoid contact with physicians, fearing that some disease might be found (Desai et al. 1999; Noyes et al. 2000). There is still controversy in the literature whether illness phobia should be distinguished from hypochondriasis (Noyes et al. 2004). Currently in DSM-IV-TR, it is considered to be a specific phobia, other type. According to DSM-IV-TR, illness phobia has to be distinguished from hypochondriasis, but some experts in this field do not agree with this distinction (e.g., Barsky 1992). This distinction is primarily based on phenomenological studies and factor-analytic studies that support separate dimensions of disease phobia and disease conviction within hypochondriasis (Côté et al. 1996; Kellner 1985). Additional research, however, supports the distinction between illness phobia and hypochondriasis (e.g., Fava and Grandi 1991; Fava et al. 1995; Salkovskis et al. 1990).

3. Similarly, the delineation of specific phobias from partly overlapping symptom clusters in social phobia and agoraphobia has not been sufficiently addressed to provide guidance as to how to solve this frequent differential diagnostic problem. However, the practical problems in differential diagnosis, as well as the longitudinal overlap, suggest the need for further studies.

TREATMENT ISSUES

Further research is needed to identify why specific phobia is so rarely treated and why specific phobias have rarely been a target for early intervention or prevention trials. There is some evidence that severity plays a role, but it is less clear what ultimately drives severity. The epidemiological evidence suggests that demoralization might play a core role, because only the presence of depressive disorders is substantially associated with increased odds of early and specific treatments. Yet core questions remain unresolved: Why do only very few individuals with specific phobia apply for treatment, and which treatments are the most effective in practice? Do specific phobias need specific treatment, or can the same treatments be applied, as in panic disorders and other anxiety disorders (Tsao et al. 2005)?

ETIOLOGICAL ISSUES

This review also highlights the need for studies that specifically examine the neuropsychological, cognitive, and neurobiological interface of specific phobias. Are there differences in the role of conditioning and cognitive processing among different subtypes of specific and social fears? Are there differences in personality traits among different subtypes of specific and social fears (Watson et al. 2005)? Functional neuroimaging studies could provide one core tool to inform us about the much-needed extensions in our etiological models.

References

Alonso J, Angermeyer MC, Bernert S, et al: Disability and quality of life impact of mental disorders in Europe: results from the European Study of the Epidemiology of Mental Disorders (ESEMeD) project. Acta Psychiatr Scand 109:38–46, 2004

American Psychiatric Association: Diagnostic and Statistical Manual of Mental Disorders, 3rd Edition, Revised. Washington, DC, American Psychiatric Association, 1987

American Psychiatric Association: Diagnostic and Statistical Manual of Mental Disorders, 4th Edition. Washington, DC, American Psychiatric Association, 1994

American Psychiatric Association: Diagnostic and Statistical Manual of Mental Disorders, 4th Edition, Text Revision. Washington, DC, American Psychiatric Association, 2000

Andrews G, Stewart G, Allen R, et al: The genetics of six neurotic disorders: a twin study. J Affect Disord 19:23–29, 1990

Antony MM, Brown TA, Barlow DH: Heterogeneity among specific phobia types in DSM-IV. Behav Res Ther 35:1089–1100, 1997

Arrindell WA, Eisemann M, Richter J, et al: Phobic anxiety in 11 nations: part I: dimensional constancy of the five-factor model. Behav Res Ther 41:461–479, 2003

Barsky AJ: Amplification, somatization, and the somatoform disorders. Psychosomatics 33:28–34, 1992

Biederman J, Rosenbaum JF, Bolduc-Murphy EA, et al: A 3-year follow-up of children with and without behavioral inhibition. J Am Acad Child Adolesc Psychiatry 32:814–821, 1993

Bienvenu OJ, Stein MB: Personality and anxiety disorders: a review. J Pers Disord 17:139–151, 2003

Bienvenu OJ, Nestadt G, Samuels JF, et al: Phobic, panic, and major depressive disorders and the five-factor model of personality. J Nerv Ment Dis 189:154–161, 2001

Bijl RV, van Zessen G, Ravelli A: Psychiatrische morbiditeit onder volwassenen in Nederland: het NEMESIS-onderzoek, II: prevalentie van psychiatrische stoornissen. Ned Tijdschr Geneeskd 141:2453–2460, 1997

Bittner A, Goodwin RD, Wittchen HU, et al: What characteristics of primary anxiety disorders predict subsequent major depression? J Clin Psychiatry 65:618–626, 2004

Bland RC, Orn H, Newman SC: Lifetime prevalence of psychiatric disorders in Edmonton. Acta Psychiatr Scand 77:24–32, 1988

Bolton D, Eley TC, O'Connor TG, et al: Prevalence and genetic and environmental influences on anxiety disorders in 6-year-old twins. Psychol Med 36:335–344, 2006

Brown DR, Eaton WW, Sussman L: Racial differences in prevalence of phobic disorders. J Nerv Ment Dis 178:434–441, 1990

Burnam MA, Hough RL, Escobar JI, et al: Six-month prevalence of specific psychiatric disorders among Mexican Americans and non-Hispanic whites in Los Angeles. Arch Gen Psychiatry 44:687–694, 1987

Chapman TF: The epidemiology of fears and phobias, in Phobias: A Handbook of Theory, Research and Treatment. Edited by Davey GCL. New York, Wiley, 1997, pp 416–434

Charney DS: Neuroanatomical circuits modulating fear and anxiety behaviors. Acta Psychiatr Scand Suppl 417:38–50, 2003

Cole DA, Peeke LG, Martin JM, et al: A longitudinal look at the relation between depression and anxiety in children. J Consult Clin Psychol 66:451–460, 1998

Côté G, O'Leary T, Barlow DH, et al: Hypochondriasis, in DSM-IV Sourcebook, Vol 2. Edited by Widiger TA, Frances AJ, Pincus HA, et al. Washington, DC, American Psychiatric Association, 1996, pp 933–947

Cox BJ, McWilliams LA, Clara IP, et al: The structure of feared situations in a nationally representative sample. J Anxiety Disord 17:89–101, 2003

Cramer V, Torgersen S, Kringlen E: Quality of life and anxiety disorders: a population study. J Nerv Ment Dis 193:196–202, 2005

Craske MG: Origins of Phobias and Anxiety Disorders: Why More Women than Men? Oxford, UK, Pergamon/Elsevier, 2003

Craske MG, Poulton R, Tsao JC, et al: Paths to panic disorder/agoraphobia: an exploratory analysis from age 3 to 21 in an unselected birth cohort. J Am Acad Child Adolesc Psychiatry 40:556–563, 2001

Curtis GC, Magee WJ, Eaton WW, et al: Specific fears and phobias: epidemiology and classification. Br J Psychiatry 173:212–217, 1998

Da Motta WR, de Lima MS, de Oliveira Soares BG, et al: An epidemic of phobic disorders in Brazil? Results from a population-based cross-sectional survey. Poster presented at the annual meeting of the American Psychiatric Association, Chicago, IL, May 2000

Davey GCL: Preparedness and phobia: specific evolved associations or a generalized expectancy bias? Behav Brain Sci 18:289–325, 1995

Davey GCL: A conditioning model of phobias, in Phobias: A Handbook of Theory, Research and Treatment. Edited by Davey GCL. New York, Wiley, 1997, pp 301–318

Desai MM, Bruce ML, Kasl SV: The effects of major depression and phobia on stage at diagnosis of breast cancer. Int J Psychiatry Med 29:29–45, 1999

Dhossche D, Ferdinand R, van der Ende J, et al: Diagnostic outcome of adolescent self-reported suicidal ideation at 8-year follow up. J Affect Disord 72:273–279, 2002

Edelmann RJ: Anxiety: Theory, Research and Intervention in Clinical and Health Psychology. Chichester, UK, Wiley, 1992

Eifert GH, Forsyth JP: Heart-focused and general illness fears in relation to parental medical history and separation experiences. Behav Res Ther 34:735–739, 1996

Emmelkamp PM: Phobic and Obsessive-Compulsive Disorders. New York, Plenum, 1982

Emmelkamp PM: Behavior therapy with adults, in Bergin and Garfield's Handbook of Psychotherapy and Behavior Change, 5th Edition. Edited by Lambert M. New York, Wiley, 2004, pp 379–427

Emmelkamp PM: Technological innovations in clinical assessment and psychotherapy. Psychother Psychosom 74:336–343, 2005

Emmelkamp PM, Felten M: The process of exposure in vivo: cognitive and physiological changes during treatment of acrophobia. Behav Res Ther 23:219–223, 1985

Emmelkamp PM, Scholing A: Anxiety disorders, in Developmental Psychopathology. Edited by Essau CA, Petermann F. Amsterdam, The Netherlands, Harwood, 1997, pp 219–263

Emmelkamp PM, Krijn M, Hulsbosch AM, et al: Virtual reality treatment vs. exposure in vivo: a comparative evaluation in acrophobia. Behav Res Ther 40:509–516, 2002

Essau CA, Conradt J, Petermann F: Frequency, comorbidity, and psychosocial impairment of specific phobia in adolescents. J Clin Child Psychol 29:221–223, 2000

Fava GA, Grandi S: Differential diagnosis of hypochondriacal fears and beliefs. Psychother Psychosom 55:114–119, 1991

Fava GA, Freyberger HJ, Bech P, et al: Diagnostic criteria for use in psychosomatic research. Psychother Psychosom 63:1–8, 1995

Fredrikson M, Annas P, Fischer H, et al: Gender and age differences in the prevalence of specific fears and phobias. Behav Res Ther 34:33–39, 1996

Fyer AJ, Mannuzza S, Martin LY, et al: Familial transmission of simple phobias and fears. Arch Gen Psychiatry 47:252–256, 1990

Fyer AJ, Mannuzza S, Chapman TF, et al: Specificity in familial aggregation of phobic disorders. Arch Gen Psychiatry 52:564–573, 1995

Goisman RM, Allsworth J, Rogers MP, et al: Simple phobia as a comorbid anxiety disorder. Depress Anxiety 7:105–112, 1998

Goodwin RD, Jacobi F, Thefeld W: Mental disorders in the community. Arch Gen Psychiatry 60:1125–1130, 2003

Hayward C, Killen JD, Kraemer HC, et al: Predictors of panic attacks in adolescents. J Am Acad Child Adolesc Psychiatry 39:207–214, 2000

Hellström K, Öst LG: One-session therapist directed exposure vs two forms of manual directed self-exposure in the treatment of spider phobia. Behav Res Ther 33:959–965, 1995

Hettema JM, Annas P, Neale MC, et al: A twin study of the genetics of fear conditioning. Arch Gen Psychiatry 60:702–708, 2003

Hettema JM, Prescott CA, Myers JM, et al: The structure of genetic and environmental risk factors for anxiety disorders in men and women. Arch Gen Psychiatry 62:182–189, 2005

Johanson A, Gustafson L, Passant U, et al: Brain function in spider phobia. Psychiatry Res 84:101–111, 1998

Kagan J: Temperament and the reactions to unfamiliarity. Child Dev 68:139–143, 1997

Karno M, Hough RL, Burnam A, et al: Lifetime prevalence of specific psychiatric disorders among Mexican Americans and non-Hispanic whites in Los Angeles. Arch Gen Psychiatry 44:695–701, 1987

Karno M, Golding JM, Burnam MA, et al: Anxiety disorders among Mexican Americans and non-Hispanic Whites in Los Angeles. J Nerv Ment Dis 177:202–209, 1989

Kawakami N, Takeshima T, Ono Y, et al: Twelve-month prevalence, severity, and treatment of common mental disorders in communities in Japan: preliminary finding from the World Mental Health Japan Survey 2002–2003. Psychiatry Clin Neurosci 59:441–452, 2005

Kellner R: Functional somatic symptoms and hypochondriasis: a survey of empirical studies. Arch Gen Psychiatry 42:821–833, 1985

Kendler KS, Neale MC, Kessler RC, et al: The genetic epidemiology of phobias in women: the interrelationship of agoraphobia, social phobia, situational phobia, and simple phobia. Arch Gen Psychiatry 49:273–281, 1992

Kessler RC, McGonagle KA, Zhao S, et al: Lifetime and 12-month prevalence of DSM-III-R psychiatric disorders in the United States. Arch Gen Psychiatry 51:8–19, 1994

Kessler RC, Berglund P, Demler O, et al: Lifetime prevalence and age-of-onset distributions of DSM-IV disorders in the National Comorbidity Survey Replication. Arch Gen Psychiatry 62:593–602, 2005a

Kessler RC, Chiu WT, Demler O, et al: Prevalence, severity, and comorbidity of 12-month DSM-IV disorders in the National Comorbidity Survey Replication. Arch Gen Psychiatry 62:617–627, 2005b

Kindt M, Brosschot JF: Phobia-related cognitive bias for pictorial and linguistic stimuli. J Abnorm Psychol 106:644–648, 1997

Kindt M, Brosschot JF: Cognitive inhibition in phobia. Br J Clin Psychol 37:103–106, 1998

Kindt M, Brosschot JF: Cognitive bias in spider-phobic children: comparison of a pictorial and a linguistic spider Stroop. J Psychopathol Behav 21:207–220, 1999

Kindt M, Bierman D, Brosschot JF: Cognitive bias in spider fear and control children: assessment of emotional interference by a card format and a single-trial format of the Stroop task. J Exp Child Psychol 66:163–179, 1997

Koch EI, Spates CR, Himle JA: Comparison of behavioral and cognitive-behavioral one-session exposure treatments for small animal phobias. Behav Res Ther 42:1483–1504, 2004

Krueger RF, Caspi A, Moffitt TE, et al: Personality traits are differentially linked to mental disorders: a multitrait–multidiagnosis study of an adolescent birth cohort. J Abnorm Psychol 105:299–312, 1996

Last CG, Strauss CC, Francis G: Comorbidity among childhood anxiety disorders. J Nerv Ment Dis 175:726–730, 1987

Lipsitz JD, Barlow DH, Mannuzza S, et al: Clinical features of four DSM-IV specific phobia subtypes. J Nerv Ment Dis 190:471–478, 2002

Lundh LG, Wikstrom J, Westerlund J, et al: Preattentive bias for emotional information in panic disorder with agoraphobia. J Abnorm Psychol 108:222–232, 1999

Magee WJ, Baton WW, Wittchen HU, et al: Agoraphobia, simple phobia, and social phobia in the National Comorbidity Survey. Arch Gen Psychiatry 53:159–168, 1996

Marks IM: Fears, Phobias and Rituals. New York, Oxford University Press, 1987

Mataix-Cols D, Cowley AJ, Hankins M, et al: Reliability and validity of the work and social adjustment scale in phobic disorders. Compr Psychiatry 46:223–228, 2005

Mineka S, Ohman A: Phobias and preparedness: the selective, automatic, and encapsulated nature of fear. Biol Psychiatry 52:927–937, 2002

Mogg K, Bradley BP, Millar N, et al: A follow-up study of cognitive bias in generalized anxiety disorder. Behav Res Ther 33:927–935, 1995

Mountz JM, Modell JG, Wilson MW, et al: Positron emission tomographic evaluation of cerebral blood flow during state anxiety in simple phobia. Arch Gen Psychiatry 46:501–504, 1989

Muris P, Merckelbach H: The etiology of childhood specific phobia: a multifactorial model, in The Developmental Psychopathology of Anxiety. Edited by Vasey MW, Dadds MR. New York, Oxford Press, 2001, pp 355–385

Muris P, Schmidt H, Merckelbach H: The structure of specific phobia symptoms among children and adolescents. Behav Res Ther 37:863–868, 1999

Muris P, Merckelbach H, Gadet B, et al: Fears, worries, and scary dreams in 4- to 12-year-old children: their content, developmental pattern, and origins. J Clin Child Psychol 29:43–52, 2000

Muris P, Merckelbach H, Schmidt H, et al: Anxiety and depression as correlates of self-reported behavioural inhibition in normal adolescents. Behav Res Ther 39:1051–1061, 2001

Myers KM, Weissman MM, Tischler GL, et al: Six-month prevalence of psychiatric disorders in three communities. Arch Gen Psychiatry 41:959–967, 1984

Neale NC, Walters EE, Eaves LJ, et al: Genetics of blood-injury fears and phobias: a population-based twin study. Am J Med Genet 54:326–334, 1994

Noyes R Jr, Hartz AJ, Doebbeling CC, et al: Illness fears in the general population. Psychosom Med 63:318–325, 2000

Noyes R Jr, Carney CP, Langbehn DR: Specific phobia of illness: search for a new subtype. J Anxiety Disord 18:531–545, 2004

Öhman A: As fast as the blink of an eye: preattentive processing and evolutionary facilitation of attention, in Attention and Motivation: Cognitive Perspectives from Psychophysiology, Reflexology, and Neuroscience. Edited by Lang PJ, Balaban M, Simons RF. Hillsdale, NJ, Erlbaum, 1997a, pp 165–184

Öhman A: On the edge of consciousness: preattentive mechanisms in the generation of anxiety, in A Century of Psychology: Progress, Paradigms, and Prospects for the New Millennium. Edited by Fuller R, Walsh P, McGinley P. London, Routledge, 1997b, pp 252–270

Öhman A: Unconscious preattentive mechanisms in the activation of phobic fear, in Phobias: A Handbook of Description, Treatment, and Theory. Edited by Davey GCL. Chichester, UK, Wiley, 1997c, pp 349–374

Ollendick T, King NJ, Muris P: Fears and phobias in children: phenomenology, epidemiology and aetiology. Child Adolesc Ment Health 7:98–106, 2002

Öst LG: Age of onset in different phobias. J Abnorm Psychol 96:223–229, 1987

Öst LG: One-session treatment for specific phobias. Behav Res Ther 27:1–7, 1989

Öst LG, Hellström K: Blood-injury-injection phobia, in Phobias: A Handbook of Theory, Research and Treatment. Edited by Davey GCL. New York, Wiley, 1997, pp 63–80

Öst LG, Hellström K, Kåver A: One vs. five sessions of exposure in the treatment of injection phobia. Behav Ther 23:263–282, 1992

Pierce KA, Kirkpatrick DR: Do men lie on fear surveys? Behav Res Ther 30:415–418, 1992

Rachman S: The conditioning theory of fear-acquisition: a critical examination. Behav Res Ther 15:375–387, 1977

Rauch SL, Savage CR, Alpert NM, et al: A positron emission tomographic study of simple phobic symptom provocation. Arch Gen Psychiatry 52:20–28, 1995

Reiman EM: The application of positron emission tomography to the study of normal and pathologic emotions. J Clin Psychiatry 16:4–12, 1997

Reznick JS, Hegeman IM, Kaufman E, et al: Retrospective and concurrent self-report of behavioral inhibition and their relation to adult mental health. Dev Psychopathol 4:301–321, 1992

Roberts SB, Kendler KS: Neuroticism and self-esteem as indices of the vulnerability to major depression in women. Psychol Med 29:1101–1109, 1999

Robins LN, Helzer JE, Weissman MM, et al: Lifetime prevalence of specific psychiatric disorders in three sites. Arch Gen Psychiatry 41:949–958, 1984

Salkovskis PM, Storer D, Atha C, et al: Psychiatric morbidity in an accident and emergency department: characteristics of patients at presentation and one-month followup. Br J Psychiatry 156:483–487, 1990

Sareen J, Cox BJ, Clara I, et al: The relationship between anxiety disorders and physical disorders in the U.S. National Comorbidity Survey. Depress Anxiety 21:193–202, 2005

Seligman ME: Phobias and preparedness. Behav Ther 2:307–320, 1971

Silverman WK, Kurtines WM, Ginsburg GS, et al: Contingency management, self-control and education support in the treatment of childhood phobic disorders: a randomized clinical trial. J Consult Clin Psychol 67:675–687, 1999

Skre L, Onstad S, Torgersen J, et al: A twin study of DSM-III-R anxiety disorders. Acta Psychiatr Scand 88:85–92, 1993

Starcevic V, Bogojevic G: Comorbidity of panic disorder with agoraphobia and specific phobia: relationship with the subtypes of specific phobia. Compr Psychiatry 38:315–320, 1997

Straube T, Glauer M, Dilger S, et al: Effects of cognitive-behavioral therapy on brain activation in specific phobia. Neuroimage 29:125–135, 2006a

Straube T, Mentzel HJ, Miltner WH: Neural mechanisms of automatic and direct processing of phobogenic stimuli in specific phobia. Biol Psychiatry 59:162–170, 2006b

Thorpe SJ, Salkovskis PM: Information processing in spider phobics: the Stroop colour naming task may indicate strategic but not automatic attentional bias. Behav Res Ther 35:131–144, 1997

Torgersen S: The nature and origin of common phobic fears. Br J Psychiatry 134:343–351, 1979

Tsao JC, Mystkowski JL, Zucker BG, et al: Impact of cognitive-behavioral therapy for panic disorder on comorbidity: a controlled investigation. Behav Res Ther 43:959–970, 2005

Turner SM, Beidel DC, Wolff PL: Is behavioural inhibition related to the anxiety disorders? Clin Psychol Rev 16:157–172, 1996

Tyrer P: Classification of Neurosis. New York, John Wiley and Sons, 1989 van den Hout M, Tenney N, Huygens K, et al: Preconscious processing bias in specific phobia. Behav Res Ther 35:29–34, 1997

Veltman DJ, Tuinebreijer WE, Winkelman D, et al: Neurophysiological correlates of habituation during exposure in spider phobia. Psychiatry Res 132:149–158, 2004

Watson D, Gamez W, Simms LJ: Basic dimensions of temperament and their relation to anxiety and depression: a symptom-based perspective. J Res Pers 39:46–66, 2005

Watson JB, Morgan JJB: Emotional reactions and psychological experimentation. Am J Psychol 28:163–174, 1917

Wik G, Fredrikson M, Ericson K, et al: A functional cerebral response to frightening visual stimulation. Psychiatry Res 50:15–24, 1993

Wikström J, Lundh LG, Westerlund J, et al: Preattentive bias for snake words in snake phobia? Behav Res Ther 42:949–970, 2004

Williams JMG, Watts FN, McLeod C, et al (eds): Cognitive Psychology and Emotional Disorders, 2nd Edition. Chichester, UK, John Wiley and Sons, 1997

Wittchen H-U: Natural course and spontaneous remissions of untreated anxiety disorders, in Panic and Phobias II: Treatments and Variables Affecting Course and Outcome. Edited by Hand I, Wittchen HU. New York, Springer, 1988, pp 3–17

Wittchen HU, Jacobi F: Size and burden of mental disorder in Europe: a critical review and appraisal of 27 studies. Eur Neuropsychopharmacol 15:357–376, 2005

Wittchen H-U, Nelson CB, Lachner G: Prevalence of mental disorders and psychosocial impairments in adolescents and young adults. Psychol Med 28:109–126, 1998

Wittchen HU, Lieb R, Schuster P, et al: When is onset? investigations into early developmental stages of anxiety and depressive disorders, in Childhood Onset of "Adult" Psychopathology: Clinical and Research Advances. Edited by Rapoport JL. Washington, DC, American Psychiatric Press, 1999, pp 259–302

Wittchen H-U, Kessler RC, Pfister H, et al: Why do people with anxiety disorders become depressed? A prospective-longitudinal community study. Acta Psychiatr Scand 102(suppl):14–23, 2000

Wittchen H-U, Lecrubier Y, Beesdo K, et al: Relationships among anxiety disorders: patterns and implications, in Anxiety Disorders. Edited by Nutt DJ, Ballenger JC. Oxford, UK, Blackwell Science, 2003, pp 25–37

World Health Organization: The ICD-10 Classification of Mental and Behavioural Disorders: Clinical Descriptions and Diagnostic Guidelines. Geneva, Switzerland, World Health Organization, 1992

Zimmerman M, Chelminski I, Young D: On the threshold of disorder: a study of the impact of the DSM-IV clinical significance criterion on diagnosing depressive and anxiety disorders in clinical practice. J Clin Psychiatry 65:1400–1405, 2004

PART 2

COURSE AND CLASSIFICATION

5

CONTINUITY AND ETIOLOGY OF ANXIETY DISORDERS

Are They Stable Across the Life Course?

Richie Poulton, Ph.D.
Daniel S. Pine, M.D.
HonaLee Harrington, B.A.

The stress-induced and fear circuitry disorders comprise posttraumatic stress disorder (PTSD), panic disorder with and without agoraphobia, specific phobia, and social phobia. These disorders are the focus of this chapter, but we also include generalized anxiety disorder (GAD) and obsessive-compulsive disorder (OCD) for comparison purposes in analyses concerned with disorder continuity. We concentrate on DSM diagnoses (i.e., categories) and do not consider symptom measures (dimensions), but we do recognize the value of this approach (M. Rutter 2003). We begin the chapter by reviewing evidence for the continuity of the stress-induced and fear circuitry disorders from childhood to adulthood. We then ask whether the etiologies of these anxiety disorders are stable across the life course before considering current and future research opportunities. The chapter concludes with a discussion of the desiderata of a developmental framework specific to the anxiety disorders that could inform DSM-V.

Continuity of Anxiety Disorders
EVIDENCE FROM PROSPECTIVE-DEVELOPMENTAL STUDIES

Most adult psychiatric disorders have their roots in early life (Kim-Cohen et al. 2003; Pine et al. 1998). Such evidence is found for the majority of psychiatric disorders, including the "stress-related and fear circuitry" disorders, as well as for a range of other syndromes, such as behavior disorders and substance-use disorders. Yet "it is apparent that the amount of life span information that is provided in DSM-IV is only the tip of the iceberg of what should in fact be known" (Widiger and Clark 2000, p.955). "A comparable means of characterizing a developmental, life span history of a patient's symptomatology should be developed for DSM-V" (Widiger and Clark 2000, p. 956).

To address the issue of continuity, we reviewed prospective-developmental studies that met five basic criteria. First, studies had to use general population samples, because clinical or convenience samples have limited generalizability (Cohen and Cohen 1984). Second, the samples had to represent both males and females, because of the known sex differences in anxiety disorders (Craske 2003). Third, sample size had to be greater than 500 to ensure adequate prevalence of disorders and sufficient statistical power. Fourth, at least one data point was required from both the juvenile (<18 years) and adult periods. Fifth, information on DSM anxiety diagnoses had to be available in adulthood to permit "disorder" continuity analyses.

Two broad types of disorder stability can be identified in longitudinal studies: 1) homotypic continuity, which refers to continuity of similar behaviors or phenotypes, and 2) heterotypic continuity (or sequential comorbidity), which is continuity of an inferred latent attribute presumed to underlie diverse phenotypes or behaviors. It is important to emphasize that heterotypic continuity refers to a *conceptual* rather than literal continuity among disorders—hence the requirement for some theory or working hypothesis as to how the different diagnoses are linked (via genes and/or environmental factors) and what latent variable(s) they reflect.

We identified five studies that met these criteria. In the first, Hofstra et al. (2002) examined adult mental health outcomes of children and adolescents recruited in 1983 at ages 6 through 16 years ($N=1,587$). At follow-up 14 years later, participants—now ages 20–30 years—were assessed for DSM-IV (American Psychiatric Association 1994) diagnoses by means of the computerized version of the Composite International Diagnostic Interview (World Health Organization 1997). Hofstra et al. found that juvenile internalizing problems measured by the Child Behavior Checklist (Achenbach 1991) at the 82nd percentile or greater predicted an increase in the likelihood of receiving an anxiety disorder diagnosis (any of GAD, OCD, panic disorder, agoraphobia, social phobia, or specific phobia) among females (OR=1.6 [1.1–2.5]) and mood disorder diagnosis among males (OR=5.2 [1.8–14.5]).

In the second study, Goodwin et al. (2004) used a similar approach to examine the relation between parent reports of anxious/withdrawn behavior at age 8 years, as assessed with scales by Rutter et al. (1970) and Conners (1969), and anxiety diagnoses at ages 18–21 ($N=957$) in the Christchurch Health and Development Study. Increasing levels of anxious/withdrawn behavior at age 8 were associated with increased rates of social phobia, specific phobia, and panic/agoraphobia but not with GAD. In adjusted models, the odds ratios for each of these disorders in persons with childhood anxious/withdrawn behavior in the highest quintile were 2.4–4.5 times higher compared to those with childhood anxious/withdrawn behavior in the lowest quintile. After adjustment for social and family factors during childhood and adolescence, the associations between childhood and adult pathology remained significant for social phobia (OR=3.37; 95% CI=1.54–7.39) and specific phobia (OR=3.89; 95% CI=1.89–8.02).

Both these studies used broadly defined dimensional measures of childhood anxiety symptoms rather than childhood anxiety diagnoses. However, it seems likely that there would have been significant overlap between those who would have met diagnostic criteria and those scoring at the high end on these dimensional measures. Moreover, methodological factors may have led to an underestimate of stability in these studies. Because these studies relied on broad classification schemes in childhood, stronger associations may have been expected with more narrowly defined syndromes, to the extent that continuity for disorders across development results from specific associations with more narrowly defined syndromes.

Wittchen et al. (2000) studied a representative sample of German 14- to 17-year-olds ($N=1,128$) and followed them up 20 months later (range=15–26 months). Using liberal criteria that included subthreshold and DSM-IV threshold cases, these investigators reported greatest continuity for panic disorder (44%) and specific phobia (30%) and least continuity for agoraphobia (13%) and social phobia (16%). However, the short duration of follow-up, and the fact that many individuals in the sample were still of adolescent age at follow-up, limit interpretation of these data.

In the fourth study, Pine et al. (1998) assessed a community sample ($N=776$) of young Americans three times, beginning in 1983 when sample members were between 9 and 18 years of age and again in 1985 and 1992, using structured interviews that provided DSM diagnoses. In simple logistical models, adolescent anxiety disorders were associated with a two- to threefold increase in risk for adult anxiety disorders. There was evidence for homotypic continuity in the course of simple and social phobia, but there was less evidence of homotypic continuity in the course of GAD or depression. Analyses in this study treated overanxious disorder and GAD as strongly related, on the basis of perspectives in DSM-IV and of data showing strong associations in symptoms of the two disorders in the sample. However, symptom scales in the two samples shared less than 50% of the variance.

In reality, overanxious disorder and GAD may capture somewhat different conditions. In analyses adjusted for age, ethnicity, social class, and sex, adolescent simple phobia predicted adult simple phobia only (OR=3.79; CI=2.37–6.05). Adolescent social phobia (OR=3.29; 95% CI=1.52–7.10), as well as overanxious disorder (OR=2.27; 95% CI=1.06–7.10), predicted adult social phobia, indicating considerable homotypic continuity. Interestingly, latent Markov analyses revealed that approximately half of adolescent anxiety disorders were no longer present in adulthood, yet the vast majority of adult anxiety disorders were preceded by some type of disorder during adolescence.

These results are consistent with more recent findings from the fifth study, the Dunedin birth cohort study, which sought to establish the extent to which adult psychiatric disorders are extensions of juvenile disorders (Kim-Cohen et al. 2003). Psychiatric diagnoses were made according to DSM criteria at ages 11, 13, 15, 18, 21, and 26 years (N=976). Among adult cases interviewed at age 26, 50% had received a diagnosis before 15 years of age and 74% before 18 years of age. Among the subset receiving treatment, similar patterns were observed, with 60% having received a diagnosis before 15 years and 78% before age 18. Follow-back analyses of adult anxiety disorder (any of panic disorder, agoraphobia, specific phobia, social phobia, PTSD, GAD, and OCD) showed evidence of homotypic continuity—that is, adults with anxiety disorders had also had anxiety disorders in childhood or adolescence. In addition, adults with anxiety were also at elevated risk of having had juvenile externalizing-spectrum diagnoses of attention-deficit/hyperactivity disorder (ADHD) and conduct disorder (CD) or oppositional defiant disorder (ODD). However, this follow-back analysis reported the seven DSM anxiety disorders as one group, potentially obscuring important differences in continuity patterns among the disorders.

These studies converge to show that continuities exist between childhood/juvenile anxiety disorder and adult anxiety diagnoses. There is evidence for both homotypic (most strongly for social phobia) and heterotypic continuity, the strength of which appears to vary among the disorders. To further explore these patterns, we "unpacked" the grouped anxiety disorder data from the Dunedin study (Kim-Cohen et al. 2003) and used the same follow-back design to examine continuity between juvenile disorders and *specific* adult anxiety disorders. The findings are presented in Table 5–1.

A more nuanced picture might be expected if the separate DSM-IV and DSM-IV-TR (American Psychiatric Association 2000) anxiety diagnostic classifications have validity as distinct conditions, which was the case here. PTSD was characterized by heterotypic continuity, with all but juvenile ADHD being associated with this outcome by age 26. This is perhaps understandable, given that PTSD requires exposure to a traumatic event, and risk for exposure may be elevated among children with CD and ODD. For panic disorder and social phobia, there was strong evidence for homotypic continuity, a finding consistent with some previous stud-

TABLE 5–1. Anxiety disorder diagnosis at age 26 and history of juvenile psychiatric diagnoses between ages 11 and 15, after control for sex

		Diagnoses at ages 11–15			
Diagnosis at age 26 (sample prevalence[a])	Anxiety disorders[b] (20.4%)	Depression (7.0%)	ADHD (6.3%)	CD/ODD (20.0%)	
Generalized anxiety disorder N=50 (5.5%)	42%, P<0.001 AOR=3.06 (1.70–5.51)	14%, P=0.048 AOR=2.34 (1.01–5.44)	6%, P=0.89 AOR=1.09 (0.32–3.66)	32%, P=0.015 AOR=2.12 (1.16–3.91)	
Obsessive-compulsive disorder N=22 (2.4%)	41%, P=0.023 AOR=2.73 (1.15–6.52)	23%, P=0.007 AOR=4.18 (1.49–11.74)	4%, P=0.88 AOR=0.85 (0.11–6.59)	41%, P=0.009 AOR=3.21 (1.33–7.76)	
Posttraumatic stress disorder N=40 (4.1%)	35%, P=0.026 AOR=2.15 (1.10–4.21)	20%, P=0.002 AOR=3.68 (1.62–8.36)	8%, P=0.54 AOR=1.47 (0.43–5.00)	38%, P=0.003 AOR=2.80 (1.43–5.49)	
Panic disorder N=36 (3.9%)	36%, P=0.022 AOR=2.28 (1.13–4.60)	14%, P=0.10 AOR=2.27 (0.85–6.05)	6%, P=0.98 AOR=1.02 (0.23–4.41)	26%, P=0.23 AOR=1.58 (0.75–3.36)	
Agoraphobia N=31 (3.5%)	52%, P<0.001 AOR=4.35 (2.10–9.00)	16%, P=0.052 AOR=2.69 (0.99–7.27)	13%, P=0.054 AOR=3.01 (0.98–9.22)	31%, P=0.058 AOR=2.13 (0.98–4.63)	
Specific phobia N=68 (7.1%)	38%, P=0.001 AOR=2.46 (1.46–4.16)	18%, P=0.001 AOR=3.27 (1.63–6.57)	9%, P=0.055 AOR=2.48 (0.98–6.26)	28%, P=0.015 AOR=2.04 (1.15–3.62)	
Social phobia N=100 (10.7%)	31%, P=0.006 AOR=1.92 (1.21–3.04)	9%, P=0.38 AOR=1.40 (0.67–2.92)	10%, P=0.052 AOR=2.06 (0.99–4.29)	23%, P=0.30 AOR=1.30 (0.79–2.12)	

Note. Boldface text indicates $P<0.05$. ADHD = attention-deficit/hyperactivity disorder; AOR=sex adjusted odds ratio; CD=conduct disorder; ODD=oppositional defiant disorder.
[a]12-month prevalence.
[b]Juvenile anxiety disorders comprise overanxious disorder, separation anxiety disorder, and phobia.
Source. Calculated from data reported by Kim-Cohen et al. 2003.

ies (Pine et al. 1998; Wittchen et al. 2000). In contrast, agoraphobia and specific phobia (accepting associations of borderline significance, all P values < 0.06) exhibited marked heterotypic continuity, with a juvenile history of anxiety (overanxious disorder, separation anxiety disorder, and phobia), depression, ADHD, and CD/ODD. Interestingly, both GAD and OCD showed the same patterns of heterotypic continuity as PTSD and were similar to agoraphobia and specific phobia.

Comparison of these findings reveals a more complex picture of continuity than observed when all adult anxiety disorder diagnoses were grouped together (Kim-Cohen et al. 2003). The findings direct attention to the processes that promote homotypic continuity in social phobia and panic disorder. They also highlight the importance of questions about sequential patterns of comorbidity (i.e., heterotypic continuity) in which a broad range of juvenile disorders reliably preceded agoraphobia, specific phobia, and, to a lesser extent, PTSD. The latter is perhaps expected given the requirement for exposure to a traumatic event, but the findings for agoraphobia and specific phobia are not so easily explained. Finally, it was noteworthy that neither GAD or OCD "looked out of place" compared with the other anxiety disorders; their patterns of continuity closely mirrored those for PTSD, which raises questions about the exclusion of these two disorders from the anxiety disorders section for DSM-V. If, as these data suggest, adult anxiety disorders have their roots in early life, then focusing on childhood and adolescence will be critical to understanding their etiology and advancing taxonomy. Developmental research on antisocial behavior (Moffitt 1993; Moffitt and Caspi 2001) and depression (Harrington et al. 1990, 1997; Jaffee et al. 2002; Wickramaratne et al. 2000) has demonstrated the value of distinguishing persistent (from child to adult) cases from those limited to specific developmental periods. This distinction may also prove useful for the stress-induced and fear circuitry disorders.

FUTURE RESEARCH ON DISORDER CONTINUITY

We identified five studies with sufficient data to test for juvenile–adult diagnostic continuity, but more data would clearly be desirable. The most obvious source of new information will remain the ongoing longitudinal studies reviewed here. Examination of the developmental history of mental disorders in these cohorts, as cohort members age, will provide more useful information, but this should also be complemented by studies in young adults with follow-up extending well beyond mid-life. Nonetheless, the present findings are important because they cover the peak period of risk for onset of most anxiety disorders (Kessler et al. 2005), perhaps with the exception of panic disorder with agoraphobia. It should also be stressed that none of the studies reviewed here included diagnostic data from early childhood. The earliest DSM diagnoses were obtained in the Dunedin study and referred to the 12-month period prior to age 11 years. Recent evidence suggests that many anxiety disorders emerge at younger ages (Costello et al. 2005). Other studies exist that, if extended, will contribute valuable data at comparatively low cost. For example, the Great Smoky Mountains Study has excellent diagnostic information about a range of childhood anxiety disorders up to the age of 16, as well as good data on homotypic and heterotypic continuity in this age group (Costello et al. 2003). Given the importance of characterizing developmental antecedents of anxiety disorders (Zahn-Waxler et al. 2000), researchers should fully interrogate existing databases before embarking on new time-consuming studies (Robins 2005).

New ways of thinking about anxiety disorder continuity are required. Dimensional data must be incorporated, and models that can be fitted to multiwave data must be developed to allow tests of competing hypotheses (e.g., are two correlated disorders distinct or simply "phenocopies" of the same underlying construct?). These approaches should help elucidate the processes giving rise to different patterns of life course continuity among similar disorders (e.g., agoraphobia, social phobia, and specific phobia). Such work may also help resolve current ambiguities in the literature. For example, modeling the factor structure and stability of depression, GAD, and phobia between ages 18 and 21 years in the Christchurch Health and Development Study revealed that the best-fitting model was consistent with both "pure" expressions of depression, GAD, and phobia and a mixed "internalizing" disorder factor in which symptoms of depression, anxiety, and phobia co-occurred. Whereas the majority of stability of depression and GAD between ages 18 and 21 was accounted for by this general mixed "internalizing" factor, less of the stability of phobias was accounted for by this factor, with approximately half attributable to disorder-specific factors (David Fergusson, personal communication, October 28, 2005).

Moreover, further insights concerning continuity may be gained by looking beyond symptom patterns. Symptom patterns are expected to reflect underlying perturbations in the capacity for the brain to process information. In recent years, paradigms derived from experimental psychology typically have been employed in neuroimaging experiments and should allow a precise linking of data from neuroimaging, experimental psychology, and clinical fields. It is also important to realize that demonstrating continuity is not the same as understanding the processes that give rise to such continuity. The major challenge is to describe *how, when, why,* and *for whom* continuity exists.

Stability of Etiology of Anxiety Disorders Over the Life Course

ETIOLOGY OF ANXIETY DISORDERS: CURRENT CONTROVERSIES

Before considering how stable etiologies are for the stress-induced and fear circuitry disorders over time, we feel obliged to discuss etiology per se. It is almost universally accepted that the capacity to experience fear and anxiety is adaptive, enabling, as it does, rapid and energetic response to imminent danger or preparation for more distal challenges. However, the nature of maladaptive fear and anxiety remains controversial, and despite many hopeful leads, there is still no consensus about the etiology of any of the anxiety disorders. Anxiety disorders could reflect perturbations in core features of an individual's responses to imminent danger. Alternatively, they could reflect an intact "core" response to danger that is elicited by inappropriate circumstances or that cannot be terminated appropriately. Moreover, distinct disorders may reflect distinct perturbations. Indeed, the current anxiety disorders in DSM-IV-TR (comprising seven disorders) and the proposed stress-induced and fear circuitry disorders grouping (made up of PTSD, panic disorder with and without agoraphobia, social phobia, and specific phobia) are characterized by enormous etiological heterogeneity, which we briefly review here.

PTSD is unique among psychiatric disorders because exposure to a traumatic event is a diagnostic criterion. PTSD is therefore the quintessential "conditioning" or stress-diathesis disorder. Risk factors for PTSD are of two types: 1) those that increase risk of exposure to trauma and 2) those that lead to the development of symptoms subsequent to that exposure. A recent report from the Dunedin study found that a number of risk factors (of both types) present in the first decade of life were associated with developing PTSD by age 32 years (Koenen et al. 2007). This suggests that PTSD is not simply a conditioned response to trauma but a more complex disorder with etiological links to capacities and conditions determined in early childhood, long before exposure to the traumatic event takes place.

With regard to phobia etiology, two major schools of thought are apparent: those suggesting dysfunctional fear arises largely as a result of associative-conditioning processes (i.e., stress-diathesis models) and those that favor more biologically based, nonassociative etiological explanations. In an interesting challenge to the applicability of the stress-diathesis model for phobias (agoraphobia, social, animal, situational, and blood-injury), Kendler et al. (2002) operationalized three hypotheses, consistent with the stress-diathesis model, in their large twin sample ($N=7,500$). Their findings were most compatible with nonassociative models postulating that vulnerability to phobias is largely innate and does not arise directly from environmental experiences. Thus, it is possible that the stress-diathesis model that applies to many psychiatric disorders is not an appropriate paradigm for some phobias. To complicate matters further, there is no consensus about etiological pathways *within* phobia categories (e.g., see the February 2002 special issue of *Behaviour Research and Therapy*). Some specific fears/phobias appear to arise completely independently of direct or indirect conditioning events (e.g., height and water fear), whereas others are strongly reliant on conditioning events for onset (e.g., dental fear) (Poulton and Menzies 2002).

With regard to panic disorder (with and without agoraphobia), etiological theories again fall into two broad camps: those emphasizing psychosocial and cognitive processes (Clark 1988) and those emphasizing more biological/physical explanations. Here the biological models specify abnormally low thresholds for suffocation symptoms as the key etiological factor (Klein 1993; Verburg et al. 1995), but findings have been mixed (Roth et al. 2005). In one report that compared etiological explanations, the findings were consistent with both cognitive and biological interpretations (Craske et al. 2001). Knowledge about the etiology of social phobia also remains rudimentary. A recent review of putative etiological factors for social phobia that considered genetic factors, temperament, childrearing, negative life events, adverse social experiences, cognitive distortions, and skill deficits highlighted "the strict limits to our current knowledge and understanding of causal origins" (Rapee and Spence 2004).

REVIEW OF THE DEVELOPMENTAL LITERATURE ON LIFE COURSE STABILITY OF ETIOLOGY

A search of the developmental literature on the life course stability of etiology among anxiety disorders turned up no studies that explicitly tested for etiological stability across the juvenile and adult period. The closest was a longitudinal investigation of early (< 18 years) and late-onset (> 18 years) dental fear in relation to conditioning experiences, service-use patterns, and personality (Poulton et al. 2001). Results showed that in addition to conditioning experiences, those with high scores on the stress-reactivity subscale of the Multidimensional Personality Questionnaire (Tellegen 1982) were approximately seven times more likely to develop a dental fear by the age of 18 than those with low scores on this scale. In contrast, the stress-reactive personality trait was unrelated to the onset of dental fear in adulthood. Consistent with other developmental findings, patients with early-onset anxiety disorders characterized by personality vulnerability appear to be more difficult to treat (Fiset et al. 1989; Locker et al. 1999).

This research approach to mapping different developmental trajectories of the supposedly same disorder is important because it can provide insights into etiology, course, and optimal intervention strategies. This is because juvenile-onset forms of disorders are known to be associated with more severe childhood risks (Geller et al. 1998; Jaffee et al. 2002; Moffitt and Caspi 2001) and worse prognosis in adulthood (Moffitt et al. 2002; Rosario-Campos et al. 2001; Weissman et al. 1999; Wickramaratne et al. 2000). It is reasonable, then, to ask why there are so few studies of developmental heterogeneity among the anxiety disorders.

There are several possible explanations. The first is historical. It was only 28 years ago that DSM-III (American Psychiatric Association 1980) standardized the definition and diagnosis of psychiatric disorders. This finally enabled researchers to systematically collect (via structured diagnostic interviews) information about children's symptoms and disorders. These children have only recently "come of age," thereby permitting investigation of juvenile–adult disorder continuities (Coleman and Jones 2004).

A second reason may be the lack of clarity about which etiological (risk) factors should be investigated for which disorders, as noted earlier. Third, a less obvious limitation has been the tendency for most studies to focus on single, or on several, risk factors only. For example, studies have examined specific risk factors for PTSD, such as child abuse (Widom 1999), prior trauma exposure (Breslau et al. 1999), pretrauma intelligence (Macklin et al. 1998; Pitman et al. 1991), personality (Schnurr et al. 1993), heart rate (Shalev et al. 1998), and family environment (Costello et al. 2002), but until recently no one had investigated a wide range of childhood risk factors starting from birth through to PTSD diagnosis in adulthood (see Koenen et al. 2007). Finally, according to clinical lore, and supported by recent findings from the National Comorbidity Survey Replication (Kessler et al. 2005), some anxiety disorders have their onset in the late twenties and early thirties. This effectively extends the ideal time frame for studying juvenile–adult disorder associations, at least for some anxiety disorders—thus, waiting until longitudinal study participants are 30 or more years of age to study developmental heterogeneity seems prudent.

FUTURE RESEARCH ON STABILITY OF ETIOLOGY

A good illustration of the way forward comes from a study able to distinguish prospectively between juvenile- and adult-onset cases of depression in a birth cohort followed to adulthood (Jaffee et al. 2002). In this study, early childhood risk factors were assessed from birth to 9 years. Diagnoses of depression were made according to DSM criteria on three occasions prior to adulthood (ages 11, 13, and 15 years) and three occasions during adulthood (ages 18, 21, and 26 years). Four groups were defined: 1) individuals first diagnosed as having depression in childhood, but not in adulthood ($n=21$); 2) individuals first diagnosed as having depression in adulthood ($n=314$); 3) individuals first diagnosed in childhood whose depression recurred in adulthood by age 26 years ($n=34$); and 4) never-depressed individuals ($n=629$). The two juvenile-onset groups had similar high-risk profiles on childhood measures. Compared with the adult-depressed group, the juvenile-onset groups experienced more perinatal insults and motor skill deficits, caretaker instability, criminality, and psychopathology in the family of origin and more behavioral and socio-emotional problems (see Figure 5–1). The adult-onset group's risk profile was similar to that of the never-depressed group, with the exception of elevated history of childhood sexual abuse.

Those people with depression in childhood had a markedly different risk profile from those who experienced depression for the first time in adulthood. Applying this approach to anxiety disorders may prove fruitful and yield interesting insights into developmental course and etiology. Future research also needs to move away from the traditional risk-factor approach, in which single or sometimes several risk factors are examined, to an approach that includes multiple risk factors

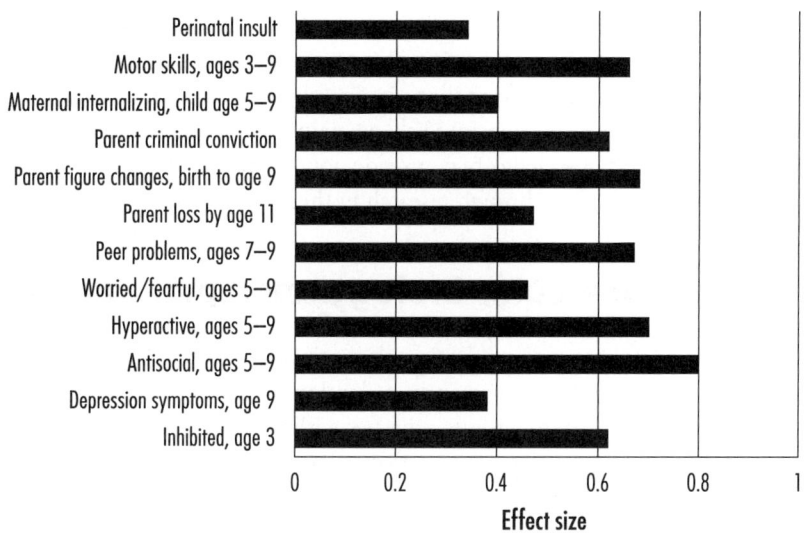

FIGURE 5–1. Comparison of adult depressed groups with juvenile and juvenile+adult depressed groups.

Positive values mean juvenile depressed groups have higher scores than adult depressed group.

Source. Adapted from Jaffee et al. 2002.

and assesses cumulative risk. For example, 58% of cohort members in the Dunedin study who experienced three or more childhood risks developed PTSD after being exposed to a trauma, as compared with only 25% of those with no childhood risks (Koenen et al. 2007). Moreover, the time is right to explore the full range of potential early life risk factors for adult anxiety disorders. This should include investigating risk factors that have not traditionally been of interest for anxiety, for example, neurodevelopmental measures of cognitive and motor abilities (Fergusson et al. 2005; Koenen et al. 2007).

Similarly, true progress in research on etiology is likely to follow an integration of clinical and basic work in the neurosciences. Such integration has been difficult to achieve because of the complexity of both research areas. Nevertheless, the current view of anxiety disorders—as perturbations in information processing—offers guidelines for research that could lead to such integration. Perturbations in core information processing functions are becoming increasingly understood from both clinical and basic neuroscience perspectives. For example, threat-related information shows a unique capacity to influence measures of attention among both children and adults with anxiety disorders (see Pine et al. 2005; Mogg and Bradley 1998), and this capacity may result from the ability of threat-related information to engage a specific neural circuit that regulates responses to threats in mammals. Imaging studies are consistent with the hypothesis that anxiety disorders result from perturbations in this core circuitry (Monk et al. 2006). Moreover, imaging studies also show that such perturbations in circuitry may arise from genetic and environmental influences in capacity to shape brain function and behavior (Pezawas et al. 2005). This knowledge may provide opportunities for integrating clinical and genetic perspectives through research in the neurosciences.

Marrying Molecular Biology and Epidemiology

DSM-IV-TR produces diagnoses that are characterized by (often great) heterogeneity *within* each disorder. Importantly, a developmental perspective explicitly posits the existence of heterogeneous subtypes within disorders that follow quite distinctive developmental trajectories, reflected in age of onset (early versus late) and subsequent course of symptoms over time (temporary versus persistent). Genetic factors are likely to be relevant to a deeper understanding of developmental subtypes and the course of disorder.

Indeed, there is increasing interest in environmental risk moderation by genetic factors, otherwise known as gene–environment interaction. This occurs whenever the relation between an environmental risk factor and a disorder depends upon (or is moderated by) naturally occurring genetic variability (polymorphisms). Recent findings have shown how the association between maltreatment and antisocial behavior is moderated by the monoamine oxidase A gene (*MAOA*) (e.g., Caspi et al. 2002; Foley et al. 2004), how the relation between life stress and adversity and subsequent depression is moderated by the serotonin transporter promoter gene (*5-HTTLPR*) (Caspi et al. 2003; Kendler et al. 2005), and how the relation between teenage cannabis use and the risk of developing adult psychosis is moderated by the catechol-O-methyltransferase gene (*COMT*) (Caspi et al. 2005). To continue moving research on genes and behavior toward pathophysiological models, it will be important to embed future research in samples where data on information processing functions have been obtained.

A good illustration of this approach for the anxiety disorders is the work by Fox et al. (2005), who reported a gene–environment interaction between maternal reports of social support and child *5-HTT* status in predicting behavioral inhibition in middle childhood (age 8). Behavioral inhibition in this sample was assessed using measures from experimental psychology that measure patterns of information processing observed by the investigators. As such, this is an example of prospective research that uses directly observed laboratory measures of temperament and provides internal replication using two parallel measures of child behavior, one derived from maternal report and the other from direct observation by examiners—both assessing aspects of social reticence.

Future studies on anxiety disorders need to select genes that prior research indicates are likely to be related to both the exposure (or environmental risk factor) and the outcome (the anxiety disorder of interest) (see Moffitt et al. 2005 for a more detailed discussion of these issues). Ideally, risk factors should be proximal and known to be "true" environmental risk factors (M. Rutter et al. 2001). Otherwise, gene–environment correlations (passive, active, and evocative) can "set up" or drive environmental risk exposure, resulting in potentially misleading conclusions about the presence of gene–environment interactions. In the absence of opportunities for concurrent external replication, internal replication should be attempted using alternate measures of the phenotype wherever possible. One aim of genetic research is to provide new etiological information and objective tests that resolve clinical heterogeneity and thereby improve diagnostic practice (Bearden et al. 2004). Some genes do not operate as pure susceptibility genes for disorder onset but rather operate as modifier genes affecting the disorder's clinical features and course (Fanous and Kendler 2005). For example, among children diagnosed with ADHD, an increasing number of "risk genotypes" (*DAT1* and *DRD4*) were associated with a subtype of ADHD characterized by low IQ. These modifier genes predicted a poorer long-term prognosis among this ADHD subtype (Mill et al. 2006). These data illustrate how genetic information might be incorporated into psychiatric nosology through biomarker testing.

Despite promising developments in the field of psychiatric genetics, we still know little about how genes and their products (RNA, polypeptides, proteins) interact with one another, let alone how they interact with a host of environmental factors impacting people at different points across the life course. Because we know so little about how the brain works to produce psychopathology, progress will require careful, systematic hypothesis testing. Such work will benefit from twin research that aims to identify the genetic and environmental sources of individual differences in endophenotypes, such as fear conditioning, including variability in habituation, acquisition, and extinction of fears (Hettema et al. 2005). These studies will, no doubt, build on work that suggests that genes may predispose to two broad groups of anxiety disorders, made up of panic-generalized-agoraphobic anxiety versus the specific phobias (Hettema et al. 2003).

We also need more studies that generate information about how risk for psychopathology is transmitted from parents to children and the conditions under which these intergenerational cycles can be broken. At present we have an incomplete understanding of 1) the effects of parents' psychopathology on children's development across a broad range of domains, including both positive and negative outcomes; 2) the mechanisms of risk transmission; 3) the reasons for discontinuities in the transmission of risk for psychopathology across generations; 4) the role of mothers' and fathers' mental health in children's development; and 5) the bidirectional nature of parents' and children's relationships—that is, children have effects on their parents just as parents have effects on their children (Jaffee and

Poulton 2006). For example, Harper (2005) pointed to epigenetic inheritance as a mechanism of interest. This refers to the transmission to offspring of parental phenotypic responses to environmental challenges—even when the young do not experience the challenges themselves. Genetic inheritance is not altered; rather, gene expression is. Weissman et al. (2005) recently confirmed the value of three-generation cohorts by illustrating cross-generation moderation. Specifically, they found that the association between parental depression and child diagnosis of anxiety was moderated by grandparental depression. Clearly, evidence from intergenerational studies of risk transmission (occurring via secular, social learning, and/or biological mechanisms) is necessary to obtain a deeper understanding of disorder continuity and etiological stability.

A Developmental Perspective for DSM-V

Reducing the burden of disease associated with psychiatric disorder (World Health Organization 1996) will require knowledge about the risk processes occurring during childhood and adolescence. Against this background, a developmental research framework is needed to inform refinement of DSM-IV in arriving at DSM-V. This need presents a challenge for the anxiety disorders, particularly because knowledge about etiology is, at best, rudimentary. Although there has been some progress toward understanding life course continuities among the anxiety disorders, there are many unanswered questions, particularly those related to heterotypic continuity (sequential comorbidity). Desiderata of a developmental framework include 1) the capacity to describe (e.g., natural history, episodic versus chronic course, and evidence for critical [sensitive] periods of risk), and 2) quantitative data (i.e., sturdiness or robustness of risk factors, and effect size).

A useful starting point might be learning ways other branches of medicine have dealt with similar challenges. For example, the American Heart Association ranks cardiovascular risk factors according to the strength of the evidence base ("major independent risk factors" vs. "predisposing risk factors" vs. "conditional risk factors") (Grundy et al. 1999; Pearson 2002).

Any developmental understanding of anxiety disorders also needs to embrace the notion of cumulative risk, in terms of both total risk-factor burden and length of time exposed. Such a framework needs to be sufficiently flexible to integrate new knowledge as it emerges. If diagnosis *is* prognosis, then it seems that too little attention has been paid to developmental aspects of anxiety disorders or to considering how the interplay of biology and environment influences course, both singularly and across disorders. The current DSM provides a multiaxial system that recognizes cross-sectional heterogeneity. DSM-V requires a developmental equivalent.

References

Achenbach TM: Manual for the Child Behavior Checklist/4–18 and 1991 Profile. Burlington, University of Vermont, Department of Psychiatry, 1991

American Psychiatric Association: Diagnostic and Statistical Manual of Mental Disorders, 3rd Edition. Washington, DC, American Psychiatric Association, 1980

American Psychiatric Association: Diagnostic and Statistical Manual of Mental Disorders, 4th Edition. Washington, DC, American Psychiatric Association, 1994

American Psychiatric Association: Diagnostic and Statistical Manual of Mental Disorders, 4th Edition, Text Revision. Washington, DC, American Psychiatric Association, 2000

Bearden CE, Reus VI, Freimer NB: Why genetic investigation of psychiatric disorders is so difficult. Curr Opin Genet Dev 14:280–286, 2004

Breslau N, Chilcoat HD, Kessler RC, et al: Previous exposure to trauma and PTSD effects of subsequent trauma: results from the Detroit Area Survey of trauma. Am J Psychiatry 156:902–907, 1999

Caspi A, McClay J, Moffitt TE, et al: Role of genotype in the cycle of violence in maltreated children. Science 297:851–854, 2002

Caspi A, Sugden K, Moffitt TE, et al: Influence of life stress on depression: moderation by a polymorphism in the 5-HTT gene. Science 301:386–389, 2003

Caspi A, Moffitt TE, Cannon M, et al: Moderation of the effect of adolescent-onset cannabis use on adult psychosis by a functional polymorphism in the COMT gene: longitudinal evidence of a gene x environment interaction. Biol Psychiatry 57:1117–1127, 2005

Clark DM: A cognitive model of panic attacks, in Panic: Psychological Perspectives. Edited by Rachman SJ, Maser JD. Hillsdale, NJ, Erlbaum, 1988, pp 71–89

Cohen P, Cohen J: The clinician's illusion. Arch Gen Psychiatry 41:1178–1182, 1984

Coleman I, Jones P: Birth cohort studies in psychiatry: beginning at the beginning. Psychol Med 34:1375–1383, 2004

Conners CK: A teacher rating scale for use in drug studies with children. Am J Psychiatry 126:884–888, 1969

Costello EJ, Erkanli A, Fairbank JA, et al: The prevalence of potentially traumatic events in childhood and adolescence. J Trauma Stress 15:99–112, 2002

Costello EJ, Mustillo S, Erkanli A, et al: Prevalence and development of psychiatric disorders in childhood and adolescence. Arch Gen Psychiatry 60:837–844, 2003

Costello EJ, Egger H, Angold A: 10-year research update review: the epidemiology of child and adolescent psychiatric disorders, I: methods and public health burden. J Am Acad Child Adolesc Psychiatry 44:972–986, 2005

Craske MG: Origins of Phobias and Anxiety Disorders: Why More Women than Men? Oxford, UK, Pergamon/Elsevier, 2003

Craske MG, Poulton R, Tsao JCI, et al: Paths to panic disorder/agoraphobia: an exploratory analysis from age 3 to 21 in an unselected birth cohort. J Am Acad Child Adolesc Psychiatry 40:556–563, 2001

Fanous AH, Kendler KS: Genetic heterogeneity, modifier genes and quantitative phenotypes in psychiatric illness: searching for a framework. Mol Psychiatry 10:6–13, 2005

Fergusson DM, Horwood LJ, Ridder EM: Show me the child at seven, II: childhood intelligence and later outcomes in adolescence and young adulthood. J Child Psychol Psychiatry 46:850–858, 2005

Fiset L, Milgrom P, Weinstein P, et al: Common fears and their relationship to dental fear and utilization of the dentist. Anesth Prog 36:258–264, 1989

Foley DL, Eaves LJ, Wormley B, et al: Childhood adversity, monoamine oxidase a genotype, and risk for conduct disorder. Arch Gen Psychiatry 61:738–744, 2004

Fox NA, Nichols KE, Henderson HA, et al: Evidence for a gene environment interaction in predicting behavioral inhibition in middle childhood. Psychol Sci 16:921–926, 2005

Geller D, Biederman J, Jones J, et al: Is juvenile obsessive-compulsive disorder a developmental subtype of the disorder? A review of the pediatric literature. J Am Acad Child Adolesc Psychiatry 37:420–427, 1998

Goodwin RD, Fergusson DM, Horwood LJ: Early anxious/withdrawn behaviours predict later internalising disorders. J Child Psychol Psychiatry 45:874–883, 2004

Grundy SM, Pasternak R, Greenland P, et al: Assessment of cardiovascular risk by use of multiple-risk-factor assessment equations: a statement for healthcare professionals from the American Heart Association and the American College of Cardiology. Circulation 100:1481–1492, 1999

Harper LV: Epigenetic inheritance and the intergenerational transfer of experience. Psychol Bull 131:340–360, 2005

Harrington R, Fudge H, Rutter M, et al: Adult outcomes of childhood and adolescent depression, I: psychiatric status. Arch Gen Psychiatry 47:465–473, 1990

Harrington R, Rutter M, Weissman M, et al: Psychiatric disorders in the relatives of depressed probands, I: comparison of prepubertal, adolescent and early adult onset cases. J Affect Disord 42:9–22, 1997

Hettema JM, Annas P, Neale MC, et al: A twin study of the genetics of fear conditioning. Arch Gen Psychiatry 60:702–708, 2003

Hettema JM, Prescott CA, Myers JM, et al: The structure of genetic and environmental risk factors for anxiety disorders in men and women. Arch Gen Psychiatry 62:182–189, 2005

Hofstra MB, van der Ende J, Verhulst FC: Child and adolescent problems predict DSM-IV disorders in adulthood: a 14-year follow-up of a Dutch epidemiological sample. J Am Acad Child Adolesc Psychiatry 41:182–189, 2002

Jaffee SR, Poulton R: Reciprocal effects of mothers' depression and children's problem behaviors from middle childhood to early adolescence, in Development Contexts in Middle Childhood. Edited by Huston AC, Ripke M. New York, Cambridge University Press, 2006, pp 107–129

Jaffee SR, Moffitt TE, Caspi A, et al: Differences in early childhood risk factors for juvenile-onset and adult-onset depression. Arch Gen Psychiatry 59:215–222, 2002

Kendler KS, Myers J, Prescott C: The etiology of phobias: an evaluation of the stress-diathesis model. Arch Gen Psychiatry 59:242–248, 2002

Kendler KS, Kuhn JW, Vittum J, et al: The interaction of stressful life events and a serotonin transporter polymorphism in the prediction of episodes of major depression: a replication. Arch Gen Psychiatry 62:529–535, 2005

Kessler RC, Berglund P, Demler O, et al: Lifetime prevalence and age-of-onset distributions of DSM-IV disorders in the National Comorbidity Survey Replication. Arch Gen Psychiatry 62:593–602, 2005

Kim-Cohen J, Caspi A, Moffitt TE, et al: Prior juvenile diagnoses in adults with mental disorder: developmental follow-back of a prospective-longitudinal cohort. Arch Gen Psychiatry 60:709–719, 2003

Klein DF: False suffocation alarms, spontaneous panics, and related conditions: an integrative hypothesis. Arch Gen Psychiatry 50:306–317, 1993

Koenen K, Moffitt TE, Poulton R, et al: Early childhood factors associated with the development of posttraumatic stress disorder: results from a longitudinal birth cohort. Psychol Med 37:181–192, 2007

Locker D, Liddell A, Dempster L, et al: Age of onset of dental anxiety. J Dent Res 78:790–796, 1999

Macklin ML, Metzger LJ, Litz BT, et al: Lower precombat intelligence is a risk factor for posttraumatic stress disorder. J Consult Clin Psychol 66:323–326, 1998

Mill J, Caspi A, Williams BS, et al: Prediction of heterogeneity in intelligence and adult prognosis by genetic polymorphisms in the dopamine system among children with attention-deficit/hyperactivity disorder: evidence from 2 birth cohorts. Arch Gen Psychiatry 63:462–469, 2006

Moffitt TE: Adolescent-limited and life-course-persistent antisocial behavior: a developmental taxonomy. Psychol Rev 100:674–701, 1993

Moffitt TE, Caspi A: Childhood predictors differentiate life-course persistent and adolescence-limited antisocial pathways among males and females. Dev Psychopathol 13:355–375, 2001

Moffitt TE, Caspi A, Harrington HL, et al: Males on the life-course persistent and adolescence-limited antisocial pathways: follow-up at age 26. Dev Psychopathol 14:179–206, 2002

Moffitt TE, Caspi A, Rutter M: Strategy for investigating interactions between measured genes and measured environments. Arch Gen Psychiatry 62:473–481, 2005

Mogg K, Bradley BP: A cognitive-motivational analysis of anxiety. Behav Res Ther 36:809–848, 1998

Monk CS, Nelson EE, McClure EB, et al: Ventrolateral prefrontal cortex activation and attentional bias in response to angry faces in adolescents with generalized anxiety disorder. Am J Psychiatry 163:1091–1097, 2006

Pearson TA: New tools for coronary assessment: what are their advantages and limitations? Circulation 105:886–892, 2002

Pezawas L, Meyer-Lindenberg A, Drabant EM, et al: 5-HTTLPR polymorphism impacts human cingulate-amygdala interactions: a genetic susceptibility mechanism for depression. Nat Neurosci 6:828–834, 2005

Pine DS, Cohen P, Gurley D, et al: The risk for early adulthood anxiety and depressive disorders in adolescents with anxiety and depressive disorders. Arch Gen Psychiatry 55:56–64, 1998

Pine DS, Mogg K, Bradley BP, et al: Attention bias to threat in maltreated children: implications for vulnerability to stress-related psychopathology. Am J Psychiatry 162:291–296, 2005

Pitman RK, Orr SP, Lowenhagen MJ, et al: Pre-Vietnam contents of posttraumatic stress disorder veterans' service medical and personnel records. Compr Psychiatry 32:416–422, 1991

Poulton R, Menzies RG: Non-associative fear acquisition: a review of the evidence from retrospective and longitudinal research. Behav Res Ther 40:127–149, 2002

Poulton R, Waldie KE, Thomson WM, et al: Determinants of early versus late-onset dental fear in a longitudinal epidemiological study. Behav Res Ther 39:777–785, 2001

Rapee RM, Spence SH: The etiology of social phobia: empirical evidence and an initial model. Clin Psychol Rev 24:737–767, 2004

Robins LN: Using survey results to improve the validity of the standard psychiatric nomenclature. Arch Gen Psychiatry 61:1188–1194, 2005

Rosario-Campos MC, Leckman JF, Mercadante MT, et al: Adults with early onset obsessive-compulsive disorder. Am J Psychiatry 158:1899–1903, 2001

Roth WT, Wilhelm FH, Pettit D: Are current theories of panic falsifiable? Psychol Bull 131:171–192, 2005

Rutter K, Tizard J, Whitmore K: Education, Health and Behaviour. London, Longmans, 1970

Rutter M: Categories, dimensions and the mental health of children and adolescents. Ann N Y Acad Sci 1008:11–21, 2003

Rutter M, Pickles A, Murray R, et al: Testing hypotheses on specific environmental causal effects on behavior. Psychol Bull 127:291–324, 2001

Schnurr PP, Friedman MJ, Rosenberg SD: Premilitary MMPI scores as predictors of combat-related PTSD symptoms. Am J Psychiatry 150:479–483, 1993

Shalev AY, Sahar T, Freedman S, et al: A prospective study of heart rate response following trauma and the subsequent development of posttraumatic stress disorder. Arch Gen Psychiatry 55:553–559, 1998

Tellegen A: Brief Manual for the Multidimensional Personality Questionnaire. Minneapolis, University of Minnesota, 1982

Verburg K, Griez E, Meijer J, et al: Respiratory disorders as a possible predisposing factor for panic disorder. J Affect Disord 33:129–134, 1995

Weissman MM, Wolk S, Wickramaratne P, et al: Children with prepubertal-onset major depressive disorder and anxiety grown up. Arch Gen Psychiatry 56:794–801, 1999

Weissman MM, Wickramaratne P, Nomura Y, et al: Families at high and low risk for depression. Arch Gen Psychiatry 62:29–36, 2005

Wickramaratne PJ, Greenwald S, Weissman MM: Psychiatric disorders in the relatives of probands with prepubertal-onset or adolescent-onset major depression. J Am Acad Child Adolesc Psychiatry 39:1396–1405, 2000

Widiger TA, Clark LA: Toward DSM-V and the classification of psychopathology. Psychol Bull 126:946–963, 2000

Widom CS: Posttraumatic stress disorder in abused and neglected children grown up. Am J Psychiatry 156:1223–1229, 1999

Wittchen HU, Lieb R, Pfister H, et al: The waxing and waning of mental disorders: evaluating the stability of syndromes of mental disorders in the population. Compr Psychiatry 41(suppl):122–132, 2000

World Health Organization: Investing in Health Research and Development: Report of the Ad Hoc Committee on Health Research Relating to Future Intervention Options. Geneva, World Health Organization, 1996

World Health Organization: Composite International Diagnostic Interview, Version 2.1. Geneva, World Health Organization, 1997

Zahn-Waxler C, Klimes-Dougan B, Slattery MJ: Internalizing problems of childhood and adolescence: prospects, pitfalls, and progress in understanding the development of anxiety and depression. Dev Psychopathol 12:443–466, 2000

6

STRESS-INDUCED AND FEAR CIRCUITRY ANXIETY DISORDERS

Are They a Distinct Group?

Abby J. Fyer, M.D.
Timothy A. Brown, Ph.D.

In this chapter we consider whether the DSM anxiety disorders form a cohesive group distinct from other psychiatric diagnoses. The objective is to contribute to decisions about the classification of these disorders in DSM-V. The particular focus here is on genetic and epidemiological data as they concern the proposed subgroup of "stress-induced and fear circuitry–related disorders": panic disorder, posttraumatic stress disorder (PTSD), and specific and social phobias (social anxiety disorder [SocAD]). Data from developmental and animal model studies and neuroimaging are reviewed elsewhere in this volume (see Chapter 10, "Role of Cognition in Stress-Induced and Fear Circuitry Disorders" and Chapter 13, "Role of Neurochemical and Neuroendocrinological Markers of Fear in Classification of Anxiety Disorders"). The classification of the two remaining anxiety disorders—obsessive-compulsive disorder (OCD) and generalized anxiety disorder (GAD)—is the subject of two separate DSM conferences, so these disorders are considered only in comparison to the stress-induced and fear circuitry–related group.

The question of overlap versus distinctness of any set of categories depends on the chosen criterion—that is, overlapping versus distinct with respect to what?

Given that the DSM anxiety disorders are descriptive categories of unknown pathophysiology, these questions cannot be answered on the basis of etiology. Here we review several types of data that are thought to be related to etiology: traditional epidemiological validators (age at onset, gender distribution, comorbidity); patterns of broadly defined heritability in family and twin studies; and analyses (e.g., latent class, factor) designed to identify shared or unshared "underlying" diatheses. An exhaustive review of the literature is outside the scope of this work. Instead, we attempt to summarize consistent findings and provide a few relevant examples as well as references to recent reviews.

For each area examined, we have found evidence for both distinctness and overlap of the current diagnostic categories. We conclude that the data, consistent with findings in other areas of medicine, suggest a more complicated interrelationship between potential etiological factors (e.g., genetics, environment, developmental course) and current clinical syndrome definitions. As has been suggested by Hyman (2003), "it appears likely that mental disorders (including depression, schizophrenia, panic disorder and [attention-deficit/hyperactivity disorder]) will each represent clusters of illnesses with overlapping or even distinct genetic and non-genetic risk factors that converge to produce patterns of pathogenesis, symptoms, and course that have a close family resemblance" (p. xii).

Epidemiology

PREVALENCE, AGE AT ONSET, AND GENDER DISTRIBUTION

As a group, anxiety disorders are among the most prevalent of mental disorders, but there is a wide range of variability in occurrence of the individual illnesses, with 1%–2% for OCD, 3%–4% for panic disorder, 6%–8% for PTSD and GAD, and 10%–15% for SocAD and specific phobias. Age at onset also varies considerably, both across and within groups. Most cases of anxiety disorder begin in childhood or early adulthood, but there are clear between-disorder differences in mean or usual age at onset. For example, the recent National Comorbidity Survey Replication (Kessler et al. 2005) found that specific phobia and SocAD usually begin in childhood or adolescence and only rarely have a first onset after age 25. The respective mean onsets for these disorders were 7 years (range, 4–23) and 13 years (5–23). In contrast, panic disorder and PTSD are most likely to start in young adulthood but also occur throughout middle age. Their mean onsets were ages 24 (range, 6–51) and 23 (6–53), respectively. OCD had a slightly earlier mean onset (19 years) and GAD a slightly later one (31 years), but both had ranges of onset from childhood to middle age. There are also several hypotheses in the literature relating within-group age at onset variation to possible diagnostic heterogeneity. For example, situational-specific phobias (e.g., claustrophobia, crowds), which have been linked to panic disorder by clinical phenomenology, also have their usual onset at an age similar to that of panic disorder and much later than that of other specific phobia subtypes (e.g., animal, blood-injury). For OCD, several studies have suggested increased familial transmission by early (<18 years) versus later (>18) onset cases (Nestadt et al. 2000; Pauls et al. 1995). Generalized SocAD is characterized by earlier onset and also differs in physiological arousal and treatment response from the non-generalized subtype (Levin et al. 1993; Liebowitz et al. 1985; Mannuzza et al. 1995).

In epidemiological samples all anxiety disorders except OCD are more common in women than in men, although this effect is strongest for specific phobia (3:1) and weakest for SocAD (1.5:1), with panic disorder, PTSD, and GAD in the middle (2:1). OCD occurs equally in men and women. Clinical studies have shown a similar distribution, with the exception that in these settings the gender ratio for SocAD is often 1:1 (Kessler et al. 2005).

COMORBIDITY

The finding of greater-than-expected comorbidity between anxiety disorders and of anxiety disorders with depression and, to a lesser extent, substance abuse has been consistently replicated in both epidemiological and clinical samples (Goldenberg et al. 1996; Kessler et al. 1994, 2005; Klerman et al. 1991; Schneier et al. 1992). It is generally accepted that there are several potential interpretations of comorbidity, including overlapping etiological mechanisms (Klein et al. 2004; Wickramaratne and Weissman 1993). There has not been a specific study to test the hypothesis that the proposed stress-induced and fear circuitry–related disorders are more likely to be comorbid among themselves than with other anxiety or affective syndromes. The few studies that have reported on comorbidity of each anxiety disorder with the other do not appear to demonstrate a consistently stronger association among panic disorder, SocAD, specific phobia, and PTSD versus other disorders. For example, the recent National Comorbidity Survey Replication study (Kessler et al. 2005) found a significant bivariate comorbidity among all anxiety disorders except OCD. However, OCD was more likely to co-occur with panic disorder with agoraphobia than with panic disorder without agoraphobia or the other four adult anxiety disorders (Kessler et al. 2005).

Several investigators have hypothesized that specific patterns of sequential comorbidity may define etiologically coherent syndromes that cross DSM diagnostic categories. For example, on the basis of their work with behavioral inhibition, Kagan et al. (1987) and Smoller et al. (2001) have defined a "D type" anxiety syndrome characterized by onset of an anxiety disorder before age 13, lifetime panic disorder, and additional adult anxiety comorbidity. Specific relationships have also been proposed between childhood separation anxiety disorder and panic disorder and SocAD and atypical depression (Alpert et al. 1997).

Heritability

Specific genes contributing to any anxiety disorder have not been identified. Information about the interrelationship of disorders is derived from 1) patterns of intergenerational transmission in family studies and 2) comparisons between observed data and predictions of hypothesized transmissional models in twin studies. These data indicate that all anxiety disorders are moderately heritable but provide evidence for both shared (i.e., a common "proneness" to develop anxiety disorder that is inherited) and specific genetic and environmental contributions (Hettema et al. 2005; Kendler et al. 2003; Smoller and Tsuang 1998).

FAMILY STUDIES

A disorder is considered to be familial if individuals who have an affected relative are at increased risk for the disorder as compared with individuals who do not have an affected relative (Klein et al. 2004; Wickramaratne and Weissman 1993). For example, if disorder A is familial, we would expect there to be a higher rate of A among the relatives of individuals who have A as compared with the relatives of individuals with disorder B. However, if we also find a significantly higher rate of another disorder (e.g., disorder B) in the family members of individuals who have disorder A but *not disorder B,* we assume that there is some overlap in the transmissible etiology of A and B. Another way to say this is that having disorder A transmits to your relatives an increased risk for disorder B, so A and B must share some risk factor or causal mechanism. It is important to note that this conclusion can only be drawn if your proband has A *and not B*. If A and B are familial, and we happen to have chosen some probands who have both A and B, then the excess rate of B in relatives of the A individuals may be due to simple familial transmission rather than overlap. Finally, the two disorders A and B would be considered as distinct, with respect to transmission, only if the lack of transmission was on both sides—that is, A does not transmit B *and* B does not transmit A.

Although existing family studies provide strong support for familial transmission of each anxiety disorder, there are few analyses that specifically address distinctness/overlap of the various syndromes. Data from studies that do not address this question are often hard to evaluate as effects of proband anxiety comorbidity or as a report of familial rates of anxiety disorders other than the one under study. Given these restrictions, the existing data show a mixed pattern. In some studies, a disorder will show a "pure" pattern, with relatives showing increased risk for only the proband's disorder, whereas in others there is a significant increased risk for one or more additional anxiety disorders. These inconsistencies may reflect variability in assessment or sampling or heterogeneity within the diagnostic category. For example, panic disorder has been the subject of well-designed direct-interview family studies (Crowe et al. 1983; Goldstein et al. 1997; Maier et al. 1993; Noyes et al.

1987; Weissman et al. 1993). The earlier studies did not show any increased familial risk for social phobia, but these findings may reflect assessment methods, because the interviews included only a few brief screening questions about social fears. However, of the three more recent studies, each of which carefully inventoried different types/situations of social anxiety, two studies found increased risk for social anxiety in relatives of panic disorder patients, whereas one did not. In contrast, for OCD, there has been a fairly consistent, although unexplained, finding of increased risk for GAD among relatives of OCD probands versus relatives of well control subjects (Fyer et al. 2005; Lipsitz et al. 2005; Nestadt et al. 2000; Pauls et al. 1995). Three studies reported a significant increase independent of proband GAD comorbidity, and a fourth found a trend ($P<0.1$).

TWIN STUDIES

Kendler and colleagues have conducted a series of analyses using multivariate structural equation modeling to address the distinctness/overlap of heritability of anxiety and affective disorders in their study of twins from the Virginia registry (Hettema et al. 2001; Kendler et al. 1992, 1993). One recent analysis by this group assessed factors contributing to the liability for six DSM anxiety disorders—panic disorder; GAD; social, situational, and animal phobias; and agoraphobia (Hettema et al. 2005). The best-fitting model included two genetic factors (each of which loaded more heavily on one subgroup of the disorders) as well as environmental (shared and unique) and disorder-specific factors. Overall, genetic heritability was estimated at 25%–35%, except for social phobia (10%). One of the two genetic factors contributed most robustly to liability for panic disorder, GAD, and agoraphobia, and the other factor contributed to specific phobias. Social phobia had modest contributions from both factors. Substantial nongenetic effects were seen, but again these also were both common (across disorders) and specific in nature. These data are consistent with the hypothesis that the DSM anxiety syndromes have both shared and distinct etiological factors. A study conducted in the Vietnam Era Twin Registry (Chantarujikapong et al. 2001) found a similar pattern of partial overlap and distinctness among three DSM anxiety disorders: panic disorder, GAD, and PTSD.

Efforts to Identify Common Underlying Diatheses

Another approach to understanding the overlap/distinctness of different anxiety disorders has been the hypothesis that these disorders share an underlying temperament or personality trait that is a potent risk factor for developing these syndromes. However, this common vulnerability is manifested heterogeneously (i.e., as different DSM disorders), based on exposure to differing environmental influences, other genetic/biological agents, and so on (Barlow 2002; Clark 2005; Hettema et al. 2005). There are two general types of studies. In the first, investigators attempt to use factor-analytic and latent-class analyses to identify "inherent" clusters of symptoms that may make up a particular diathesis. In the second, investigators test a specific hypothesis of association of a "trait" or other diathesis with one or more disorders. Here the hypothesized diathesis may be derived from several sources, for example, a previous latent-class or factor analysis; child development or other observational temperament research; or human- or animal-model psychophysiological research. A complete review of this literature is outside the scope of this chapter. To illustrate this approach, we discuss briefly work concerning two genetically based dimensions of temperament: neuroticism/negative affectivity and extraversion/positive affectivity, both of which have been posited to be instrumental in the etiology and course of the emotional disorders. For further examples, the reader is referred to the work of Krueger (1999) and the recent latent-class analyses in the National Comorbidity Survey Replication data set (Kessler et al. 2006).

The concepts of neuroticism and extraversion were first suggested in the work of Eysenck (1947; Eysenck and Eysenck 1985). Although the theoretical frameworks were developed independently (Eysenck 1981; Tellegen 1985), neuroticism/negative affectivity and extraversion/positive affectivity are closely related to Gray's (1987) constructs of behavioral inhibition and behavioral activation, respectively (e.g., Campbell-Sills et al. 2004; Carver and White 1994; Kasch et al. 2002). Neuroticism/negative affectivity is considered to be etiologically relevant to the full range of emotional disorders; the influence of extraversion/positive affectivity is more specific to depression and social phobia (e.g., Brown et al. 1998; Mineka et al. 1998).

A number of studies indicate moderate heritability of these constructs (e.g., Fanous et al. 2002; Hettema et al. 2004; Viken et al. 1994) and suggest that these vulnerability dimensions may contribute to the overlap of DSM anxiety disorders (e.g., Brown et al. 1998; Gershuny and Sher 1998; Kasch et al. 2002). For example, in a sample of 350 outpatients, Brown et al. (1998) found that virtually all the considerable covariance among latent variables corresponding to the DSM-IV (American Psychiatric Association 1994) constructs of unipolar depression, SocAD, GAD, OCD, and panic disorder/agoraphobia was explained by the higher-order dimensions of negative affect and positive affect (replicated by Brown 2007). Although the results were consistent with the notion of neuroticism/negative affect as a broadly relevant dimension of vulnerability, the DSM-IV disorder constructs were differentially related to negative affect, with depression and GAD evidencing the strongest associations. In accord with a reformulated hierarchical model of anxiety and depression (Mineka et al. 1998), positive affect was predictive of depression and SocAD only. More recent comorbidity and structural genetic findings also reveal a differential relationship between mood disorders and social phobia, which could be seen as consistent with the existence of a temperamental vulnerability dimension specific to these two disorders (e.g., Brown et al. 2001).

Brown (2007), in an extension of previous work (Brown et al. 1998), examined the temporal course and temporal structural relationships of dimensions of temperament (neuroticism/behavioral inhibition [N/BI]; behavioral activation/positive affect [BA/P]) and DSM-IV disorder constructs in 606 patients who were assessed at intake and 1- and 2-year follow-ups. Findings indicated that N/BI operated differently than the DSM-IV disorder constructs in several ways. For instance, latent growth models of each DSM-IV disorder construct revealed inverse relations between the intercept and slope ($r_s = -42$ to -0.48)—that is, higher initial disorder severity was associated with greater change over time. However, the intercept and slope of N/BI were positively correlated ($r = 0.47$), indicating that patients with higher initial levels of N/BI tended to show less change in this dimension over time and patients with lower initial levels of N/BI tended to evidence greater change. Thus, the stability of N/BI, unlike the DSM-IV disorders, increased as a function of initial severity. This may indicate that the influence of mood-state distortion/general distress on the measurement of N/BI is most pronounced at the lower end of its continuum. It is the lower range of N/BI that is less temporally stable and presumably more apt to covary with temporal change in disorder severity.

In addition, parallel-process latent growth models were employed to examine the directional effects among temperament and psychopathology constructs over time. Higher initial levels of N/BI were associated with less change in the DSM-IV constructs of GAD and SocAD but not depression. Lower BA/P predicted poorer outcome of SocAD, although this effect only approached statistical significance when N/BI was in the analysis. Consistent with prediction and theory, initial levels of the DSM-IV disorders did not predict increases in temperament over time. Moreover, temporal change in depression, SocAD, and GAD was significantly related to change in N/BI. Of particular interest is the finding that all the temporal covariance of the DSM-IV disorder constructs was accounted for by change in N/BI—that is, when N/BI was specified as a predictor, the temporal overlap among disorder constructs was reduced to zero. The correlational nature of these findings precludes firm conclusions about the direction of these effects. Although counter to earlier initial evidence and conceptualization (Brown et al. 1995; Kasch et al. 2002), N/BI may be therapeutically malleable, and this, in fact, mediates the extent of change in the emotional disorders. Alternatively or additively, a reduction in disorder severity is associated with a decrease in generalized distress, a feature that is shared by the emotional disorders and that is partially reflected in the measurement of N/BI. At any rate, these findings extend the extant literature by demonstrating, in a longitudinal context, the role of N/BI as a unifying construct accounting for the covariance among the emotional disorders.

Conclusion

The available genetic/epidemiological data provide clear evidence of both commonalities and distinctions among the DSM-IV anxiety disorders. In addition, the pattern of interrelationships between the categories is not consistent. Findings vary across studies, and the groupings themselves change depending on which type of data are used as the criterion. For example, categorizing by genetic data creates one set of groupings; using age at onset creates a second set; and latent-class analysis creates a third. There is also considerable within-disorder heterogeneity. These observations suggest that the DSM anxiety categories do not map neatly onto simple, consistent, and distinct etiological pathways. Instead, it seems most likely that many different specific developmental trajectories—each of which incorporates a variety of influences (genetic, environmental, interpersonal)—can lead to the final common pathway that is a particular DSM anxiety diagnosis. Given this complexity and our current extremely incomplete stage of knowledge, we are unlikely, at this point in time, to define a significantly "truer" anxiety nosology. Plans to make major modifications in the classification should probably be undertaken with some degree of caution. Although many patients have symptoms that do not fit neatly into the DSM categories, the use of these categories has clearly been helpful, both in describing variation in patients' subjective experiences and in enabling research that has improved both the efficacy and, at least in some areas (e.g., cognitive-behavioral therapy, interpersonal psychotherapy), the specificity of treatment.

References

Alpert JE, Ueblacker LA, McLean NE, et al: Social phobia, avoidant personality disorder and atypical depression: co-occurrence and clinical implications. Psychol Med 27:627–633, 1997

American Psychiatric Association: Diagnostic and Statistical Manual of Mental Disorders, 4th Edition. Washington, DC, American Psychiatric Association 1994

Barlow DH: Anxiety and Its Disorders: The Nature and Treatment of Anxiety and Panic, 2nd Edition. New York, Guilford, 2002

Brown TA: Temporal course and structural relationships among dimensions of temperament and DSM-IV anxiety and mood disorder constructs. J Abnorm Psychol 116:313–328, 2007

Brown TA, Marten PA, Barlow DH: Discriminant validity of the symptoms constituting the DSM-III-R and DSM-IV associated symptom criterion of generalized anxiety disorder. J Anxiety Disord 9:317–328, 1995

Brown TA, Chorpita BF, Barlow DH: Structural relationships among dimensions of the DSM-IV anxiety and mood disorders and dimensions of negative affect, positive affect, and autonomic arousal. J Abnorm Psychol 107:179–192, 1998

Brown TA, Campbell LA, Lehman CL: Current and lifetime comorbidity of the DSM-IV anxiety and mood disorders in a large clinical sample. J Abnorm Psychol 110:585–599, 2001

Campbell-Sills L, Livernat GI, Brown TA: Psychometric evaluation of the Behavioral Inhibition/Behavioral Activation scales in a large sample of outpatients with anxiety and mood disorders. Psychol Assess 16:244–254, 2004

Carver CS, White TL: Behavioral inhibition, behavioral activation, and affective responses to impending reward and punishment: the BIS/BAS Scales. J Pers Soc Psychol 67:319–333, 1994

Chantarujikapong S, Scherrer JF, Xian H: A twin study of generalized anxiety disorder symptoms, panic disorder symptoms and post-traumatic stress disorder in men. Psychiatry Res 103:133–145, 2001

Clark LA: Temperament as a unifying basis for personality and psychopathology. J Abnorm Psychol 114:505–521, 2005

Crowe RR, Noyes R, Pauls DL, et al: A family study of panic disorder. Arch Gen Psychiatry 40:1065–1069, 1983

Eysenck HJ: Dimensions of Personality. New York, Praeger, 1947

Eysenck HJ: A Model for Personality. Berlin, Germany, Springer, 1981

Eysenck HJ, Eysenck MW: Personality and Individual Differences. New York, Plenum, 1985

Fanous A, Gardner CO, Prescott CA, et al: Neuroticism, major depression and gender: a population-based twin study. Psychol Med 32:719–728, 2002

Fyer AJ, Lipsitz JD, Mannuzza S, et al: A direct interview family study of obsessive-compulsive disorder, I. Psychol Med 35:1611–1621, 2005

Gershuny BS, Sher KJ: The relation between personality and anxiety: findings from a 3-year prospective study. J Abnorm Psychol 107:252–262, 1998

Goldenberg IM, White K, Yonkers K, et al: The infrequency of pure culture diagnoses among the anxiety disorders. J Clin Psychiatry 57:528–533, 1996

Goldstein RB, Wickramaratne PJ, Horwath E, et al: Familial aggregation and phenomenology of 'early'-onset (at or before age 20 years) panic disorder. Arch Gen Psychiatry 54:271–278, 1997

Gray JA: The neuropsychology of emotion and personality, in Cognitive Neurochemistry. Edited by Stahl SM, Iversen SD, Goodman EC. Oxford, UK, Oxford University Press, 1987, pp 171–190

Hettema JM, Prescott CA, Kendler KS: A population-based twin study of generalized anxiety disorder in men and women. J Nerv Ment Dis 189:413–420, 2001

Hettema JM, Prescott CA, Kendler KS: Genetic and environmental sources of covariation between generalized anxiety disorder and neuroticism. Am J Psychiatry 161:1581–1587, 2004

Hettema JM, Prescott CA, Myers JM, et al: The structure of genetic and environmental risk factors for anxiety disorders in men and women. Arch Gen Psychiatry 62:182–189, 2005

Hyman SE: Foreword, in Advancing DSM: Dilemmas in Psychiatric Diagnosis. Edited by Phillips KA, First MB, Pincus HA. Washington, DC, American Psychiatric Association, 2003

Kagan J, Reznick JS, Snidman N: The physiology and psychology of behavioral inhibition in children. Child Dev 58:1459–1473, 1987

Kasch KL, Rottenberg J, Arnow BA, et al: Behavioral activation and inhibition systems and the severity and course of depression. J Abnorm Psychol 111:589–597, 2002

Kendler KS, Neale MC, Kessler RC, et al: Major depression and generalized anxiety disorder: same genes, (partly) different environments? Arch Gen Psychiatry 49:716–722, 1992

Kendler KS, Neale MC, Kessler RC, et al: Panic disorder in women: a population-based twin study. Psychol Med 23:397–406, 1993

Kendler KS, Prescott CA, Myers J, et al: The structure of genetic and environmental risk factors for common psychiatric and substance use disorders in men and women. Arch Gen Psychiatry 60:929–937, 2003

Kessler RC, McGonagle KA, Zhao S, et al: Lifetime and 12-month prevalence of DSM-III-R psychiatric disorders in the United States: results from the National Comorbidity Survey. Arch Gen Psychiatry 51:8–19, 1994

Kessler RC, Chiu WT, Demler O, et al: Prevalence, severity, and comorbidity of 12-month DSM-IV disorders in the National Comorbidity Survey Replication. Arch Gen Psychiatry 62:617–627, 2005

Kessler RC, Akiskal HS, Ames M, et al: Prevalence and effects of mood disorders on work performance in a nationally representative sample of U.S. workers. Am J Psychiatry 163:1561–1568, 2006

Klein DN, Shankman SA, Lewinsohn PM, et al: Family study of chronic depression in a community sample of young adults. Am J Psychiatry 161:646–653, 2004

Klerman G, Weissman M, Ouellette R, et al: Panic attacks in the community: social morbidity and health care utilization. JAMA 265:742–746, 1991

Krueger RF: The structure of common mental disorders. Arch Gen Psychiatry 56:921–926, 1999

Levin AP, Saoud JB, Strauman T, et al: Response of "generalized" and "discrete" social phobics during public speaking. J Anxiety Disord 7:207–221, 1993

Liebowitz MR, Gorman JM, Fyer AJ, et al: Social phobia: review of a neglected anxiety disorder. Arch Gen Psychiatry 42:729–736, 1985

Lipsitz JD, Mannuzza S, Chapman TF: A direct interview family study of obsessive-compulsive disorder, II: contribution of proband informant information. Psychol Med 35:1623–1631, 2005

Maier W, Lichtermann D, Minges J, et al: A controlled family study in panic disorder. J Psychiatr Res 27(suppl):79–87, 1993

Mannuzza S, Schneier FR, Chapman TF, et al: Generalized social phobia: reliability and validity. Arch Gen Psychiatry 52:230–237, 1995

Mineka S, Watson D, Clark LA: Comorbidity of anxiety and unipolar mood disorders. Annu Rev Psychol 49:377–412, 1998

Nestadt G, Samuels J, Riddle M, et al: A family study of obsessive compulsive disorder. Arch Gen Psychiatry 57:358–363, 2000

Noyes R, Moroz G, Davidson JRT, et al: A family study of generalized anxiety disorder. Am J Psychiatry 144:1019–1024, 1987

Pauls DL, Alsobrook JP, Goodman W, et al: A family study of obsessive-compulsive disorder. Am J Psychiatry 152:76–84, 1995

Schneier FR, Johnson J, Hornig CD, et al: Social phobia: comorbidity and morbidity in an epidemiologic sample. Arch Gen Psychiatry 49:282–288, 1992

Smoller JW, Tsuang MT: Panic and phobic anxiety: defining phenotypes for genetic studies. Am J Psychiatry 155:1152–1162, 1998

Smoller JW, Acierno JS Jr, Rosenbaum JF, et al: Targeted genome screen of panic disorder and anxiety disorder proneness using homology to murine QTL regions. Am J Med Genet 105:195–206, 2001

Tellegen A: Structures of mood and personality and their relevance to assessing anxiety with an emphasis on self-report, in Anxiety and the Anxiety Disorders. Edited by Tuma A, Maser J. Hillsdale, NJ, Erlbaum, 1985, pp 681–706

Viken RJ, Rose RJ, Kaprio J, et al: A developmental genetic analysis of adult personality: extraversion and neuroticism from 18 to 59 years of age. J Pers Soc Psychol 66:722–730, 1994

Weissman MM, Wickramaratne P, Adams PB, et al: The relationship between panic disorder and major depression: a new family study. Arch Gen Psychiatry 50:767–780, 1993

Wickramaratne PJ, Weissman MM: Using family studies to understand comorbidity. Eur Arch Psychiatry Clin Neurosci 243:150–157, 1993

PART 3

SPECIAL TOPICS

7

ANXIETY DISORDERS IN AFRICAN AMERICANS AND OTHER ETHNIC MINORITIES

William B. Lawson, M.D., Ph.D.

The United States is becoming more ethnically diverse. It is projected that, 50 years from now, people of European American ancestry will make up less than 50% of the population (U.S. Census Bureau 2006). For this reason alone, we need to study the presentation, etiology, and outcome of mental disorders in ethnically diverse populations.

Prevalence of Anxiety Disorders in Diverse Populations

Large population studies using the more reliable structured-interview methodology have provided mixed results about whether there are racial differences in the prevalence of anxiety disorders. The Epidemiologic Catchment Area (ECA) study found higher rates of anxiety disorders in African Americans and Latinos than in non-Latino whites (Robins et al. 1991). The ECA study examined only five cities and used an assessment instrument whose reliability has been criticized. However, it also oversampled ethnic minorities. The more recent National Comorbidity Survey (NCS) has included two waves, and both times, lower rates of anxiety disorders were found in racial and ethnic minorities than in the majority population

(Breslau et al. 2006; Kessler et al. 1994). The NCS studies used structured interviews that led to DSM-III-R (American Psychiatric Association 1987) and DSM-IV (American Psychiatric Association 1994) diagnoses, but these studies did not oversample minorities. Also, individuals from institutional settings were not included, whereas ethnic minorities tend to be overrepresented in such settings (Lawson 1999).

DIAGNOSTIC DIFFERENCES

Studies of affective disorders show that mood states are often underdiagnosed or misdiagnosed in ethnic minority groups, and this is especially true for African Americans (Lawson 1999; Strakowski et al. 2003). Anxiety disorders also appear to be underdiagnosed in clinical populations of African Americans. As in the mood disorders literature, African Americans with various anxiety disorders are more likely to have the diagnosis missed or to be misdiagnosed with another psychiatric disorder than are other groups (Neal and Turner 1991). Panic disorder and phobic disorders are often underdiagnosed in African Americans, despite evidence that these disorders may be more common in ethnic minorities than other groups (Brown et al. 1990; Neal and Turner 1991; Paradis et al. 1994). Similarly, obsessive-compulsive disorder is rarely diagnosed in African Americans (Friedman et al. 1993; Hatch et al. 1992; Paradis et al. 1994). The problem does not appear to be a lower incidence of the disorder, but rather, underrecognition by clinicians (Friedman et al. 1993; Hatch et al. 1992). Posttraumatic stress disorder (PTSD) in African Americans may also be misdiagnosed or underdiagnosed, despite independent evidence that PTSD may occur more frequently in African Americans in combat because of greater combat exposure (Neal and Turner 1991; Penk et al. 1989).

DIFFERENCES IN TREATMENT RESPONSE

In recent years, the usefulness of the concept of race has been questioned, with race often assumed to be a marker for socioeconomic status. However, the approval of the drug BiDil has caused a reevaluation of the race concept. BiDil emerged from studies conducted on the effectiveness on congestive heart failure of the combination of two older agents, hydralazine and isosorbide dinitrate, which were not approved for congestive heart failure. No significant effect was seen in a general Veterans Administration hospital population, but a later analysis showed efficacy for an African American subset, which was confirmed in a subsequent larger study of only African Americans (Carson et al. 1999; Taylor et al. 2004). The U.S. Food and Drug Administration for the first time approved a medication for a specific racial group. There has been a great deal of controversy about this approval, but the clinical findings that led to the approval showed that, in some instances, race may have empirical significance (Sankar and Kahn 2005). The findings from these trials provided evidence that race and ethnicity can make a clinical difference in treatment response.

Complexities of Understanding Differences in Prevalence

Anxiety disorders may, indeed, have different prevalences in African Americans compared with other groups, as indicated by several studies (Breslau et al. 2006; Neal and Turner 1991), yet other important factors in interpreting such differences also should be considered.

DIAGNOSTIC INTERPRETATION

It is possible that these disorders have the same prevalence but different symptoms; that they have the same prevalence and the same symptoms but clinicians may err because of misconceptions or bias; or that the prevalence may actually be the same but that cultural or unknown factors may affect the presentation of ancillary symptoms but not the core symptoms (Neal and Turner 1991).

Improved assessment instruments could be a factor in reducing potential errors in diagnosis. For example, a reassessment of an older population of African Americans found no difference in phobias; in contrast, the older ECA study had found higher rates in African Americans (Cohen et al. 2006).

CULTURAL FACTORS

Anxiety disorders also may be affected by cultural factors, which may be manifested as environmental stressors that differ by race (Neal and Turner 1991). Culture may affect a willingness to discuss syndromal versus subsyndromal symptoms. Different apparent rates of prevalence of these disorders for African Americans might reflect a failure by clinicians to recognize subsyndromal symptoms (Cohen et al. 2005). Disorders such as PTSD are, by definition, triggered by environmental factors, and, as noted earlier, African Americans may be differentially exposed to combat, compared with other groups, which could thereby differentially affect the incidence of this disorder. In addition, African Americans are more likely to be exposed to the stressors of an inner city, which can be viewed as a combat zone and a risk for PTSD (Alim et al. 2006).

SYMPTOM DIFFERENCES

There is evidence suggesting that core symptoms may remain the same but that other symptoms may differ, thereby muddying up the picture. Symptom presentation can differ in African Americans with combat-related PTSD compared with Caucasians and Latinos (Allen 1996; Penk and Allen 1991). African American substance abusers who had heavy combat exposure were reported to be more disturbed than a similar group of whites and also scored higher on the Minnesota Multiphasic Personality Inventory (MMPI) scales for paranoid and psychotic symptoms (Penk et al. 1989).

In the mood disorders literature, African Americans are far more likely to have psychotic symptoms, although the prevalence and core symptoms of mood disorders do not differ from other ethnic groups (Kirov and Murray 1999; Patel et al. 2006; Strakowski et al. 1996). African Americans with anxiety disorders also appear more likely to have psychotic features, which certainly could lead to the diagnosis of other disorders, such as paranoia or schizophrenia (Neal and Turner 1991). Similarly, studies of PTSD found higher levels of psychotic symptoms and paranoid ideation for blacks versus whites (Frueh et al. 1996, 2002). These observations were made even with the Minnesota Multiphasic Personality Inventory–2, which, unlike the older MMPI, was based on normative data from diverse ethnic groups.

Conclusion

Fundamental questions remain that require additional research. Both large population studies and smaller clinical studies show that African Americans are underdiagnosed and that there may be ethnic differences in presentation. Moreover, various anxiety subtypes have been understudied in diverse populations. Although there is an emerging literature in PTSD that has looked closely at phenomenology, there are virtually no studies in recent years that have examined other anxiety subtypes. Issues such as the relationship between neurobiological correlates and genetic risk factors simply have not been studied. As development of DSM-V proceeds, a special effort should be made to add to our knowledge base about the nation's growing ethnic minority populations and their vulnerabilities to anxiety disorders.

References

Alim TN, Graves E, Mellman TA, et al: Trauma exposure, posttraumatic stress disorder and depression in an African-American primary care population. J Natl Med Assoc 98:1630–1636, 2006

Allen IM: PTSD among African Americans, in Ethnocultural Aspects of Posttraumatic Stress Disorder: Issues, Research, and Clinical Applications. Edited by Marsella AJ, Friedman MJ, Gerrity ET, et al. Washington, DC, American Psychological Association, 1996, pp 209–238

American Psychiatric Association: Diagnostic and Statistical Manual of Mental Disorders, 3rd Edition, Revised. Washington, DC, American Psychiatric Association, 1987

American Psychiatric Association: Diagnostic and Statistical Manual of Mental Disorders, 4th Edition. Washington, DC, American Psychiatric Association, 1994

Breslau J, Aguilar-Gaxiola S, Kendler KS, et al: Specifying race-ethnic differences in risk for psychiatric disorder in a USA national sample. Psychol Med 36:57–68, 2006

Brown DR, Eaton WW, Sussman L: Racial differences in prevalence of phobic disorders. J Nerv Ment Dis 178:434–441, 1990

Carson P, Ziesche S, Johnson G, et al: Racial differences in response to therapy for heart failure: analysis of the vasodilator-heart failure trials. J Card Fail 5:178–187, 1999

Cohen CI, Magai C, Yaffee R, et al: Racial differences in syndromal and subsyndromal depression in an older urban population. Psychiatr Serv 56:1556–1563, 2005

Cohen CI, Magai C, Yaffee R, et al: The prevalence of phobia and its associated factors in a multiracial aging urban population. Am J Geriatr Psychiatry 14:507–514, 2006

Friedman S, Hatch ML, Paradis C, et al: Obsessive-compulsive disorder in two Black ethnic groups: incidence in an urban dermatology clinic. J Anxiety Disord 7:343–348, 1993

Frueh BC, Smith DW, Libet JM: Racial differences on psychological measures in combat veterans seeking treatment for PTSD. J Pers Assess 66:41–53, 1996

Frueh BC, Hamner MB, Bernat JA, et al: Racial differences in psychotic symptoms among combat veterans with PTSD. Depress Anxiety 16:157–161, 2002

Hatch ML, Paradis C, Friedman S, et al: Obsessive-compulsive disorder in patients with chronic pruritic conditions: case studies and discussion. J Am Acad Dermatol 26:549–551, 1992

Kessler RC, McGonogle KA, Zhao S, et al: Lifetime and 12-month prevalence of DSM-III-R psychiatric disorders in the United States. Arch Gen Psychiatry 51:8–19, 1994

Kirov G, Murray RM: Ethnic differences in the presentation of bipolar disorder. Eur Psychiatry 14:199–204, 1999

Lawson WB: Psychiatric diagnosis of African Americans, in Cross Cultural Psychiatry. Edited by Herrara JM, Lawson WB, Sramek JJ. Chichester, UK, Wiley, 1999, pp 135–142

Neal AM, Turner SM: Anxiety disorders research with African Americans: current status. Psychol Bull 109:400–410, 1991

Paradis CM, Hatch M, Friedman S: Anxiety disorders in African Americans: an update. J Natl Med Assoc 86:609–612, 1994

Patel NC, Delbello MP, Strakowski SM: Ethnic differences in symptom presentation of youths with bipolar disorder. Bipolar Disord 8:95–99, 2006

Penk WE, Allen IM: Clinical assessment of post-traumatic stress disorder (PTSD) among American minorities who served in Vietnam. J Trauma Stress 4:41–66, 1991

Penk WE, Robinowitz R, Black J, et al: Ethnicity: post-traumatic stress disorder (PTSD) differences among black, white, and Hispanic veterans who differ in degrees of exposure to combat in Vietnam. J Clin Psychol 45:729–735, 1989

Robins LN, Locke B, Regier DA: An overview of psychiatric disorders in America, in Psychiatric Disorders in Americans: The Epidemiologic Catchment Area Study. Edited by Robins LN, Regier DA. New York, The Free Press, 1991, pp 328–366

Sankar P, Kahn J: BiDil: race medicine or race marketing? Health Aff (Millwood) (suppl web exclusives):W5-455–W5-463, 2005. Available online at http://shc.stanford.edu/hrn/SankarKahn2005Bidil.pdf. Accessed February 11, 2006.

Strakowski SM, McElroy SL, Keck PE Jr, et al: Racial influence on diagnosis in psychotic mania. J Affect Disord 39:157–162, 1996

Strakowski SM, Keck PE Jr, Arnold LM, et al: Ethnicity and diagnosis in patients with affective disorders. J Clin Psychiatry 64:747–754, 2003

Taylor AL, Ziesche S, Yancy C, et al: Combination of isosorbide dinitrate and hydralazine in blacks with heart failure. N Engl J Med 351:2049–2057, 2004

U.S. Census Bureau: Table 1a: Projected Population of the United States, by Race and Hispanic Origin: 2000 to 2050. Available online at http://www.census.gov/ipc/www/usinterimproj/. Accessed June 17, 2008.

8

THE GENETIC BASIS OF ANXIETY DISORDERS

Thalia C. Eley, Ph.D.

In this overview I summarize behavioral genetic work on anxiety disorders and related symptoms in *children and adolescents*. In particular, my aim is to go beyond simply identifying the level of genetic influence to asking more interesting questions.

Specifically, I first consider whether there are distinct patterns of genetic and environmental influences on different types of anxiety in young people. Second, by considering multivariate genetic analyses, I examine the extent to which the same genetic and environmental factors influence different types of anxiety. Third, I summarize extremes analyses, which consider the roles of genes and environment on high scores for symptoms, and how these compare with findings for the full range. Fourth, I look at what we have learned with respect to two areas of genetic-environmental interplay: gene–environment correlations and gene–environment interactions. Finally, I examine the roles of cognitive processing and biased cognitions as possible mediators of genetic and environmental influences on the development of anxiety in childhood.

Behavioral Genetic Methodology

There are three main types of behavioral genetic study: family, twin, and adoption studies. The last-mentioned approach has not been used as yet to examine childhood anxiety and so is not described here. The first, and historically the most broadly applied of these approaches, is the family study. It has long been recognized that family members resemble one another for a wide variety of characteristics, ranging from cognitive ability or personality to emotional and behavioral symptoms. This resemblance may be due to shared genetic influence and thus can be taken as a maximum level of potential genetic effect. However, this resemblance can also be due to the shared environment that family members experience. The family method is unable to distinguish between these two types of influence. This limitation means that results from family studies are best considered in combination with other behavioral genetic designs.

Twin studies make use of the natural experiment provided by the existence of two types of twins: monozygotic twins (MZ), who share all of their genes, and dizygotic twins (DZ), who share, on average, half of their segregating genes—those that vary in the human population (A). As with other family members, they share their family environment. Aspects of this environment that make twins (and other family members) resemble one another are defined as *shared environment* (C). Aspects of the environment (including family and nonfamily influences) that make family members different from one another are termed *nonshared environment* (E). MZ twins therefore share all their genes and all their shared environment (i.e., $rMZ = A + C$). In contrast, DZ twins share just half their genes but all of the effects of shared environment (i.e., $rDZ = \frac{1}{2}A + C$). The difference in correlation between a group of MZ and DZ twins therefore provides a rough estimate of heritability (i.e., $A = 2[rMZ - rDZ]$). Shared environment is the difference between MZ resemblance and heritability (i.e., $C = rMZ - A$). Nonshared environment, or E, is calculated as the difference between the MZ twin correlation and 1 (i.e., $E = 1 - rMZ$). Thus this approach allows the variance in a trait to be divided into that due to each of these three factors. Model-fitting analyses allow the estimation of precise variance components—that is, the contribution to variance in the measure of genes, shared environment, and nonshared environment, along with confidence intervals. Furthermore, such models can be extended to examine more sophisticated hypotheses such as the role of genes and shared and nonshared environment on the covariation between two measures or on continuity over time.

However, there are limitations to the twin study, and these include the equal environments assumption, chorionicity, assortative mating, and generalizability. The equal environment assumption states that both MZ and DZ twin pairs experience shared environment to the same degree. Some authors question this assumption on the basis that twins who resemble one another more closely physically are more likely to be treated alike, inflating their experience of shared environment. In fact, studies exploring the equal environments assumption have found that for most aspects of psychopathology it holds true, and that although MZ twins *are* treated more similarly, it is because they behave in a more similar fashion and thus elicit more similar responses from others. This effect is thus due to their genes (and therefore accurately modeled as such) rather than the environment (Martin et al. 1997). *Chorionicity* refers to the number of chorions, the sack within which, in singletons, the fetus develops. In all DZ twins there are two chorions, but in two-thirds of MZ twins there is just one chorion, which leads to the possibility that increased MZ resemblance may be due to chorion sharing. There are few data on this issue because it requires skilled work, but the data that are available indicate that monochorionic MZ twins may be a little more similar to one another than dichorionic MZ twins, an effect that would slightly inflate heritability estimates (Martin et al. 1997; Plomin et al. 2001). *Assortative mating* refers to the well-replicated finding that "birds of a feather flock together" or that individuals mate with those similar to themselves. This leads to an increase in genetic variance in the population and to increased genetic resemblance in DZ twin-pairs, which leads to a resultant decrease of genetic estimates (Plomin et al. 2001). Finally, there is the question of the degree to which twins are representative of the nontwin population. Extant data indicate that with the exception of a slight initial delay in language development, which disappears by school age, twins are largely indistinguishable from non-twins (Rutter and Redshaw 1991). These limitations mean that values of, for example, heritability from twin studies should not be regarded as absolute but as an indication of the approximate role of genes on the measured trait.

Genetic and Environmental Influences

It is clear, from more than two decades of literature, that there are substantial genetic influences on almost all aspects of human psychological development. Anxiety is no exception to this rule, and heritability estimates tend to be around 20%–30% (for a review, see Eley and Gregory 2004). Exceptions to this pattern include obsessive-compulsive symptoms, which may have rather higher genetic influence (Eley et al. 2003). In addition to genetic influence, the majority of the remaining variance (~60%–70%) is due to nonshared environment, which is child specific. However, it is interesting that although for most aspects of developmental psychopathology there is minimal shared environmental influence, for certain aspects of anxiety this is not the case. For example, separation anxiety disorder (Feigon et al. 2001; Silberg et al. 2001b), separation anxiety symptoms (Silove et al. 1995; Topolski et al. 1997), and fear symptoms (Lichtenstein and Annas 2000; Rose and Ditto 1983; Stevenson et al. 1992) have all been found to have significant shared environmental influences, although there are exceptions to this pattern of results (Eaves et al. 1997; Silberg et al. 2001a). This higher shared environment may reflect processes such as modeling of parental behaviors or the fact that, for separation anxiety, the parent is as involved as the child and thus the behavior may be more likely to apply to both children.

Multivariate Genetic Analyses

Most of the multivariate studies of anxiety in samples of young people have examined the covariation between trait anxiety and depression, but they confirm that, as in adults (Kendler et al. 1992), there is substantial genetic overlap between anxiety and depression, both when self-report (Eley and Stevenson 1999) and when parent report (Thapar and McGuffin 1997) are used. As a result of this high genetic overlap between depression and anxiety, I review literature pertaining to depression as well as anxiety. Far fewer studies have examined subtypes of anxiety (in any age range), and those available are somewhat contradictory. A longitudinal study over early adolescence and late adolescence found that depression before 14 years had an etiology distinct from depression with onset after 14, which shared genetic vulnerability with overanxious disorder and simple phobia (Silberg et al. 2001a). Although there was strong genetic continuity across time for overanxious disorder and simple phobia, depression in early adolescence was not influenced by genetic factors. This suggests that the genetic vulnerability to depression manifests as anxiety early in adolescence, playing a role on depression only during middle to late adolescence. A study of adult female twins found genetic overlap between phobia and panic disorder, which was largely distinct from that shared by generalized anxiety disorder (GAD) and depressive disorder (Kendler et al. 1995). Indeed, in this and other studies, genetic overlap seems to be particularly marked between GAD and depressive disorder (Kendler et al. 2003). In contrast, a more recent analysis using both this sample and a sample of male twins found evidence for genetic overlap among GAD, panic disorder, agoraphobia, and social phobia, with a second set of genes largely influencing animal phobia and situational phobia (Hettema et al. 2005).

In my own work with preschool children and adolescents, I have found moderate genetic overlap between most aspects of anxiety. First, in a study of anxiety-related behaviors in preschool children, my colleagues and I assessed general distress (worry and sadness), fears, separation anxiety, shyness, and obsessive-compulsive symptoms (Eley et al. 2003). Genetic overlap was found for all five scales, accounting for around half the covariation between each pair of scales and being particularly pronounced for the overlap between general distress and all other scales. Genetic variance for obsessive-compulsive symptoms was largely distinct from that on the other scales. In our adolescent sample, confirmatory factor analyses of the symptoms confirmed the presence of six anxiety disorder–related factors (generalized anxiety, obsessions-compulsions, panic/agoraphobia, separation anxiety, specific fears, and social anxiety) in addition to a depression factor. Genetic influences ranged from 34% to 52% and accounted for more than half the overlap between each pair of variables. The remaining variance in each measure and covariation between measures was due to nonshared environmental overlap between these scales. In summary, it is clear that there is substantial genetic overlap between differing aspects of anxiety and depression.

Extremes Analyses

Extremes analyses can establish the level of genetic and environmental influence on high scores on a measure, as compared with the full range. Analyses of this kind have found little of note. Fear symptoms appear to have similar genetic and environmental influences whether assessed by questionnaire (Stevenson et al. 1992) or as part of temperament (Robinson et al. 1992). Similarly, mixed anxiety/depression symptoms (Deater-Deckard et al. 1997) and pure depression symptoms (Eley 1997; Rende et al. 1993; Rice et al. 2002) also showed nonsignificant differences between extreme high scores and the full range. However, for depression symptoms, there did appear to be some indication of greater shared environmental influence for those with high scores.

Gene–Environment Correlation

Perhaps surprisingly, a key finding from behavioral genetic studies concerns the environment; many environmental measures are genetically influenced. Genetic influence on measured aspects of the environment is described by the term *gene–environment correlation*. There are three routes by which gene–environment correlations may arise.

1. Biological family members share both genes and environment. So, for example, antisocial parents are likely not only to pass on genes related to such behaviors to their children but also to expose the children to such behaviors, which may then be modeled and learned. This is called a *passive gene–environment correlation* (Scarr and McCartney 1983).
2. *Evocative gene–environment correlations* refer to the fact that the behavior of a child will evoke certain reactions from others, thus influencing the experienced environment. For example, a sociable, smiley baby will evoke positive responses from those around it, whereas one with high irritability and low soothability will elicit quite different responses from others. This can have the effect of producing a vicious circle whereby the more positive or negative a child's behavior, the more their environment reflects that, and thus the better or worse their chances of optimal psychological development.
3. Finally, *active gene–environment correlation* refers to the fact that as children grow, and particularly once they enter adolescence or adulthood, they make choices about their worlds. For example, a child who is bright may choose to join after-school clubs of an educational nature, thus increasing his or her learning and potential. A child who is struggling may not feel comfortable with any extra exposure to learning situations and will thus lose out on this opportunity to help his or her development.

Such gene–environment correlations result in influences, previously thought of as purely environmental, that are now considered to have a heritable component. Of note, almost every study to date has found genetic influence on measures of family life, including family connectedness (Jacobson and Rowe 1999); parent–child interaction, as assessed by questionnaire (Plomin et al. 1994), observation (O'Connor et al. 1995) or both (Pike et al. 1996); sibling interactions assessed by questionnaire alone (Plomin et al. 1994) or combined with observation (Pike et al. 1996); parental divorce (O'Connor et al. 2000); and life events (Silberg et al. 1999; Thapar and McGuffin 1996; Thapar et al. 1998). This astonishing array of family environment variables on which there is significant genetic influence indicates that there is far more complexity to the origins of the family environment than had previously been thought.

An even more interesting area of research is that regarding the origins of the links *between* family environment and psychopathology. Studies in this area have all found not only that there are genetic influences on these measured aspects of the environment but also that these overlap to some degree with the genetic influences on psychological outcomes in the child. For example, genetic overlap has been identified on the associations between parenting and depression (Lau et al. 2006; Pike et al. 1996), parental divorce and many aspects of child adjustment (O'Connor et al. 2000), and between life events and depression (Rice et al. 2003; Silberg et al. 1999; Thapar et al. 1998). These results reveal that the same genes are involved not only in the etiology of aspects of the child's environment but also in the development of his or her symptoms. This means that the child may, in some way, be driving his or her own environment more than has previously been thought (e.g., behavior influences the way he or she is disciplined) or that the genes the child has inherited from the parent, which influence the development of symptoms, also affect the parents' own life choices (e.g., divorce).

Gene–Environment Interaction

The first stage of work in this area has been to explore interaction effects between differing types of risk on psychopathology within the family design. For example, one study found that the offspring of adult women with depression, who also had chronic interpersonal difficulties, were more depressed than the offspring of those with depression but no interpersonal difficulties or of nondepressed women (Hammen et al. 2003). In another study, a composite index of parental familial vulnerability to anxiety, depression, and neuroticism was used to predict depression scores in their adolescent offspring (Eley et al. 2004a). The composite index of vulnerability was previously created using quantitative genetic modeling techniques that maximized familial liability to depression, anxiety, and neuroticism in an adult sample of siblings (Sham et al. 2000) and is likely to reflect the effects of shared genes among family members. A significant interaction was found between this parental familial vulnerability composite and parental educational level on self-reported symptoms in the adolescent offspring. Specifically, individuals whose parents lacked educational qualifications and who displayed high levels of familial risk were the most likely to have high depression scores (see Figure 8–1). This implies that adolescents in families with a high rate of depression are particularly at risk for depression themselves if their parents lack qualifications. This effect may be mediated by coping strategies and ability to seek help, because these may all be improved in families where educational qualifications have been obtained. However, it should be noted that the familial vulnerability measure could reflect either genetic or shared environmental influences or both.

In order to disentangle these two sources of influence, twin studies are again required. One study utilizing this method found evidence for an interaction between genetic risk and a composite measure of three life events on depression in adolescent females (Silberg et al. 2001b). However, the requirement that the life events not be genetically influenced led to an unusual selection of events for the composite scale (i.e., new stepsibling, sibling leaving home, father losing job—all of which should apply equally to both members of a twin pair). A more sophisticated approach is to model gene–environment correlation alongside gene–environment interaction (Purcell 2002). This approach has been used to examine

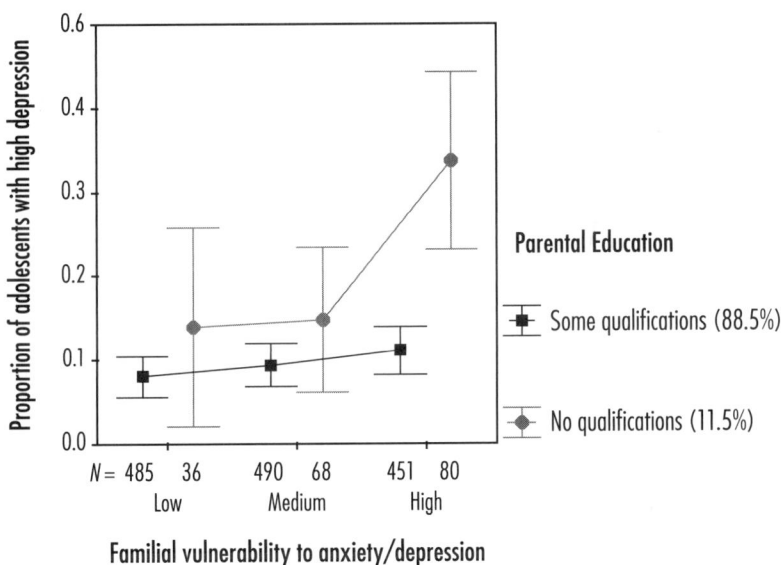

FIGURE 8–1. Interaction between parental education and familial vulnerability to anxiety/depression on adolescent depression.

the role of gene–environment interaction in the presence or absence of gene–environment correlation for adolescent depression (Lau and Eley 2008). The environmental measures were parental negative disciplinary style and life events, and both were found to be influenced by a combination of gene–environment correlation *and* gene–environment interaction. Thus, genetic influences on adolescent depression are not only shared with those on negative disciplinary style or life events but are also moderated by the presence of negative discipline or life events. In both cases, the variation in depression increased substantially with higher levels of the moderator, and genetic differences were important in this increase. In other words, there was a greater range of depression scores in those at the "at-risk" end of the environmental distribution, and this was partly due to a greater "expression" of genetic influence on those individuals. This indicates that when individuals experience high levels of life events or negative parenting, the genes they have that are influential on depression have a greater opportunity to show their effect.

The most precise way to examine gene–environment interactions is to obtain specific measures not only of the environment but of individual sources of genetic risk—in other words, to identify specify candidate genes and to include these in the analysis (for introductory guides to the language and statistics of molecular genetics, see Eley and Craig 2005 and Eley and Rijsdijk 2005). A groundbreaking study from our department first showed an interaction between a functional polymorphism in the serotonin transporter (5-HTT) promoter region and the effect of life events in relation to depression symptoms in adults (Caspi et al. 2003). The 5-HTT gene is involved in regulatory processes during stress (Hariri et al. 2002), making it an excellent candidate for interaction with environmental stress. The polymorphism exists in two forms, a "long" and a "short" form. The short allele is less efficient than the longer allele, thus leading to differences in available serotonin in the brain (Lesch et al. 1996). Analyses revealed a significant interaction between the 5-HTT gene and self-reported life events over the past 5 years on depression symptoms. The effects of stressful life events were significantly stronger among individuals carrying one or two copies of the short form of the allele, s, as shown by an increase in symptom frequencies and severity. Furthermore, this allele also moderated the longitudinal prediction from childhood maltreatment to adult depression. We subsequently replicated this finding in adolescent females, with an interaction between the same 5-HTT regulatory region and a family based measure of environmental risk—including social adversity, family life events, and parental employment level (Eley et al. 2004b). The effects of family based environmental risk were significantly stronger among female adolescents who possessed at least one short allele (see Figure 8–2). This interaction has now been subjected to numerous replication attempts, and meta-analyses indicate that it appears to be a true finding. Identification of specific effects of this kind will aid our understanding of vulnerabilty to stress and the development of associated disorders.

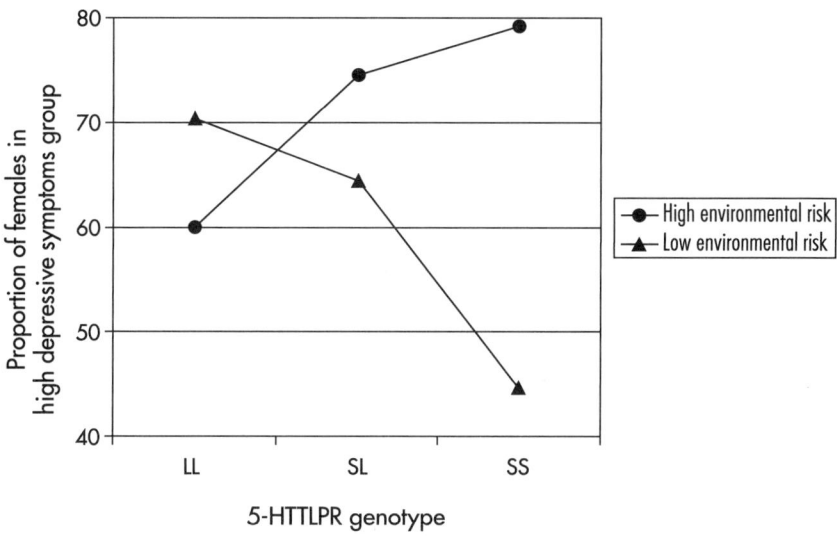

FIGURE 8–2. Interaction between serotonin transporter genotype and environmental risk on female adolescent depression.

LL=long-long genotype; SL=short-long genotype; SS=short-short genotype.

Cognitive Biases As Mediators of Genetic and Environmental Risk

It is clear that we have reached a stage now where we need to know *how* genes influence anxiety. One approach to this question is to examine cognitive biases as potential mediators of genetic risk. Recently, geneticists working on complex traits have begun to be interested in aspects of cognitive or brain functioning that may be better markers of the underlying genetic risks. These have been referred to as *endophenotypes*, and it is hoped that they will be more proximal to the underlying genetic risk than actual symptoms (Gottesman and Gould 2003). Ideally, such markers should be developmental precursors of the disorder of interest, be heritable, and share genetic influences with the disorder of interest (for examples in hyperactivity, see Doyle et al. 2005; Waldman 2005).

To date there has been little work in this area, although it is expanding rapidly. With regard to anxiety specifically, there have now been three studies of the cognitive style "anxiety sensitivity." This construct reflects fear of physical symptoms described by individuals with panic disorder and the belief that these are harmful (McNally 2002; Reiss 1986). Heritability of anxiety sensitivity has been estimated at around 50%, with the remaining variance due to nonshared environment in adults (Stein et al. 1999) and adolescents (Eley and Brown 2004), and slightly lower in children (Eley et al. 2008). Furthermore, in the child sample, this genetic risk was found to overlap with that for panic symptoms. Also in our child sample, we found genetic overlap between depression symptoms and interpretation of ambiguity (Eley et al. 2007), and in our adolescent sample we found genetic overlap between attributional style and depression (Lau et al. 2006). Thus all of these aspects of cognitive bias may prove useful for molecular genetic studies of the development of anxiety and depression.

Conclusion

It is an exciting time for the genetics of complex disorders. We are starting to move beyond asking *whether* there is genetic influence to asking *how* this influence operates. There is much still to learn, but I predict that incorporating measures of the environment and assessing relevant cognitive biases will all be crucial to the next stage of understanding genetic influences on the development of anxiety disorders.

References

Caspi A, Sugden K, Moffitt TE, et al: Influence of life stress on depression: moderation by a polymorphism in the 5-HTT gene. Science 301:386–389, 2003

Deater-Deckard K, Reiss D, Hetherington EM, et al: Dimensions and disorders of adolescent adjustment: a quantitative genetic analysis of unselected samples and selected extremes. J Child Psychol Psychiatry 38:515–525, 1997

Doyle AE, Willcutt EG, Seidman LJ, et al: Attention-deficit/hyperactivity disorder endophenotypes. Biol Psychiatry 57:1324–1335, 2005

Eaves LJ, Silberg JL, Meyer JM, et al: Genetics and developmental psychopathology, 2: the main effects of genes and environment on behavioral problems in the Virginia Twin Study of Adolescent Behavioral Development. J Child Psychol Psychiatry 38:965–980, 1997

Eley TC: Depressive symptoms in children and adolescents: etiological links between normality and abnormality: a research note. J Child Psychol Psychiatry 38:861–866, 1997

Eley TC, Brown TA: Phenotypic and genetic/environmental structure of anxiety sensitivity in adolescents. Behav Genet 34:637, 2004

Eley TC, Craig IW: Introductory guide to the language of molecular genetics. J Child Psychol Psychiatry 46:1039–1041, 2005

Eley TC, Gregory AM: Behavioral genetics, in Anxiety Disorders in Children and Adolescents, 2nd Edition. Edited by Morris TL, March JS. New York, Guilford, 2004, pp 71–97

Eley TC, Rijsdijk FV: Introductory guide to the statistics of molecular genetics. J Child Psychol Psychiatry 46:1042–1044, 2005

Eley TC, Stevenson J: Using genetic analyses to clarify the distinction between depressive and anxious symptoms in children and adolescents. J Abnorm Child Psychol 27:105–114, 1999

Eley TC, Bolton D, O'Connor TG, et al: A twin study of anxiety-related behaviours in preschool children. J Child Psychol Psychiatry 44:945–960, 2003

Eley TC, Liang H, Plomin R, et al: Parental familial vulnerability, family environment, and their interactions as predictors of depressive symptoms in adolescents. J Am Acad Child Adolesc Psychiatry 43:298–306, 2004a

Eley TC, Sugden K, Gregory AM, et al: Gene-environment interaction analysis of serotonin system markers with adolescent depression. Mol Psychiatry 9:908–915, 2004b

Eley TC, Gregory AM, Clark DM, et al: Feeling anxious: a twin study of panic/somatic symptoms, anxiety sensitivity and heart-beat perception in children. J Child Psychol Psychiatry 48:1184–1191, 2007

Eley TC, Gregory AM, Lau JYF, et al: In the face of uncertainty: a twin study of ambiguous information, anxiety and depression in children. J Abnorm Child Psychol 36:55–65, 2008

Feigon SA, Waldman ID, Levy F, et al: Genetic and environmental influences on separation anxiety disorder symptoms and their moderation by age and sex. Behav Genet 31:403–411, 2001

Gottesman II, Gould TD: The endophenotype concept in psychiatry: etymology and strategic intentions. Am J Psychiatry 160:636–645, 2003

Hammen C, Shih JS, Altman T, et al: Interpersonal impairment and the prediction of depressive symptoms in adolescent children of depressed and nondepressed mothers. J Am Acad Child Adolesc Psychiatry 42:571–577, 2003

Hariri AR, Mattay VS, Tessitore A, et al: Serotonin transporter genetic variation and the response of the human amygdala. Science 297:400–403, 2002

Hettema JM, Prescott CA, Myers JM, et al: The structure of genetic and environmental risk factors for anxiety disorders in men and women. Arch Gen Psychiatry 62:182–189, 2005

Jacobson KC, Rowe DC: Genetic and environmental influences on the relationships between family connectedness, school connectedness, and adolescent depressed mood: sex differences. Dev Psychol 35:926–939, 1999

Kendler KS, Neale MC, Kessler RC, et al: Major depression and generalized anxiety disorder: same genes, (partly) different environments? Arch Gen Psychiatry 49:716–722, 1992

Kendler KS, Walters EE, Neale MC, et al: The structure of the genetic and environmental risk factors for six major psychiatric disorders in women: phobia, generalized anxiety disorder, panic disorder, bulimia, major depression, and alcoholism. Arch Gen Psychiatry 52:374–383, 1995

Kendler KS, Prescott CA, Myers J, et al: The structure of genetic and environmental risk factors for common psychiatric and substance use disorders in men and women. Arch Gen Psychiatry 60:929–937, 2003

Lau JYF, Eley TC: Disentangling gene-environment correlations and interactions on adolescent depressive symtpoms. J Child Psychol Psychiatry 49:142–150, 2008

Lau JYF, Rijsdijk FV, Eley TC: I think, therefore I am: a twin study of attributional style in adolescents. J Child Psychol Psychiatry 47:696–793, 2006

Lesch KP, Bengel D, Heils A, et al: Association of anxiety-related traits with a polymorphism in the serotonin transporter gene regulatory region. Science 274:1527–1531, 1996

Lichtenstein P, Annas P: Heritability and prevalence of specific fears and phobia in childhood. J Child Psychol Psychiatry 41:927–937, 2000

Martin N, Boomsma DI, Machin G: A twin-pronged attack on complex traits. Nat Genet 17:387–392, 1997

McNally RJ: Anxiety sensitivity and panic disorder. Biol Psychiatry 52:938–946, 2002

O'Connor TG, Hetherington EM, Reiss D, et al: A twin-sibling study of observed parent–adolescent interactions. Child Dev 66:812–829, 1995

O'Connor TG, Caspi A, DeFries JC, et al: Are associations between parental divorce in children's adjustment genetically mediated? an adoption study. Dev Psychol 36:429–437, 2000

Pike A, McGuire S, Hetherington EM, et al: Family environment and adolescent depressive symptoms and antisocial behavior: a multivariate genetic analysis. Dev Psychol 32:590–603, 1996

Plomin R, Reiss D, Hetherington EM, et al: Nature and nurture: genetic contributions to measures of the family environment. Dev Psychol 30:32–43, 1994

Plomin R, DeFries JC, McClearn GE, et al: Behavioral Genetics, 4th Edition. New York, Worth Publishers, 2001

Purcell S: Variance components models for gene-environment interaction in twin analysis. Twin Res 5:554–571, 2002

Reiss S: Anxiety sensitivity, anxiety frequency and the predictions of fearfulness. Behav Res Ther 24:1–8, 1986

Rende RD, Plomin R, Reiss D, et al: Genetic and environmental influences on depressive symptomatology in adolescence: individual differences and extreme scores. J Child Psychol Psychiatry 34:1387–1398, 1993

Rice F, Harold GT, Thapar A: Assessing the effects of age, sex and shared environment on the genetic aetiology of depression in childhood and adolescence. J Child Psychol Psychiatry 43:1039–1051, 2002

Rice F, Harold GT, Thapar A: Negative life events as an account of age-related differences in the genetic aetiology of depression in childhood and adolescence. J Child Psychol Psychiatry 44:977–987, 2003

Robinson JL, Kagan J, Reznick JS, et al: The heritability of inhibited and uninhibited behavior: a twin study. Dev Psychol 28:1030–1037, 1992

Rose RJ, Ditto WB: A developmental-genetic analysis of common fears from early adolescence to early adulthood. Child Dev 54:361–368, 1983

Rutter M, Redshaw J: Annotation: growing up as a twin: twin-singleton differences in psychological development. J Child Psychol Psychiatry 32:885–895, 1991

Scarr S, McCartney K: How people make their own environments: a theory of genotype greater than environmental effects. Child Dev 54:424–435, 1983

Sham PC, Sterne A, Purcell S, et al: GENESiS: creating a composite index of the vulnerability to anxiety and depression in a community-based sample of siblings. Twin Res 3:316–322, 2000

Silberg J, Pickles A, Rutter M, et al: The influence of genetic factors and life stress on depression among adolescent girls. Arch Gen Psychiatry 56:225–232, 1999

Silberg JL, Rutter M, Eaves L: Genetic and environmental influences on the temporal association between earlier anxiety and later depression in girls. Biol Psychiatry 49:1040–1049, 2001a [erratum appears in Biol Psychiatry 50:393, 2001]

Silberg J, Rutter M, Neale M, et al: Genetic moderation of environmental risk for depression and anxiety in adolescent girls. Br J Psychiatry 179:116–121, 2001b

Silove D, Manicavasagar V, O'Connell D, et al: Genetic factors in early separation anxiety: implications for the genesis of adult anxiety disorders. Acta Psychiatr Scand 92:17–24, 1995

Stein MB, Jang KL, Livesley WJ: Heritability of anxiety sensitivity: a twin study. Am J Psychiatry 156:246–251, 1999

Stevenson J, Batten N, Cherner M: Fears and fearfulness in children and adolescents: a genetic analysis of twin data. J Child Psychol Psychiatry 33:977–985, 1992

Thapar A, McGuffin P: Genetic influences on life events in childhood. Psychol Med 26:813–820, 1996

Thapar A, McGuffin P: Anxiety and depressive symptoms in childhood: a genetic study of comorbidity. J Child Psychol Psychiatry 38:651–656, 1997

Thapar A, Harold G, McGuffin P: Life events and depressive symptoms in childhood: shared genes or shared adversity? A research note. J Child Psychol Psychiatry 39:1153–1158, 1998

Topolski TD, Hewitt JK, Eaves LJ, et al: Genetic and environmental influences on child reports of manifest anxiety and symptoms of separation anxiety and overanxious disorders: a community-based twin study. Behav Genet 27:15–28, 1997

Waldman ID: Statistical approaches to complex phenotypes: evaluating neuropsychological endophenotypes for attention-deficit/hyperactivity disorder. Biol Psychiatry 57:1347–1356, 2005

9

SEROTONIN, SENSITIVE PERIODS, AND ANXIETY

Mark D. Alter, M.D., Ph.D.
Rene Hen, Ph.D.

Much research with animals points to the early life experience of an animal as an important determinant of adult neural functioning, whereas in humans, early life stress has been linked to a multitude of psychiatric disorders. Genetic variation has also been demonstrated to be an important factor in risk of psychopathology. Furthermore, recent studies have highlighted the interaction of genetic variation and early life stress acting together to influence an individual's risk for psychopathology. These observations have led to the hypothesis that both genetic variation and experience may impact the formation of neural circuits during a developmentally sensitive period and that disruptions of neural circuit formation during this sensitive period are mediators of increased risk of psychopathology later in life. In this review we discuss the evidence for this hypothesis and, in more depth, the role of serotonin in neural circuit formation and how changes in the genetics of the serotonin system can lead to disruption of this formation and increased risk of psychiatric disorders—in particular, anxiety.

Early Life Stress and Mental Health

A multitude of research studies associate early life stress with the development of mental health problems. Increased morbidity and mortality from a wide array of medical and mental illnesses are increased in abused children (Bremner 2003; Felitti et al. 1998; Heim and Nemeroff 2001, 2002; Nemeroff 2004). Even less severe forms of early life stress have been associated with an increase in adverse outcomes. Children brought up in families characterized by a lack of parental warmth or either over- or underregulation of children's behavior are more likely to have medical or psychiatric problems (Repetti et al. 2002; Serbin and Karp 2004).

Still, not all children exposed to these stressful environments have adverse outcomes. A particularly interesting line of research has demonstrated that at least a portion of these effects is mediated by genetic variability. In a landmark study, Caspi et al. (2002) demonstrated that boys with a hypofunctioning polymorphism in the monoamine oxidase A gene *(MAO-A)* are at increased risk for adolescent and adult antisocial behavior if they were abused during childhood. In a separate study in the same prospective cohort, which utilized both males and females, individuals homozygous (s/s) or heterozygous (l/s) for the short allele of a hypofunctioning polymorphism in the serotonin transporter gene *(SERT)* were found to have a markedly increased risk for depression if subjected to child abuse, whereas individuals homozygous for the normal functioning long allele (l/l) had no increase in depression when exposed to abuse (Caspi et al. 2003).

The logical question, when one examines the multiple studies demonstrating the detrimental effects of early life stress and genetic variance on mental health, is how are these detrimental effects being mediated? An attractive hypothesis is that early life represents a particularly sensitive period for the development of neural circuits, the disruption of which makes a person more vulnerable to the development of psychopathology.

Sensitive Periods of Development: A Role for Serotonin?

A "sensitive period" is a general term that applies whenever experience has a particularly strong and lasting effect over a limited time (Ito 2004; Knudsen 2004) (Figure 9–1). A classic example is that of filial imprinting, which occurs shortly after birth when a young animal learns to recognize and bond with its parent (Lorenz 1937). Sensitive periods are of particular interest to researchers and clinicians because they represent periods in development during which certain capacities are readily shaped or altered by experience. Another important characteristic of sensitive periods is that the effects of experience are not readily amenable to change after the sensitive period has occurred. For example, once an animal has undergone imprinting, the attachment to the parent will be strong and persistent; moreover, attachment to an alternative parental figure will be much more difficult to achieve. Why is this true? Although sensitive periods are marked by specific behaviors, such as attachment to a parent or speaking a language, the periods are ac-

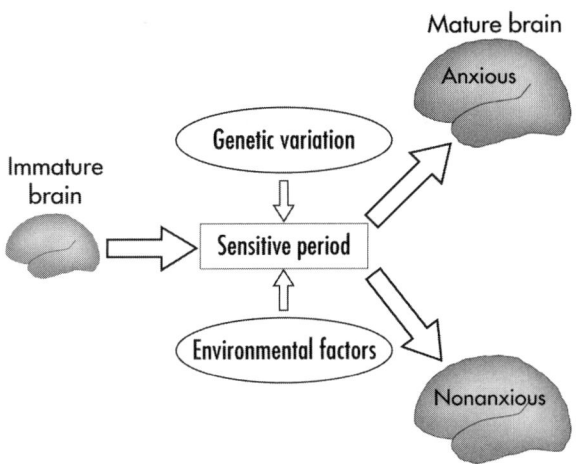

FIGURE 9–1. Sensitive period of brain development.
The immature brain goes through a sensitive period of development during which the brain is particularly sensitive to environmental and genetic factors. Changes that occur during this period are persistent and are reflected as differences in adult behavior.

tually properties of neural circuits (Hensch et al. 1998; Horn 2004; Knudsen 2004).

Neural circuit properties that are shaped by experience during the sensitive period are important. Neural circuits, once formed, may be modulated but do not easily change their basic structure (Knudsen 2004). Furthermore, because behaviors—in particular, complex behaviors such as language or anxiety—represent the coordination of many neural circuits, the true effects, or the persistence, of circuit-level changes that occur during a sensitive period will tend to be underestimated (Knudsen 2004).

Research on the serotonin system has underscored an important role of serotonin in the development of anxiety. Many regions innervated by the serotonin system—including the amygdala, hippocampus, anterior and posterior cingulate, and prefrontal cortex—have been suggested to play a role in anxiety and anxiety behavior (Charney 2003; Lopez et al. 1999; Miczek et al. 2002). Studying the genetics of the serotonin system has helped to outline circuits important in anxiety and to further suggest that serotonin impacts these circuits during sensitive periods of their development. This work has again pointed to the involvement of the amygdala and hippocampus as regions of importance and to early life as a sensitive period of development (Gingrich and Hen 2000; Gingrich et al. 2003; Gordon and Hen 2004; Grailhe et al. 1999; Zhuang et al. 1999). Together, these lines of research are lending insight into how a molecule traditionally believed to be only involved in synaptic transmission can have multiple roles in shaping brain development and function.

Multiple Roles of Serotonin

Serotonin has traditionally been viewed as a modulatory neurotransmitter. Through its diverse projections, the serotonin system plays a role in modulating sleep, appetite, memory/cognitive function, impulsivity, sexual behavior, motor function, and limbic/affective responsiveness (Ressler and Nemeroff 2000). In addition to this traditional understanding of serotonin as a neuromodulator, increasing evidence demonstrates that neurotransmitters, including serotonin, have important roles in development (Azmitia 2001; Levitt et al. 1997; Whitaker-Azmitia 2001). Serotonin has been well studied in this regard. Pharmacological studies have shown that serotonin can modulate a number of developmental events, including cell division, neuronal migration, cell differentiation, and synaptogenesis (Gaspar et al. 2003).

How can serotonin have such diverse modulatory functions and also play a role in the complex regulation of circuit formation? The serotonin system is itself quite complex and appears ideally suited for multiple roles. Serotonin exerts its effect through a multitude of receptors. Fifteen distinct genes encode for serotonin receptors that are classified into five families based on their second messenger systems (Harrington et al. 1992; Hartig 1994; Noda et al. 2004; Rho and Storey 2001). Splice variants and posttranslational processing expand the repertoire of viable receptor products to 30 (Bruss et al. 2000; Krobert et al. 2001; Olsen et al. 1999; Pindon et al. 2002). These serotonin receptors are located throughout the body and brain. Their expression is both temporally and spatially dynamic (del Olmo and Pazos 2001; Flugge 2000; Gaspar et al. 2003; Gross and Hen 2004a, 2004b; Kent et al. 2002). Depending on the receptor type, location, and developmental timing, stimulation of the receptors can be excitatory or inhibitory (Baumgarten and Lachenmayer 1985; Gaspar et al. 2003; Kelly et al. 1991; Walker et al. 1996; B. Zhang and Harris-Warrick 1994; Zhou and Hablitz 1999). In addition to the complexity of the receptor system, serotonin function is further regulated at the levels of serotonin synthesis, reuptake, and degradation. Disruption at each of these dynamically controlled levels of serotonin regulation has been demonstrated to have longstanding effects on anxiety behavior (Gaspar et al. 2003; Struder and Weicker 2001). These effects appear to be mediated at least in part through changes that occur during development.

Disruption of Serotonin Homeostasis During Development

Excessive extracellular serotonin during development is associated with increased aggressive and anxiety behavior. Deletion of *MAOA* or *SERT* leads to an accumulation of extracellular serotonin in the brain (Cases et al. 1995, 1998). Knockout mice with deletion of either *MAOA* or *SERT* have marked alterations in behavior characterized by increased anxiety and aggressiveness. Additionally, these mice have been found to have defects in the formation of brain circuits involved in sensory processing (Hendricks et al. 2003).

MAO-A is the principal enzyme responsible for degradation of monoamines in early postnatal life. MAO-B compensates for the deletion later in life, but mice lacking MAO-A have a ninefold increase in brain serotonin levels during the first postnatal week (Hendricks et al. 2003). In *SERT* knockout mice, the serotonin transporter is absent. Serotonin continues to be released but cannot be removed and accumulates in the synaptic cleft (Gingrich and Hen 2001). Interestingly, both these mutations lead to abnormal development of thalamocortical axons important in formation of barrel receptive fields and retinal axons important in visual processing (Persico et al. 2001; Salichon et al. 2001; Upton et al. 1999; Vitalis et al. 2002). This abnormal development was shown to be mediated by the serotonin 5-HT_{1B} receptor. Double knockouts of *MAOA* and *HTR1B* or triple knockouts of *MAOA*, *SERT*, and *HTR1B* resulted in normal axonal development (Salichon et al. 2001).

Despite the clear anxiety-behavioral phenotype, putative anxiety circuits have not been carefully examined in these mice. It is tempting, however, to speculate that excessive serotonin might mediate abnormal development of anxiety circuits in a manner similar to the serotonin-dependent disruption of thalamocortical and retinal circuits in these knockout mice. Disruption of anxiety circuits would help to explain the persistence of anxiety-like behavior in these mice throughout their lifespan (Gingrich and Hen 2001).

Reduced levels of serotonin can also be problematic. Pet-1 is a transcription factor that regulates transcription of several genes important in serotonergic function (Cheng et al. 2003; Hendricks et al. 2003). Pet-1 knockout mice have an 80% reduction in brain serotonin levels (Hendricks et al. 1999, 2003). Interestingly, although the levels of serotonin move in opposite directions to those of the *MAOA* and *SERT* knockout mice, at a behavioral level, these mice resemble *MAOA* and *SERT* knockout mice in terms of their increased anxiety and aggressive behavior (Hendricks et al. 2003).

The recent identification of a neuronal-specific form of tryptophan hydroxylase provides another example of the effects of reduced serotonin (X. Zhang et al. 2004, 2005). Functionally significant polymorphisms in the gene that encodes for this neuron-specific form, *TPH2*, have been found in humans and mice. In humans, the hypofunctioning allele is markedly overrepresented in depressed individuals (X. Zhang et al. 2005). In mice, the hypofunctioning allele is found in the hyperanxious BALB strain but not in the less anxious strain, C57 (X. Zhang et al. 2004). There is good evidence that the effects of decreased serotonin may be mediated through effects on development. Pharmacological depletion of serotonin in the mother or embryo results in alterations in neurogenesis (Lauder and Krebs 1978; Vitalis and Parnavelas 2003), neuronal migration (Choi et al. 1997), and dendritic maturation (Durig and Hornung 2000; Levitt et al. 1997; Mazer et al. 1997; Vitalis and Parnavelas 2003).

Taken together, the evidence shows that disruption of serotonergic homeostasis, in either direction, can have clear effects on anxiety behavior. There is also good evidence that serotonergic dysregulation can have developmental effects on circuit formation, neurogenesis, neuronal migration, and dendritic maturation. Putting these observations together, the idea that serotonin's effects on development, at least in part, underlie serotonin's effects on behavior seems quite plausible.

Development of Anxiety Phenotype in Early Life

In the models just described, it is not clear when the gene deletions are mediating their effects. For example, germline deletions of *MAOA* and *SERT* result in changes in serotonin levels throughout the life of the animal, thus making it difficult to determine when these changes might be most influential. In order to address this issue of timing, researchers utilized fluoxetine, a selective inhibitor of serotonin transporter activity, to mimic the effects of disrupting *SERT* during a restricted time period. Newborn mice were given fluoxetine for only the first 3 weeks of life. In this way, the effects on serotonin levels were only present postnatally for a limited time period. Nonetheless, behaviorally, these mice were indistinguishable from the *SERT* knockout mice in respect to exploration in novel environments throughout the lifespan (Ansorge et al. 2004).

In a complementary line of evidence, Gross et al. (2002) examined mice deficient in the serotonin $5\text{-}HT_{1A}$ receptor. Mice deficient in the $5\text{-}HT_{1A}$ receptor have been demonstrated to have increased anxiety-related behavior. In an elegant study to address the timing of this effect, they showed that, only during the first 3 weeks of life, genetic replacement of the serotonin $5\text{-}HT_{1A}$ receptor was able to completely rescue normal anxiety behavior in mice deficient in $5\text{-}HT_{1A}$. On the other hand, replacement of the $5\text{-}HT_{1A}$ receptor throughout life, with the exception of the first 3 weeks, did not restore normal behavior (Gross et al. 2002). Mice deficient in $5\text{-}HT_{1A}$ receptor only during the first 3 weeks of life continued to display the characteristic $5\text{-}HT_{1A}$ knockout anxiety phenotype that is similar to the anxiety phenotype of *MAOA* and *SERT* knockout mice (Gross et al. 2000, 2002).

There is also substantial evidence that experience has potent effects during this same period. Rats exposed to high levels of maternal care during the first 3 weeks of life have decreased levels of anxiety relative to rats that receive low levels of maternal care (Caldji et al. 1998; Champagne et al. 2003; Francis and Meaney 1999; Francis et al. 1999; Liu et al. 1997, 2000; Meaney 2001). Conversely, lengthy maternal separation during the same period results in increased anxiety-related behavior (Boccia and Pedersen 2001; Daniels et al. 2004; Hofer 1981; Janus 1987). In humans and primates, this developmental period appears somewhat longer, with research suggesting a time course beginning during the third trimester of pregnancy and extending to periadolescence (Andersen 2003). Nonetheless, as discussed previously, early life appears to be a particularly potent period for the effects of experience and genetic variation (Heim and Nemeroff 2001, 2002; McEwen 2003; Nemeroff 2004).

Early Life: What's Going On at the Circuit Level?

It is important to consider what is occurring in brain development during this developmentally sensitive period. Numerous studies have demonstrated that different brain regions develop and mature at different rates and different times (Andersen 2003; Gogtay et al. 2004). In a general sense, phylogenetically primitive regions, such as the hippocampus or amygdala, develop earlier than the phylogenetically more advanced regions, such as the human frontal cortex (Andersen 2003). Therefore, it is important to consider not only timing but also location when trying to understand the effects of experience on development. The rat hippocampus has been particularly well studied in regard to its developmental course, and as discussed previously, the hippocampus has also been well demonstrated to be involved in anxiety and anxiety-related behavior. Looking at this anxiety-related structure within the first 3 weeks in the rat hippocampus, there is a dramatic rise and fall of dendritic growth and dendritic spine formation that is integral to the formation of synapses and circuits (Figure 9–2). At this same time, other events occur that are also indicative of the development of brain circuits. For example, during this time in the rat hippocampus, there is a dramatic increase in spontaneous synchronous firing of neurons, which is a hallmark of developing neuronal networks. The timing of this spontaneous network activity directly precedes the emergence of hippocampal-dependent functions, such as context-dependent learning (Ben-Ari 2001).

In concordance with the extended period of vulnerability, in humans, these processes are proposed to occur over an extended period of time beginning earlier in the third trimester and continuing much later throughout much of childhood (Andersen 2003). In summary, the period during which animals are most vulner-

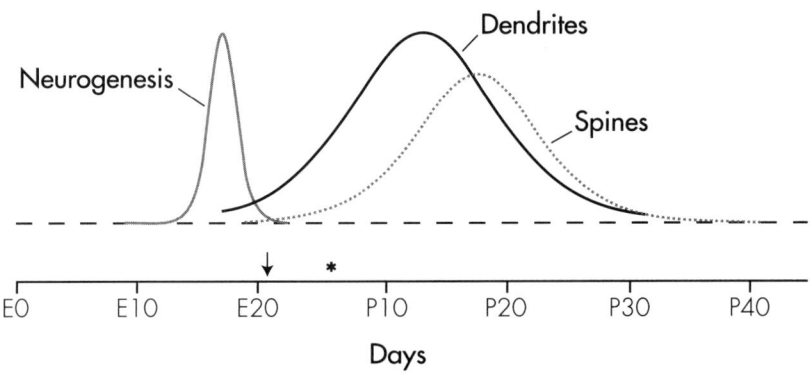

FIGURE 9–2. Development of the rat hippocampus.
Development of the rat hippocampus proceeds in a stepwise fashion in which late-prenatal neurogenesis is followed by early postnatal dendritic outgrowth and spine development. These postnatal changes are coincident with the sensitive period for the development of an anxiety phenotype.
Source. Adapted from Ben-Ari 2001.

able to experience and genetic variability is the same period during which brain circuits important in anxiety are developing.

Disruption of Anxiety Circuits

We have seen, then, that early life represents a period of increased vulnerability to the effects of both experience and genetic variation. Furthermore, it also is clear that this period is an important time in brain development and circuit formation. Yet what about the final piece of the hypothesis? Do changes in serotonin function during early postnatal life affect circuit formation in the anxiety system? The developmentally sensitive period for the development of an anxiety phenotype that persists into adulthood is highly suggestive of an effect at the circuit level. Examination of 5-HT_{1A} knockout mice adds support to this hypothesis. When examined at the level of neuronal circuits, the 5-HT_{1A} knockout mouse has an interesting, and perhaps anxiety-related, developmental alteration in the hippocampal circuit. At this level, hippocampal CA1 pyramidal neurons in 5-HT_{1A} knockout mice have increased dendritic arborization in the proximal, but not apical, dendrites. These differences have been shown to be functionally relevant in that stimulation of axons that synapse onto the region of increased dendrites is associated with a corresponding increase in activation of the neurons possessing the increased dendritic arbors. Lesion studies have implicated this hippocampal circuit in anxiety-related behaviors (Deacon and Rawlins 2005; Gray 1983; Treit and

Menard 1997), and behaviorally, $5\text{-}HT_{1A}$ knockout mice display more anxiety-related behaviors (Groenink et al. 2003; Gross et al. 2000; Lesch and Mossner 1999; Olivier et al. 2001). In humans, a functional polymorphism in the *HTR1A* promoter is associated with increased anxiety-related personality traits (Strobel et al. 2003) and an increased incidence of a subtype of panic disorder characterized by the additional presence of agoraphobia (Rothe et al. 2004).

Also in line with the hypothesis that changes in serotonin system gene expression can modulate anxiety circuits, Hariri and Weinberger (2003) have shown that in humans a polymorphism in *SERT* is associated with changes in the sensitivity of the amygdala to fearful or threatening stimuli. This change was particularly robust. Individuals with the hypofunctioning (s/s) allele had a fivefold increase in amygdala activation in response to fearful stimuli. Another group also found this increased amygdala activation, and further suggesting changes in circuitry, they also found that individuals with at least one copy of the short allele had increased coupling of amygdala and prefrontal activity (Heinz et al. 2005). Given the relation between fear and anxiety previously discussed, this change in fear responsiveness may underlie an increased risk for anxiety disorders in these individuals (McNaughton and Corr 2004). Importantly, these differences were much more readily apparent than overt behavioral differences in these individuals, underscoring the point that a change in neural circuit function does not necessarily result in a behavioral phenotype, in the case of an animal model, or result in an anxiety disorder, in the case of humans.

Sensitive Period Revisited: Gene–Environment Interactions

Upon examination of the current evidence, anxiety circuits appear to be subject to a sensitive period of development. Gene-knockout studies and phenotypic characterization of individuals with functional polymorphisms have highlighted several genes of the serotonin system that affect the developmental course of circuits involved in anxiety. Evidence for this is both direct, as with the changes in dendritic arborization in $5\text{-}HT_{1A}$ knockout mice or in functional neuroimaging of individuals with *SERT* polymorphisms, and indirect, as evidenced by the lifelong persistence of anxiety phenotypes based on genetic variation and early experience. The existence of a sensitive period in the development of neural circuits involved in anxiety becomes particularly interesting when the myriad influences are examined for their combined effects. These effects can be antagonistic, as seen when the $5\text{-}HT_{1B}$ receptor is removed in the *MAOA* and *SERT* knockout mice. Removal of this receptor blocks the detrimental effects of increased serotonin on the formation of thalamocortical and retinal circuits (Salichon et al. 2001). The combined effects can also be additive, exemplified by an exacerbation of the anxiety phenotype in

SERT knockout mice when brain-derived neurotrophic factor, another molecule important in circuit formation, is also removed (Ren-Patterson et al. 2005).

Importantly, these combined effects are not limited to gene–gene interactions. The normal functioning (l/l) allele of the *SERT* polymorphism appears to be protective against many of the behavioral consequences of early life stress in humans (Caspi et al. 2003; Jorm et al. 2000) and in primates (Barr et al. 2003, 2004; Suomi 2003), whereas those that are homozygous (s/s) or heterozygous (l/s) for the hypofunctioning short allele are affected by early life experience.

Conclusion

Understanding that psychopathology, and in particular anxiety, can represent developmentally mediated changes in neural circuits is not an end, but rather a beginning. This insight affords an opportunity to more carefully dissect not only the factors involved in psychopathology but also the resilience factors that protect individuals with circuit-level dysfunction from developing illness. Understanding brain function and pathology as an intermingling of individual circuits, each subject to their own developmental trajectory, also serves as a framework to probe for deeper understanding of the processes. Defining circuits on which to focus research opens the door for a careful dissection of genetic and environmental influences on neural function that is not available when using the gross outcome measures of behavior or disease.

Moving deeper, it is possible that dysfunction in neural circuit formation may represent a more fundamental dysfunction of molecular circuits. This certainly may be the case in the 5-HT_{1A} knockout mouse, where the 5-HT_{1A} receptor represents a critical regulator of negative feedback on serotonin function. Understanding dysfunction of molecular circuits would not only enhance understanding of the fundamentals of brain function but also may provide a yet more sensitive phenotypic marker of risk of psychopathology and a potential marker for treatment responsiveness. Ultimately, however, attempts have to be made to relate neural changes to behaviors or cognitive functions. Having defined neural changes in molecular or neural circuits, one then has a carefully defined subset of individuals to probe for subtle differences in neural function. It is through this iterative process that progress in understanding brain function and pathology can be made.

References

Andersen SL: Trajectories of brain development: point of vulnerability or window of opportunity? Neurosci Biobehav Rev 27:3–18, 2003

Ansorge MS, Zhou M, Lira A, et al: Early life blockade of the 5-HT transporter alters emotional behavior in adult mice. Science 306:879–881, 2004

Azmitia EC: Modern views on an ancient chemical: serotonin effects on cell proliferation, maturation, and apoptosis. Brain Res Bull 56:413–424, 2001

Barr CS, Newman TK, Becker ML, et al: The utility of the non-human primate; model for studying gene by environment interactions in behavioral research. Genes Brain Behav 2:336–340, 2003

Barr CS, Newman TK, Lindell S, et al: Interaction between serotonin transporter gene variation and rearing condition in alcohol preference and consumption in female primates. Arch Gen Psychiatry 61:1146–1152, 2004

Baumgarten HG, Lachenmayer L: Anatomical features and physiological properties of central serotonin neurons. Pharmacopsychiatry 18:180–187, 1985

Ben-Ari Y: Developing networks play a similar melody. Trends Neurosci 24:353–360, 2001

Boccia ML, Pedersen CA: Brief vs. long maternal separations in infancy: contrasting relationships with adult maternal behavior and lactation levels of aggression and anxiety. Psychoneuroendocrinology 26:657–672, 2001

Bremner JD: Long-term effects of childhood abuse on brain and neurobiology. Child Adolesc Psychiatr Clin North Am 12:271–292, 2003

Bruss M, Barann M, Hayer-Zillgen M, et al: Modified 5-HT3A receptor function by coexpression of alternatively spliced human 5-HT3A receptor isoforms. Naunyn Schmiedebergs Arch Pharmacol 362:392–401, 2000

Caldji C, Tannenbaum B, Sharma S, et al: Maternal care during infancy regulates the development of neural systems mediating the expression of fearfulness in the rat. Proc Natl Acad Sci U S A 95:5335–5340, 1998

Cases O, Seif I, Grimsby J, et al: Aggressive behavior and altered amounts of brain serotonin and norepinephrine in mice lacking MAOA. Science 268:1763–1766, 1995

Cases O, Lebrand C, Giros B, et al: Plasma membrane transporters of serotonin, dopamine, and norepinephrine mediate serotonin accumulation in atypical locations in the developing brain of monoamine oxidase A knock-outs. J Neurosci 18:6914–6927, 1998

Caspi A, McClay J, Moffitt TE, et al: Role of genotype in the cycle of violence in maltreated children. Science 297:851–854, 2002

Caspi A, Sugden K, Moffitt TE, et al: Influence of life stress on depression: moderation by a polymorphism in the 5-HTT gene. Science 301:386–389, 2003

Champagne FA, Francis DD, Mar A, et al: Variations in maternal care in the rat as a mediating influence for the effects of environment on development. Physiol Behav 79:359–371, 2003

Charney DS: Neuroanatomical circuits modulating fear and anxiety behaviors. Acta Psychiatr Scand Suppl 417:38–50, 2003

Cheng L, Chen CL, Luo P, et al: Lmx1b, Pet-1, and Nkx2.2 coordinately specify serotonergic neurotransmitter phenotype. J Neurosci 23:9961–9967, 2003

Choi DS, Ward SJ, Messaddeq N, et al: 5-HT2B receptor-mediated serotonin morphogenetic functions in mouse cranial neural crest and myocardiac cells. Development 124:1745–1755, 1997

Daniels WM, Pietersen CY, Carstens ME, et al: Maternal separation in rats leads to anxiety-like behavior and a blunted ACTH response and altered neurotransmitter levels in response to a subsequent stressor. Metab Brain Dis 19:3–14, 2004

Deacon RM, Rawlins JN: Hippocampal lesions, species-typical behaviours and anxiety in mice. Behav Brain Res 156:241–249, 2005

del Olmo E, Pazos A: Aminergic receptors during the development of the human brain: the contribution of in vitro imaging techniques. J Chem Neuroanat 22:101–114, 2001

Durig J, Hornung JP: Neonatal serotonin depletion affects developing and mature mouse cortical neurons. Neuroreport 11:833–837, 2000

Felitti VJ, Anda RF, Nordenberg D, et al: Relationship of childhood abuse and household dysfunction to many of the leading causes of death in adults: the Adverse Childhood Experiences (ACE) Study. Am J Prev Med 14:245–258, 1998

Flugge G: Regulation of monoamine receptors in the brain: dynamic changes during stress. Int Rev Cytol 195:145–213, 2000

Francis DD, Meaney MJ: Maternal care and the development of stress responses. Curr Opin Neurobiol 9:128–134, 1999

Francis D, Diorio J, Liu D, et al: Nongenomic transmission across generations of maternal behavior and stress responses in the rat. Science 286:1155–1158, 1999

Gaspar P, Cases O, Maroteaux L: The developmental role of serotonin: news from mouse molecular genetics. Nat Rev Neurosci 4:1002–1012, 2003

Gingrich JA, Hen R: The broken mouse: the role of development, plasticity and environment in the interpretation of phenotypic changes in knockout mice. Curr Opin Neurobiol 10:146–152, 2000

Gingrich JA, Hen R: Dissecting the role of the serotonin system in neuropsychiatric disorders using knockout mice. Psychopharmacology (Berl) 155:1–10, 2001

Gingrich JA, Ansorge MS, Merker R, et al: New lessons from knockout mice: the role of serotonin during development and its possible contribution to the origins of neuropsychiatric disorders. CNS Spectr 8:572–577, 2003

Gogtay N, Giedd JN, Lusk L, et al: Dynamic mapping of human cortical development during childhood through early adulthood. Proc Natl Acad Sci U S A 101:8174–8179, 2004

Gordon JA, Hen R: The serotonergic system and anxiety. Neuromolecular Med 5:27–40, 2004

Grailhe R, Waeber C, Dulawa SC, et al: Increased exploratory activity and altered response to LSD in mice lacking the 5-HT(5A) receptor. Neuron 22:581–591, 1999

Gray JA: A theory of anxiety: the role of the limbic system. Encephale 9:161B–166B, 1983

Groenink L, van Bogaert MJ, van der Gugten J, et al: 5-HT1A receptor and 5-HT1B receptor knockout mice in stress and anxiety paradigms. Behav Pharmacol 14:369–383, 2003

Gross C, Hen R: The developmental origins of anxiety. Nat Rev Neurosci 5:545–552, 2004a

Gross C, Hen R: Genetic and environmental factors interact to influence anxiety. Neurotox Res 6:493–501, 2004b

Gross C, Santarelli L, Brunner D, et al: Altered fear circuits in 5-HT(1A) receptor KO mice. Biol Psychiatry 48:1157–1163, 2000

Gross C, Zhuang X, Stark K, et al: Serotonin1A receptor acts during development to establish normal anxiety-like behaviour in the adult. Nature 416:396–400, 2002

Hariri AR, Weinberger DR: Functional neuroimaging of genetic variation in serotonergic neurotransmission. Genes Brain Behav 2:341–349, 2003

Harrington MA, Zhong P, Garlow SJ, et al: Molecular biology of serotonin receptors. J Clin Psychiatry Suppl 53:8–27, 1992

Hartig PR: Molecular pharmacology of serotonin receptors. EXS 71:93–102, 1994

Heim C, Nemeroff CB: The role of childhood trauma in the neurobiology of mood and anxiety disorders: preclinical and clinical studies. Biol Psychiatry 49:1023–1039, 2001

Heim C, Nemeroff CB: Neurobiology of early life stress: clinical studies. Semin Clin Neuropsychiatry 7:147–159, 2002

Heinz A, Braus DF, Smolka MN, et al: Amygdala-prefrontal coupling depends on a genetic variation of the serotonin transporter. Nat Neurosci 8:20–21, 2005

Hendricks T, Francis N, Fyodorov D, et al: The ETS domain factor Pet-1 is an early and precise marker of central serotonin neurons and interacts with a conserved element in serotonergic genes. J Neurosci 19:10348–10356, 1999

Hendricks TJ, Fyodorov DV, Wegman LJ, et al: Pet-1 ETS gene plays a critical role in 5-HT neuron development and is required for normal anxiety-like and aggressive behavior. Neuron 37:233–247, 2003

Hensch TK, Fagiolini M, Mataga N, et al: Local GABA circuit control of experience-dependent plasticity in developing visual cortex. Science 282:1504–1508, 1998

Hofer MA: Toward a developmental basis for disease predisposition: the effects of early maternal separation on brain, behavior, and cardiovascular system. Res Publ Assoc Res Nerv Ment Dis 59:209–228, 1981

Horn G: Pathways of the past: the imprint of memory. Nat Rev Neurosci 5:108–120, 2004

Ito M: 'Nurturing the brain' as an emerging research field involving child neurology. Brain Dev 26:429–433, 2004

Janus K: Early separation of young rats from the mother and the development of play fighting. Physiol Behav 39:471–476, 1987

Jorm AF, Prior M, Sanson A, et al: Association of a functional polymorphism of the serotonin transporter gene with anxiety-related temperament and behavior problems in children: a longitudinal study from infancy to the mid-teens. Mol Psychiatry 5:542–547, 2000

Kelly JS, Larkman P, Penington NJ, et al: Serotonin receptor heterogeneity and the role of potassium channels in neuronal excitability. Adv Exp Med Biol 287:177–191, 1991

Kent JM, Mathew SJ, Gorman JM: Molecular targets in the treatment of anxiety. Biol Psychiatry 52:1008–1030, 2002

Knudsen EI: Sensitive periods in the development of the brain and behavior. J Cogn Neurosci 16:1412–1425, 2004

Krobert KA, Bach T, Syversveen T, et al: The cloned human 5-HT7 receptor splice variants: a comparative characterization of their pharmacology, function and distribution. Naunyn Schmiedebergs Arch Pharmacol 363:620–632, 2001

Lauder JM, Krebs H: Serotonin as a differentiation signal in early neurogenesis. Dev Neurosci 1:15–30, 1978

Lesch KP, Mossner R: Knockout corner: 5-HT(1A) receptor inactivation. Anxiety or depression as a murine experience. Int J Neuropsychopharmacol 2:327–331, 1999

Levitt P, Harvey JA, Friedman E, et al: New evidence for neurotransmitter influences on brain development. Trends Neurosci 20:269–274, 1997

Liu D, Diorio J, Tannenbaum B, et al: Maternal care, hippocampal glucocorticoid receptors, and hypothalamic-pituitary-adrenal responses to stress. Science 277:1659–1662, 1997

Liu D, Diorio J, Day JC, et al: Maternal care, hippocampal synaptogenesis and cognitive development in rats. Nat Neurosci 3:799–806, 2000

Lopez JF, Akil H, Watson SJ: Neural circuits mediating stress. Biol Psychiatry 46:1461–1471, 1999

Lorenz K: Imprinting. Auk 54:245–273, 1937

Mazer C, Muneyyirci J, Taheny K, et al: Serotonin depletion during synaptogenesis leads to decreased synaptic density and learning deficits in the adult rat: a possible model of neurodevelopmental disorders with cognitive deficits. Brain Res 760:68–73, 1997

McEwen BS: Early life influences on life-long patterns of behavior and health. Ment Retard Dev Disabil Res Rev 9:149–154, 2003

McNaughton N, Corr PJ: A two-dimensional neuropsychology of defense: fear/anxiety and defensive distance. Neurosci Biobehav Rev 28:285–305, 2004

Meaney MJ: Maternal care, gene expression, and the transmission of individual differences in stress reactivity across generations. Annu Rev Neurosci 24:1161–1192, 2001

Miczek KA, Fish EW, De Bold JF, et al: Social and neural determinants of aggressive behavior: pharmacotherapeutic targets at serotonin, dopamine and gamma-aminobutyric acid systems. Psychopharmacology (Berl) 163:434–458, 2002

Nemeroff CB: Neurobiological consequences of childhood trauma. J Clin Psychiatry 65(suppl):18–28, 2004

Noda M, Higashida H, Aoki S, et al: Multiple signal transduction pathways mediated by 5-HT receptors. Mol Neurobiol 29:31–39, 2004

Olivier B, Pattij T, Wood SJ, et al: The 5-HT(1A) receptor knockout mouse and anxiety. Behav Pharmacol 12:439–450, 2001

Olsen MA, Nawoschik SP, Schurman BR, et al: Identification of a human 5-HT6 receptor variant produced by alternative splicing. Brain Res Mol Brain Res 64:255–263, 1999

Persico AM, Mengual E, Moessner R, et al: Barrel pattern formation requires serotonin uptake by thalamocortical afferents, and not vesicular monoamine release. J Neurosci 21:6862–6873, 2001

Pindon A, van Hecke G, van Gompel P, et al: Differences in signal transduction of two 5-HT4 receptor splice variants: compound specificity and dual coupling with Galphas- and Galphai/o-proteins. Mol Pharmacol 61:85–96, 2002

Ren-Patterson RF, Cochran LW, Holmes A, et al: Loss of brain-derived neurotrophic factor gene allele exacerbates brain monoamine deficiencies and increases stress abnormalities of serotonin transporter knockout mice. J Neurosci Res 79:756–771, 2005

Repetti RL, Taylor SE, Seeman TE: Risky families: family social environments and the mental and physical health of offspring. Psychol Bull 128:330–366, 2002

Ressler KJ, Nemeroff CB: Role of serotonergic and noradrenergic systems in the pathophysiology of depression and anxiety disorders. Depress Anxiety 12(suppl):2–19, 2000

Rho JM, Storey TW: Molecular ontogeny of major neurotransmitter receptor systems in the mammalian central nervous system: norepinephrine, dopamine, serotonin, acetylcholine, and glycine. J Child Neurol 16:271–280, 2001

Rothe C, Gutknecht L, Freitag C, et al: Association of a functional 1019C>G 5-HT1A receptor gene polymorphism with panic disorder with agoraphobia. Int J Neuropsychopharmacol 7:189–192, 2004

Salichon N, Gaspar P, Upton AL, et al: Excessive activation of serotonin (5-HT) 1B receptors disrupts the formation of sensory maps in monoamine oxidase a and 5-HT transporter knock-out mice. J Neurosci 21:884–896, 2001

Serbin LA, Karp J: The intergenerational transfer of psychosocial risk: mediators of vulnerability and resilience. Annu Rev Psychol 55:333–363, 2004

Strobel A, Gutknecht L, Rothe C, et al: Allelic variation in 5-HT1A receptor expression is associated with anxiety- and depression-related personality traits. J Neural Transm 110:1445–1453, 2003

Struder HK, Weicker H: Physiology and pathophysiology of the serotonergic system and its implications on mental and physical performance: part I. Int J Sports Med 22:467–481, 2001

Suomi SJ: Gene-environment interactions and the neurobiology of social conflict. Ann N Y Acad Sci 1008:132–139, 2003

Treit D, Menard J: Dissociations among the anxiolytic effects of septal, hippocampal, and amygdaloid lesions. Behav Neurosci 111:653–658, 1997

Upton AL, Salichon N, Lebrand C, et al: Excess of serotonin (5-HT) alters the segregation of ipsilateral and contralateral retinal projections in monoamine oxidase A knock-out mice: possible role of 5-HT uptake in retinal ganglion cells during development. J Neurosci 19:7007–7024, 1999

Vitalis T, Parnavelas JG: The role of serotonin in early cortical development. Dev Neurosci 25:245–256, 2003

Vitalis T, Cases O, Gillies K, et al: Interactions between TrkB signaling and serotonin excess in the developing murine somatosensory cortex: a role in tangential and radial organization of thalamocortical axons. J Neurosci 22:4987–5000, 2002

Walker RJ, Brooks HL, Holden-Dye L: Evolution and overview of classical transmitter molecules and their receptors. Parasitology Suppl 113:S3–S33, 1996

Whitaker-Azmitia PM: Serotonin and brain development: role in human developmental diseases. Brain Res Bull 56:479–485, 2001

Zhang B, Harris-Warrick RM: Multiple receptors mediate the modulatory effects of serotonergic neurons in a small neural network. J Exp Biol 190:55–77, 1994

Zhang X, Beaulieu JM, Sotnikova TD, et al: Tryptophan hydroxylase-2 controls brain serotonin synthesis. Science 305:217, 2004

Zhang X, Gainetdinov RR, Beaulieu JM, et al: Loss-of-function mutation in tryptophan hydroxylase-2 identified in unipolar major depression. Neuron 45:11–16, 2005

Zhou FM, Hablitz JJ: Activation of serotonin receptors modulates synaptic transmission in rat cerebral cortex. J Neurophysiol 82:2989–2999, 1999

Zhuang X, Gross C, Santarelli L, et al: Altered emotional states in knockout mice lacking 5-HT1A or 5-HT1B receptors. Neuropsychopharmacology 21:52S–60S, 1999

10

ROLE OF COGNITION IN STRESS-INDUCED AND FEAR CIRCUITRY DISORDERS

Jonathan D. Huppert, Ph.D.
Edna B. Foa, Ph.D.
Richard J. McNally, Ph.D.
Shawn P. Cahill, Ph.D.

In this chapter, we review research on the cognitive aspects of panic disorder, post-traumatic stress disorder (PTSD), social anxiety disorder (SocAD), and specific phobia. We refer readers to the comprehensive review by Harvey et al. (2004) for greater detail than we can present in this chapter. We concentrate here on studies concerning cognitive biases favoring the processing of threat-related information. For each disorder, we examine cross-sectional, longitudinal, treatment, and experimental studies to ascertain whether biases may play a causal role in the maintenance and etiology of these syndromes. We conclude by summarizing what is known about the role of cognition in anxiety and providing suggestions for further research.

Definitions, Experimental Paradigms, and Assumptions

DEFINITIONS

We define *cognitions* as information structures that result from perception, learning, memory, or reasoning and that include representations of stimuli, responses, and their meaning. Cognitions are distinct from physiological anxiety symptoms and are often assessed through self-report inventories or questionnaires. *Cognitive processes* are mechanisms underlying cognitions that are involved in the detection, encoding, storage, retrieval, and utilization of information such as attention, interpretation, and memory.

Cognitive research comprises two approaches (McNally 2001). One relies on interviews and questionnaires to ascertain the content of conscious cognitions, such as beliefs that certain bodily sensations signify catastrophic consequences. The other approach eschews self-report and relies on reaction time and other methods from cognitive science to reveal underlying biased cognitive attentional, memory, and interpretive processes that relate to the signs and symptoms of anxiety disorders. Although often presented as such, these two approaches need not be contradictory and are likely complementary.

Cognitive processes range from *automatic,* which are used without effort or awareness, to *strategic,* which are used purposefully with awareness (Bargh 1989), and cognitions also may be in or out of awareness. Biases in cognitions and cognitive processes—as they relate to anxiety disorders—refer to differences between anxious and nonanxious individuals on measures of cognitions or cognitive processes in response to ambiguous, threat-relevant, or threat-neutral stimuli. The most common focus of investigations has been biases in attention allocation, memory, and interpretation.

EXPERIMENTAL PARADIGMS

The human information-processing system has limited capacity, and any bias for attending to threat-related information should result in heightened anxiety. To test whether individuals with anxiety disorders are, indeed, characterized by an attentional bias that favors threat, researchers have devised paradigms such as the emotional Stroop (see J.M.G. Williams et al. 1996 for a review) and the dot probe (MacLeod et al. 1986). The emotional Stroop requires subjects to name the colors of words that vary in disorder relevance (e.g., "suffocate" in panic disorder) as quickly and as accurately as possible while ignoring the meanings of the words. Delays in color naming occur when the meaning of the word captures the subject's attention despite the subject's attempt to focus on its color. Attentional bias toward threat is inferred from slower naming of the color for threat words than for nonthreat words. Many researchers believe that the task is not a pure measure of attentional bias and have increasingly relied on the dot probe paradigm.

In the dot probe, a central fixation cross is followed by two stimuli (either words or pictures) presented simultaneously (one threat and one nonthreat), and then a probe (e.g., an E or an F) replaces one of the two stimuli. The subject is asked to press a key describing the probe (E or F) as quickly as possible. Attentional bias toward threat is reflected in faster responding to a probe that replaces the threat stimulus than to a probe replacing the nonthreat stimulus. Attentional bias away from threat is inferred from faster responding to the probe that replaces the nonthreat stimulus.

If information about threat were more accessible from memory than nonthreatening information, then individuals exhibiting such a memory bias would be especially prone to experience heightened anxiety. Several memory paradigms have been used to examine memory biases in anxiety disorders. In explicit memory tasks, individuals are asked to remember word lists, and then the numbers of threat versus nonthreat words recalled are examined. In implicit memory tasks, individuals are asked to engage in tasks related to words and then are asked to complete sentences or word fragments to determine whether prior exposure to threat words facilitates greater use of these words in comparison with control words (for more information on measures of memory, see Coles and Heimberg 2002; MacLeod and Mathews 2004). Memory bias for threat information is inferred from greater recall or use of threat-related words compared with control words.

In everyday life, people encounter many situations in which the implications and meanings behind what people say are ambiguous. Individuals engaging in conversations do not usually provide explicit constant approval and may even censor themselves if they think critically. Any bias for interpreting such ambiguous stimuli or situations (e.g., an ambiguous facial expression or comment during a conversation) in a threatening manner should heighten anxiety. Paradigms for assessing an interpretive bias for threat require subjects to interpret ambiguous scenarios or other stimuli. In self-report or other explicit measures, interpretation bias for threat is inferred from a more frequent resolution of ambiguous information corresponding with a threat/negative interpretation. In other methods that do not rely on explicit answers to determine interpretations, bias toward threat is inferred from shorter decision times for threat-related words in word associations, grammatical decisions, or other tasks.

ASSUMPTIONS

Most cognitive theories of anxiety disorders embody several guiding assumptions, including the following: 1) cognitions play a causal role in the etiology and/or maintenance of the anxiety disorders through cognitive biases in focusing on negative and/or ignoring positive information and through negative evaluations; 2) individuals differ in the degree to which they focus on negative or positive information; and 3) the tendency to focus on negative information increases vulnerability to anxiety, whereas the tendency to focus on positive information increases resiliency.

Cross-Sectional Studies

There have been many cross-sectional studies on cognitions (e.g., evaluations, thoughts, beliefs) or cognitive processes (e.g., attention, memory, interpretations). For comprehensive reviews of these studies in anxiety disorders, see Harvey et al. 2004 and M. Williams et al. 1997. Overall, these studies show that self-report measures tend to reveal content-specific negative evaluations among individuals with a given anxiety concern compared with nonanxious control groups and individuals with different anxiety concerns. Furthermore, several studies suggest that the greater the strength and frequency of the negative evaluations, the more severe are the anxiety symptoms reported. Finally, experimental paradigms often reveal cognitive biases in anxious individuals (M. Williams et al. 1997). In the following sections we summarize the most robust findings for each specific anxiety disorder.

PANIC DISORDER

Individuals with panic disorder have catastrophic interpretations/evaluations of bodily sensations (see Casey et al. 2004 and Clark 1996 for reviews). Overall, these individuals also tend to have more negative thoughts than positive thoughts about agoraphobic situations (Schwartz and Michelson 1987) and hold strong beliefs about their inability to cope with panic (Telch et al. 1989). Specifically, individuals with panic disorder interpret changes in bodily sensations associated with a panic attack (e.g., increased heart rate, trembling, sweating) to mean that they are dying, going crazy, or losing control. Panic disorder patients also reveal a tendency to respond fearfully to anxiety-related sensations because of their supposed harmfulness; such anxiety sensitivity is discussed by Reiss and McNally 1985 and Reiss et al. 1986. Also, panic disorder patients are likely to overestimate the probability of having physical symptoms and exaggerate the cost of having them (McNally and Foa 1987; Uren et al. 2004).

In addition to findings of negative evaluations on self-report measures in individuals with panic disorder, data from interpretation-bias paradigms show that these individuals are more likely than nonanxious control subjects to resolve ambiguous stimuli related to physical sensations in a threat-congruent fashion (Harvey et al. 2004). Attentional bias studies have shown that individuals with panic disorder are hypervigilant to bodily sensations as well as to physical threat words (Harvey et al. 2004; M. Williams et al. 1997). Explicit memory biases for threat occur in these individuals, whereas less consistent findings emerge from tasks of implicit memory (MacLeod and Mathews 2004).

POSTTRAUMATIC STRESS DISORDER

Negative views about oneself (i.e., inability to cope, incompetence) and about others or about the world (as threatening/dangerous) are higher in individuals with PTSD compared with nonanxious control subjects (Ehlers et al. 2005; Foa et al. 1999; Nasby and Russell 1997). Furthermore, evidence is accumulating regarding the specificity of the cognitive predictors of PTSD compared with predictors of other anxiety disorders (Ehring et al. 2006). Experimental paradigms have shown that individuals with PTSD are faster to respond to threat meanings of ambiguous words (Amir et al. 2002) and to complete sentences with threat meanings (Kimble et al. 2002), reflecting a negative interpretation bias. Emotional Stroop studies suggest an attentional bias for trauma cues in PTSD patients (Foa et al. 1991; McNally 1998; McNally et al. 1990). One dot-probe study indicated an attentional bias for threat (Bryant and Harvey 1997), whereas another did not (Elsesser et al. 2004). Data on explicit memory biases also indicate biased memory, whereas implicit memory paradigms have yielded conflicting findings for this disorder (McNally 1998).

SOCIAL ANXIETY DISORDER

Individuals with SocAD, especially those with the generalized subtype, exhibit negative self-evaluations and fear of negative evaluations by others (Glass et al. 1982; Stopa and Clark 1993; Sturmer et al. 2002). These negative evaluations are related to the "social self," or how one performs in interpersonal situations (e.g., "I will sound stupid when I meet someone new"; "I will freeze during my speech."). These individuals also overestimate the probability of negative social interactions and exaggerate the cost of such interactions (Foa et al. 1996). Some studies have suggested that individuals with SocAD also have biased beliefs about the interpretations of their symptoms by others, about how their performance is related to their character, and about the long-term consequences of negative performance (J.K. Wilson and Rapee 2005). Socially anxious individuals also exhibit negative interpretations of ambiguous social situations on self-report measures (Amir et al. 1998; Hirsch and Clark 2004).

Experimental procedures have also shown a lack of a positive interpretation bias in socially anxious individuals (Hirsch and Mathews 2000), and one study found both the presence of a negative bias and the lack of a positive bias (Huppert et al. 2007). Attentional biases for threat occur in the dot-probe and emotional Stroop tasks. There is also evidence of vigilance to threat faces over neutral faces (Mogg et al. 2004) and to threat words over neutral words (Heinrichs and Hofmann 2001). However, another study found more avoidance of faces than objects (Chen et al. 2002). Some theorists have suggested that the primary difficulty of individuals with SocAD is disengaging from threat stimuli, rather than a bias for attending to them (Amir et al. 2003). Studies of memory biases in social anxiety have yielded mixed results (Coles and Heimberg 2002).

SPECIFIC PHOBIA

Individuals with specific phobia overestimate the likelihood of danger posed by the feared stimulus. Studies support the notion that people with specific phobias have biased estimations of the likelihood of danger and the extent of injury or harm (Jones and Menzies 1995; Menzies and Clarke 1995). There are no data on interpretation bias in specific phobia. In a number of studies, these individuals have shown attentional bias toward threat in emotional Stroop (Watts et al. 1986a) and visual search paradigms (Öhman et al. 2001). Furthermore, eye-tracking paradigms have suggested that attention is biased towards threat stimuli (Pflugshaup et al. 2005). However, no attentional bias emerged from a study using threat words in the dot-probe paradigm (Wenzel and Holt 1999), perhaps because the words did not sufficiently activate the fears. Studies also suggest selective recall and other memory biases in specific phobias (Watts et al. 1986b).

In summary, studies of individuals with anxiety disorders consistently reveal negative evaluations, as well as negative attentional and interpretation biases, that are specific to the concern of their disorder. The data on memory bias are less consistent. It is important to note that these findings may, or may not, mean that negative cognitive biases cause the disorders.

Longitudinal Studies

Longitudinal studies offer a stronger level of evidence regarding the causal role of a given cognitive factor in an anxiety disorder. If the negative cognitions precede the onset of the disorder, then the alternative explanation that the cognitions are part of the disorder itself can be eliminated. However, it remains possible that an underlying predisposition (genetic or otherwise) may cause the cognitions and the subsequent disorder, rather than the cognitions themselves causing the disorder. These considerations notwithstanding, longitudinal studies are quite informative. However, it is difficult and costly to collect longitudinal data, and only a few studies have been conducted on cognitions and anxiety. In fact, there are no longitudinal studies for any anxiety disorder other than PTSD, although some studies have examined the ability of specific evaluations of bodily sensations (i.e., anxiety sensitivity) to predict panic attacks. No published study yet has examined whether cognitive processes predict the onset of any anxiety disorder, but some studies are in progress (e.g., those by Mineka and Craske in the United States and by Margraf in Germany). Moreover, even in PTSD, researchers have been able to collect data only prior to the emergence of disorder, not prior to the exposure to trauma.

PANIC DISORDER

Self-reported negative evaluations of bodily sensations, as measured by elevated scores on the Anxiety Sensitivity Inventory, predict subsequent spontaneous panic attacks (Reiss et al. 1986). Two of these studies examined panic attacks during basic training in a military setting (Schmidt et al. 1997, 1999), and two examined whether these negative evaluations predicted the onset of panic attacks in adolescents (Hayward et al. 2000; Weems et al. 2002). Even after controlling for a number of relevant variables (e.g., previous history of panic attacks, baseline anxiety levels), researchers found that elevated anxiety sensitivity increased vulnerability for having panic attacks, other anxiety symptoms, and/or general impairment. Other studies have shown that elevated anxiety sensitivity predicts the onset or maintenance of panic attacks over time (Ehlers 1995). Only one study to date has examined whether anxiety sensitivity predicts onset of anxiety disorders: Individuals with elevated anxiety sensitivity had a fivefold increased risk for developing an anxiety disorder 3 years later. This included an eightfold risk for panic disorder (Maller and Reiss 1992). In a recent replication and extension of this study, Schmidt et al. (2006) found that elevated Anxiety Sensitivity Inventory scores were related to a twofold increase in the incidence of anxiety disorders and a 2.5-fold increased risk for panic attacks at a 1- to 2-year follow-up. There was also an increased risk for panic disorder per se. Schmidt and Bates (2003) have suggested that anxiety sensitivity varies significantly within panic disorder patients and is therefore likely to affect how the disorder manifests (the types of symptoms, comorbidity, medication use) in addition to whether it occurs.

POSTTRAUMATIC STRESS DISORDER

Because the diagnostic criteria for PTSD require a traumatic event, as well as a set of symptoms related to that event, and because only some trauma survivors develop chronic PTSD, this disorder lends itself readily to examining longitudinal risk factors for the disorder. Specifically, studies have evaluated individuals shortly after a traumatic event to examine which individuals subsequently recover compared with which develop chronic PTSD. Findings of these studies suggest that negative views about the self and world (e.g., "I am incompetent"; "The world is dangerous"); negative interpretations of initial symptoms (e.g., "Experiencing intrusive thoughts means I am weak"); negative interpretations of others' responses (e.g., "They think I am weak for having nightmares"); and perceived permanent change all predict PTSD severity 6 months to 1 year after the trauma (r values range from 0.35 to 0.66). Organization of the memory and appraisals of the trauma memory also predicted PTSD severity 6 months after assessment, even when researchers controlled for initial symptom severity (Halligan et al. 2003). Another study found that perceived "nowness" of a memory (viewing a memory as a current occurrence instead of in the past), distress due to the memory, and lack of context of the memory were strong predictors of later PTSD severity. This occurred even after researchers controlled for initial symptom severity (Michael et al. 2005). Results of another longitudinal study have suggested that ex-consequentia reasoning (e.g., "If I feel anxious, there must be danger") is related to later PTSD severity, although this relationship became nonsignificant after initial PTSD severity was controlled for (Engelhard et al. 2002). Some recent work has begun to examine cognitive processes as predictors. For example, Michael et al. (2005) found that primed word stems were related to symptom severity soon after the trauma and were predictive of subsequent symptom severity 3 and 6 months later. However, this association was no longer significant after controlling for initial PTSD symptoms, except for predicting later flashbacks.

In summary, anxiety sensitivity predicts later panic attacks in adults and adolescents. Accumulating data suggest a relationship between anxiety sensitivity and later development of psychopathology, although the relationship with panic disorder is less established. With PTSD, certain negative cognitive evaluations predict later severity of PTSD symptoms. However, the evaluations of many individuals who participated in these studies took place weeks and even months after the trauma had occurred, and it is possible that these negative cognitions developed as a result of factors that had occurred after the trauma and before the evaluation. Indeed, several cognitive predictors of chronic PTSD involve negative appraisals of PTSD symptoms, the reactions of others, and perceived change as a result of the trauma. Prospective studies of at-risk groups (e.g., soldiers in training) should determine whether cognitive abnormalities precede exposure to trauma and thus constitute causal risk factors for PTSD.

Treatment Studies

Many cognitive-behavioral therapies (CBTs) are designed to correct negatively distorted cognitions and cognitive biases. If the presence of negative cognitions and cognitive biases are, indeed, the mechanisms causing the disorder, then a change in cognitions and cognitive biases should mediate the reduction of symptoms after treatment. However, few data corroborate the idea that changes in cognitions/cognitive biases precede reduction in symptoms. This is partially due to the difficulty in establishing the temporal order of cognitive changes and symptom changes. Nonetheless, treatment studies across the anxiety disorders have indicated that cognitions and cognitive processes tend to change with successful treatment. Moreover, some studies have shown that 1) cognitions and cognitive processes after treatment are similar to those among individuals without anxiety disorders, 2) change in the processes is related to symptom change, and 3) change in cognitions predicts maintenance of gains. Significantly more data exist for evaluations on self-report measures of cognitions than on behavioral tasks of cognitive processes.

PANIC DISORDER

In one of the first studies on cognitions in panic, McNally and Foa (1987) found that panic disorder patients who were successfully treated with CBT did not differ from nonpatients in estimating probabilities and costs of interoceptive sensations, whereas untreated patients had higher estimated probabilities and costs than the other two groups. Interestingly, Stoler and McNally (1991) showed that treated panic disorder patients continued to report elevated estimations of threat in a sentence completion task. However, although these biased interpretations remained, the way of coping with panic-related thoughts had changed. Future studies should determine whether less-biased thoughts lead to less relapse or whether such biases decrease further over time. Such data may help account for the superior maintenance of symptom remission when CBT for panic is withdrawn compared with medications being withdrawn (Barlow et al. 2000). Not only do negative cognitions change with treatment but such changes also are related to symptom reduction. Specifically, change in anxiety sensitivity and in catastrophic interpretations of physical sensations has been related to change in many aspects of panic disorder (Clark et al. 1997; McNally and Lorenz 1987; Schmidt and Bates 2003; Westling and Öst 1995). Additionally, posttreatment cognitions have been predictive of maintenance of treatment gains (Clark et al. 1994, 1999; Otto and Reilly Harrington 1999; Schmidt and Bates 2003; Westling and Öst 1995). There are no data that we are aware of that report changes in attentional biases after therapy.

POSTTRAUMATIC STRESS DISORDER

Fewer studies have examined the relation between PTSD-related cognitions and treatment effects in patients with PTSD. Resick et al. (2002) reported that guilt-related cognitions, hindsight bias, wrongdoing, and lack of justification all changed significantly with CBT treatments. Foa and Rauch (2004) found that changes in beliefs about the self and the world were strongly related to changes in PTSD symptoms after prolonged exposure. Posttreatment cognitions were also correlated with symptom severity at 1-year follow-up (S. Rauch, personal communication, May, 2006). Ehlers et al. (2005), using CBT, reported that change in cognitions was related to change in symptom severity. Only one study involving the emotional Stroop examined changes in cognitive processes with treatment in PTSD before and after CBT (Devineni et al. 2004). In this study, no relationship between changes in attentional bias and changes in symptom severity occurred in a sample of motor vehicle accident victims who had received treatment for PTSD.

SOCIAL ANXIETY DISORDER

Most studies of SocAD have examined changes in self-report measures or self-statements as a result of treatment. Results indicate that overestimations of the probability and cost of mildly negative events are reduced pre- to posttreatment and that these changes are strongly correlated with changes in symptom severity (Foa et al. 1996; McManus et al. 2000; J.K. Wilson and Rapee 2005). Furthermore, J.K. Wilson and Rapee (2005) found that reductions in beliefs that negative social events reflect negative personal characteristics were positively related to maintenance of treatment gains at 3-month follow-up. Heimberg et al. (1990) found that positive cognitions increased and negative cognitions decreased after group CBT. Chambless et al. (1997) found that changes in cognition were strongly related to SocAD symptoms immediately after treatment but not at follow-up. Inconsistent with the Heimberg et al. (1990) findings, Bruch et al. (1991) did not find a large increase in positive thoughts at posttreatment, although such changes had occurred by follow-up. Heinrichs and Hofmann (2005) also found a relationship between increases in positive self-statements and decreases in negative self-statements and symptom reduction after treatment. In addition to the multiple studies demonstrating changes in negative thoughts, judgments, and evaluations after treatment, studies have also found changes in interpretation bias (Franklin et al. 2005) and attentional bias (Lundh and Ost 2001; Mattia et al. 1993) after treatment. For example, Mattia et al. (1993) found that Stroop interference for social threat words declined following either successful CBT or successful pharmacotherapy. Patients who failed to respond to either treatment continued to exhibit the attentional bias for threat cues.

SPECIFIC PHOBIA

Three studies have shown decreases in attentional bias after exposure treatment for specific phobias. All three studies involved the emotional Stroop and demonstrated reductions in response time to threat-related color naming after treatment, reflecting reduction in attentional bias (Lavy and van den Hout 1993; Lavy et al. 1993; Watts et al. 1986a).

In summary, it is well documented that negative cognitions related to specific disorders may be reduced with successful treatment and that this change is related to symptom change. Some studies have also shown that these changes are related to maintenance of gains at follow-up. Fewer data exist on the changes in cognitive processing biases with treatment, although there is some evidence regarding changes in attentional bias in social anxiety disorder and specific phobia. More information is needed in this area. Overall, these data suggest that changes in cognitions/cognitive biases reduce symptoms, thereby implying that biases may at least be maintaining symptoms. However, the data do not speak directly to whether cognitions and biases cause the disorders in the first place.

Experimental Studies

The strongest evidence for a causal role of cognition/cognitive bias on anxiety comes from experimental manipulation of cognitions/biases, demonstrating that these manipulations influence symptom manifestation or severity.

PANIC DISORDER

Several studies have involved manipulations of cognitions related to panic and then tested whether the manipulations influence the occurrence of panic during a subsequent induction procedure. Other studies examined the relationship between perception of control over the environment and panic attacks during a CO_2 challenge. In a classic study (Sanderson et al. 1989), individuals diagnosed with panic disorder were told that when a light appeared, they could turn a dial to decrease the concentration of CO_2 that they had inhaled, although in reality the dial did not change the CO_2 concentration. In half the subjects, the light turned on during the trial, but for the other half, it never turned on. Significantly more patients reported panic attack and negative cognitions in the group that did not have the chance to use the dial. This experiment has been replicated a number of times with similar results, suggesting that thoughts or beliefs of control over anxiety symptoms are related to panic attacks.

SOCIAL ANXIETY DISORDER

Fewer studies have examined cognitive manipulations in SocAD to determine their effects on performance. However, a number of recent studies by Hirsch et al. (2003, 2005) have begun to examine the impact of manipulating negative imagery on social anxiety. They found that holding the image of another person displaying confidence decreased interpretation bias (Hirsch et al. 2005), whereas holding a negative self-image increased anxiety and negative observer ratings of performance (Hirsch et al. 2003).

SPECIFIC PHOBIA

Attempts to manipulate cognition in specific phobias and to determine what impact this manipulation has on severity of symptoms or fear have been reported. However, some researchers have attempted to manipulate one's sense of self-efficacy—that is, the expectations about one's abilities to successfully perform a specific task (Bandura 1977). In one series of studies, Bandura et al. (1982, experiments 2 and 3) used vicarious modeling (observing a study confederate interact with a spider) to manipulate levels of self-efficacy to different levels either across independent groups (experiment 2) or for different tasks within subjects (experiment 3) among highly avoidant patients with spider phobia. After self-efficacy was raised to the prespecified levels, subjects were tested for actual performance and accompanying distress and physiological arousal (experiment 3 only) on a carefully graded behavioral-avoidance task. Results indicated that behavioral performance corresponded with levels of induced self-efficacy and that higher levels of self-efficacy were associated with lower levels of self-reported distress and physiological reactivity.

TRAINING COGNITIVE BIASES

Some of the strongest evidence that cognitive biases may play a causal role in the manifestation of anxiety comes from experiments that manipulate cognitive biases and assess how the manipulations influence anxiety and emotional vulnerability (MacLeod et al. 2002; Mathews 2004; Mathews and MacLeod 2002; Yiend and Mackintosh 2004). Although these studies used nonclinical populations, the results are quite compelling.

MacLeod et al. (2002) have used a modified dot-probe paradigm to manipulate attentional bias. The probe predominantly replaced either a threat (to induce negative bias) or a nonthreat (to induce positive bias) word. The results of their studies showed that bias changed in the intended direction after training and that individuals who were trained to have a negative bias rated a separate stressor task as more anxiety-provoking than did individuals who were trained to have a positive bias.

In a second study, MacLeod et al. (2002) found a strong relationship between induced attentional bias and the level of anxiety during the stressor task. These results led to a series of additional studies in which individuals selected for high trait anxiety were successfully trained over a number of sessions to have a positive bias. This change in bias has been associated with a change in trait anxiety. Similar results have emerged for individuals with high levels of social anxiety, with training leading to decreased levels of social anxiety when compared with a neutral training control condition (MacLeod et al. 2002). Some researchers have used attentional bias training with socially anxious patients, with initial reports of success (Amir et al. 2004), although Harris and Menzies (1998) reported no change in symptoms in attentional training with individuals with specific phobias.

Similarly, exciting evidence has been found in a line of research manipulating interpretation biases (Grey and Mathews 2000; Mathews and Mackintosh 2000; E. Wilson et al. 2006; Yiend et al. 2005). This work has shown that individuals with moderate levels of anxiety can be trained to interpret ambiguous scenarios as either negative or positive through solicitation of "correct" answers to sentence completion tasks (or other similar methods) that guide the individual to either positive or negative resolutions. This line of work has shown that individuals trained to have negative interpretations tend to present with elevated levels of trait anxiety after training (Mathews and Mackintosh 2000); that a single-session training of the bias can last for 24 hours (Yiend et al. 2005); and that individuals with an induced negative bias rate video clips of anxiety-provoking scenarios as more distressing than those induced with a positive bias (E. Wilson et al. 2006; Yiend and Mackintosh 2004).

Conclusion

Hundreds of studies have examined the relationship of cognitions and cognitive biases to anxiety and to anxiety disorders. The majority of the studies suggest that cognitions and cognitive processes are biased in patients with anxiety disorders. With some exceptions, the general pattern emerging is that patients are biased toward negative or threat aspects of content-specific concerns in evaluations, interpretation, attention, and memory and that these biases tend to decrease with successful treatment. Longitudinal data are limited, although some large studies are in progress. Furthermore, recent studies have shown increased vulnerability to anxiety when these biases are induced.

Future research should examine the effects of directly reducing these negative biases among individuals with anxiety disorders or whether such training can prevent individuals from developing an anxiety disorder. Although research on the neurobiological correlates of these disorders has already begun, much more needs to be learned about the interplay of neuroendocrine response and cognition (Abelson et al. 2005; Gaab et al. 2005; van Honk et al. 2000), neuroimaging and cognition (van den Heuvel et al. 2005), neurophysiology and cognition (Pauli et al. 2005), and genetics and cognition (Schmidt et al. 2000). The question of whether cognitions and cognitive processes are *constitutive* (i.e., essential aspects of the disorder that are not etiological in nature) or *causal* (i.e., distinct processes that precede the disorder and inevitably lead to it) needs further examination. Regardless of their etiological role, cognitions and cognitive processes constitute a central aspect of stress and fear-related disorders.

References

Abelson JL, Liberzon I, Young EA, et al: Cognitive modulation of the endocrine stress response to a pharmacological challenge in normal and panic disorder subjects. Arch Gen Psychiatry 62:668–675, 2005

Amir N, Foa EB, Coles ME: Negative interpretation bias in social phobia. Behav Res Ther 36:945–957, 1998

Amir N, Coles ME, Foa EB: Automatic and strategic activation and inhibition of threat-relevant information in posttraumatic stress disorder. Cognit Ther Res 26:645–655, 2002

Amir N, Elias J, Klumpp H, et al: Attentional bias to threat in social phobia: facilitated processing of threat or difficulty disengaging attention from threat? Behav Res Ther 41:1325–1335, 2003

Amir N, Beard C, Klumpp H, et al: Modification of attentional bias in social phobia: change in attention, generalizability across paradigms, and change in symptoms. Symposium presented at the annual meeting of the European Association for Behavioural and Cognitive Therapies, Manchester, UK, 2004

Bandura A: Self-efficacy: toward a unifying theory of behavioral change. Psychol Rev 84:191–215, 1977

Bandura A, Reese L, Adams NE: Microanalysis of action and fear arousal as a function of differential levels of perceived self-efficacy. J Pers Soc Psychol 431:5–21, 1982

Bargh JA: Conditional automaticity: varieties of automatic influence in social perception and cognition, in Unintended Thought. Edited by Uleman JS, Bargh JA. New York, Guilford, 1989, pp 3–51

Barlow DH, Gorman JM, Shear MK, et al: Cognitive-behavioral therapy, imipramine, or their combination for panic disorder: a randomized controlled trial. JAMA 283:2529–2536, 2000

Bruch MA, Heimberg RG, Hope DA: States of mind model and cognitive change in treated social phobics. Cognit Ther Res 15:429–441, 1991

Bryant RA, Harvey AG: Attentional bias in posttraumatic stress disorder. J Trauma Stress 10:635–644, 1997

Casey LM, Oei TPS, Newcombe PA: An integrated cognitive model of panic disorder: the role of positive and negative cognitions. Clin Psychol Rev 24:529–555, 2004

Chambless DL, Tran GQ, Glass CR: Predictors of response to cognitive-behavioral group therapy for social phobia. J Anxiety Disord 11:221–240, 1997

Chen YP, Ehlers A, Clark DM, et al: Patients with generalized social phobia direct their attention away from faces. Behav Res Ther 40:677–687, 2002

Clark DM: Panic disorder: from theory to therapy, in Frontiers in Cognitive Therapy. Edited by Salkovskis PM. New York, Guilford, 1996, pp 318–344

Clark DM, Salkovskis PM, Hackmann A, et al: A comparison of cognitive therapy, applied relaxation and imipramine in the treatment of panic disorder. Br J Psychiatry 164:759–769, 1994

Clark DM, Salkovskis PM, Ost L, et al: Misinterpretation of body sensations in panic disorder. J Consult Clin Psychol 65:203–213, 1997

Clark DM, Salkovskis PM, Hackmann A, et al: Brief cognitive therapy for panic disorder: a randomized controlled trial. J Consult Clin Psychol 67:583–589, 1999

Coles ME, Heimberg RG: Memory biases in the anxiety disorders: current status. Clin Psychol Rev 22:587–627, 2002

Devineni T, Blanchard EB, Hickling EJ, et al: Effect of psychological treatment on cognitive bias in motor vehicle accident-related posttraumatic stress disorder. J Anxiety Disord 18:211–231, 2004

Ehlers A: A 1-year prospective study of panic attacks: clinical course and factors associated with maintenance. J Abnorm Psychol 104:164–172, 1995

Ehlers A, Clark DM, Hackmann A, et al: Cognitive therapy for post-traumatic stress disorder: development and evaluation. Behav Res Ther 43:413–431, 2005

Ehring T, Ehlers A, Glucksman E: Contribution of cognitive factors to the prediction of post-traumatic stress disorder, phobia and depression after motor vehicle accidents. Behav Res Ther 44:1699–1716, 2006

Elsesser K, Sartory G, Tackenberg A: Attention, heart rate, and startle response during exposure to trauma-relevant pictures: a comparison of recent trauma victims and patients with posttraumatic stress disorder. J Abnorm Psychol 113:289–301, 2004

Engelhard IM, van den Hout MA, Arntz A, et al: A longitudinal study of "intrusion-based reasoning" and posttraumatic stress disorder after exposure to a train disaster. Behav Res Ther 40:1415–1434, 2002

Foa EB, Rauch SAM: Cognitive changes during prolonged exposure versus prolonged exposure plus cognitive restructuring in female assault survivors with posttraumatic stress disorder. J Consult Clin Psychol 72:879–884, 2004

Foa EB, Feske U, Murdock TB, et al: Processing of threat-related information in rape victims. J Abnorm Psychol 100:156–162, 1991

Foa EB, Franklin ME, Perry KJ, et al: Cognitive biases in generalized social phobia. J Abnorm Psychol 105:433–439, 1996

Foa EB, Ehlers A, Clark DM, et al: The posttraumatic cognitions inventory (PTCI): development and validation. Psychol Assess 11:303–314, 1999

Franklin ME, Huppert J, Langner R, et al: Interpretation bias: a comparison of treated social phobics, untreated social phobics, and controls. Cognit Ther Res 29:289–300, 2005

Gaab J, Rohleder N, Nater UM, et al: Psychological determinants of the cortisol stress response: the role of anticipatory cognitive appraisal. Psychoneuroendocrinology 30:599–610, 2005

Glass CR, Merluzzi TV, Biever JL, et al: Cognitive assessment of social anxiety: development and validation of a self-statement questionnaire. Cognit Ther Res 6:37–55, 1982

Grey S, Mathews A: Effects of training on interpretation of emotional ambiguity. Q J Exp Psychol Hum Exp Psychol 53A:1143–1162, 2000

Halligan SL, Michael T, Clark DM, et al: Posttraumatic stress disorder following assault: the role of cognitive processing, trauma memory, and appraisals. J Consult Clin Psychol 71:419–431, 2003

Harris LM, Menzies RG: Changing attentional bias: can it effect self-reported anxiety? Anxiety, Stress and Coping: An International Journal 11:167–179, 1998

Harvey A, Watkins E, Mansell W, et al: Cognitive Behavioural Processes Across Psychological Disorders. New York, Oxford University Press, 2004

Hayward C, Killen JD, Kraemer HC, et al: Predictors of panic attacks in adolescents. J Am Acad Child Adolesc Psychiatry 39:207–214, 2000

Heimberg RG, Bruch MA, Hope DA, et al: Evaluating the states of mind model: comparison to an alternative model and effects of method of cognitive assessment. Cognit Ther Res 14:543–557, 1990

Heinrichs N, Hofmann SG: Information processing in social phobia: a critical review. Clin Psychol Rev 21:751–770, 2001

Heinrichs N, Hofmann SG: Cognitive assessment of social anxiety: a comparison of self-report and thought listing methods. Cogn Behav Ther 34:3–15, 2005

Hirsch CR, Clark DM: Information-processing bias in social phobia. Clin Psychol Rev 24:799–825, 2004

Hirsch CR, Mathews A: Impaired positive inferential bias in social phobia. J Abnorm Psychol 109:705–712, 2000

Hirsch CR, Clark DM, Mathews A, et al: Self-images play a causal role in social phobia. Behav Res Ther 41:909–921, 2003

Hirsch CR, Clark DM, Williams R, et al: Interview anxiety: taking the perspective of a confident other changes inferential processing. Behavioural and Cognitive Psychotherapy 33:1–12, 2005

Huppert JD, Pasupuleti RV, Foa EB, et al: Interpretation biases in social anxiety: response generation, response selection, and self-appraisals. Behav Res Ther 45:1505–1515, 2007

Jones MK, Menzies RG: The etiology of fear of spiders. Anxiety, Stress and Coping: An International Journal 8:227–234, 1995

Kimble MO, Kaufman ML, Leonard LL, et al: Sentence completion test in combat veterans with and without PTSD: preliminary findings. Psychiatry Res 113:303–307, 2002

Lavy E, van den Hout M: Selective attention evidenced by pictorial and linguistic Stroop tasks. Behav Ther 24:645–657, 1993

Lavy EH, van den Hout M, Arntz A: Attentional bias and spider phobia: conceptual and clinical issues. Behav Res Ther 31:17–24, 1993

Lundh L, Öst L: Attentional bias, self-consciousness and perfectionism in social phobia before and after cognitive-behaviour therapy. Scandinavian Journal of Behaviour Therapy 30:4–16, 2001

MacLeod C, Mathews A: Selective memory effects in anxiety disorders: an overview of research findings and their implications, in Memory and Emotion: Series in Affective Science. Edited by Reisberg D, Hertel P. London, Oxford University Press, 2004, pp 155–185

MacLeod C, Mathews A, Tata P: Attentional bias in emotional disorders. J Abnorm Psychol 95:15–20, 1986

MacLeod C, Rutherford E, Campbell L, et al: Selective attention and emotional vulnerability: assessing the causal basis of their association through the experimental manipulation of attentional bias. J Abnorm Psychol 111:107–123, 2002

Maller RG, Reiss S: Anxiety sensitivity in 1984 and panic attacks in 1987. J Anxiety Disord 6:241–247, 1992

Mathews A: On the malleability of emotional encoding. Behav Res Ther 42:1019–1036, 2004

Mathews A, Mackintosh B: Induced emotional interpretation bias and anxiety. J Abnorm Psychol 109:602–615, 2000

Mathews A, MacLeod C: Induced processing biases have causal effects on anxiety. Cogn Emot 16:331–354, 2002

Mattia JI, Heimberg RG, Hope DA: The revised Stroop color-naming task in social phobics. Behav Res Ther 31:305–313, 1993

McManus F, Clark DM, Hackmann A: Specificity of cognitive biases in social phobia and their roles in recovery. Behavioural and Cognitive Psychotherapy 28:201–209, 2000

McNally RJ: Experimental approaches to cognitive abnormality in posttraumatic stress disorder. Clin Psychol Rev 18:971–982, 1998

McNally RJ: On the scientific status of cognitive appraisal models of anxiety disorder. Behav Res Ther 39:513–521, 2001

McNally RJ, Foa EB: Cognition and agoraphobia: bias in the interpretation of threat. Cognit Ther Res 11:567–581, 1987

McNally RJ, Lorenz M: Anxiety sensitivity in agoraphobics. J Behav Ther Exp Psychiatry 18:3–11, 1987

McNally RJ, Kaspi SP, Riemann BC, et al: Selective processing of threat cues in posttraumatic stress disorder. J Abnorm Psychol 99:398–402, 1990

Menzies RG, Clarke JC: Danger expectancies and insight in acrophobia. Behav Res Ther 33:215–221, 1995

Michael T, Ehlers A, Halligan SL: Enhanced priming for trauma-related material in posttraumatic stress disorder. Emotion 5:103–112, 2005

Mogg K, Philippot P, Bradley BP: Selective attention to angry faces in clinical social phobia. J Abnorm Psychol 113:160–165, 2004

Nasby W, Russell M: Posttraumatic stress disorder and the states-of-mind model: evidence of specificity. Cognit Ther Res 21:117–133, 1997

Öhman A, Flykt A, Esteves F: Emotion drives attention: detecting the snake in the grass. J Exp Psychol Gen 130:466–478, 2001

Otto MW, Reilly Harrington NA: The impact of treatment on anxiety sensitivity, in Anxiety Sensitivity: Theory, Research, and Treatment of the Fear of Anxiety. Edited by Mahwah, TS. Florence, KY, Lawrence Erlbaum Associates, 1999, pp 321–336

Pauli P, Amrhein C, Mühlberger A, et al: Electrocortical evidence for an early abnormal processing of panic-related words in panic disorder patients. Int J Psychophysiol 57:33–41, 2005

Pflugshaupt T, Mosimann UP, von Wartburg R: Hypervigilance-avoidance pattern in spider phobia. J Anxiety Disord 19:105–116, 2005

Reiss S, McNally RJ: The expectancy model of fear, in Theoretical Issues in Behavior Therapy. Edited by Reiss S, Bootzin RR. New York, Academic Press, 1985, pp 107–121

Reiss S, Peterson RA, Gursky DM, et al: Anxiety sensitivity, anxiety frequency and the predictions of fearfulness. Behav Res Ther 24:1–8, 1986

Resick PA, Nishith P, Weaver TL, et al: A comparison of cognitive-processing therapy with prolonged exposure and a waiting condition for the treatment of chronic posttraumatic stress disorder in female rape victims. J Consult Clin Psychol 70:867–879, 2002

Sanderson WC, Rapee RM, Barlow DH: The influence of an illusion of control on panic attacks induced via inhalation of 5.5% carbon dioxide-enriched air. Arch Gen Psychiatry 46:157–162, 1989

Schmidt NB, Bates MJ: Evaluation of a pathoplastic relationship between anxiety sensitivity and panic disorder. Anxiety, Stress and Coping: An International Journal 16:17–30, 2003

Schmidt NB, Lerew DR, Jackson RJ: The role of anxiety sensitivity in the pathogenesis of panic: prospective evaluation of spontaneous panic attacks during acute stress. J Abnorm Psychol 106:355–364, 1997

Schmidt NB, Lerew DR, Jackson RJ: Prospective evaluation of anxiety sensitivity in the pathogenesis of panic: replication and extension. J Abnorm Psychol 108:532–537, 1999

Schmidt NB, Storey J, Greenberg BD, et al: Evaluating gene × psychological risk factor effects in the pathogenesis of anxiety: a new model approach. J Abnorm Psychol 109:308–320, 2000

Schmidt NB, Zvolensky MJ, Maner JK: Anxiety sensitivity: prospective prediction of panic attacks and Axis I pathology. J Psychiatr Res 40:691–699, 2006

Schwartz RM, Michelson L: States-of-mind model: cognitive balance in the treatment of agoraphobia. J Consult Clin Psychol 55:557–565, 1987

Stoler LS, McNally RJ: Cognitive bias in symptomatic and recovered agoraphobics. Behav Res Ther 29:539–545, 1991

Stopa L, Clark DM: Cognitive processes in social phobia. Behav Res Ther 31:255–267, 1993

Sturmer PJ, Bruch MA, Haase RF, et al: Convergent validity in cognitive assessment of social anxiety: endorsement versus production methods in deriving states of mind ratio. Cognit Ther Res 26:487–503, 2002

Telch MJ, Brouillard M, Telch CF, et al: Role of cognitive appraisal in panic-related avoidance. Behav Res Ther 27:373–383, 1989

Uren TH, Szabó M, Lovibond PF: Probability and cost estimates for social and physical outcomes in social phobia and panic disorder. J Anxiety Disord 18:481–498, 2004

van den Heuvel OA, Veltman DJ, et al: Disorder-specific neuroanatomical correlates of attentional bias in obsessive-compulsive disorder, panic disorder and hypochondriasis. Arch Gen Psychiatry 62:922–933, 2005

van Honk J, Tuiten A, van den Hout M, et al: Conscious and preconscious selective attention to social threat: different neuroendocrine response patterns. Psychoneuroendocrinology 25:577–591, 2000

Watts FN, McKenna FP, Sharrock R, et al: Colour naming of phobia-related words. Br J Psychol 77:97–108, 1986a

Watts FN, Trezise L, Sharrock R: Processing of phobic stimuli. Br J Clin Psychol 25:253–259, 1986b

Weems CF, Hayward C, Killen J, et al: A longitudinal investigation of anxiety sensitivity in adolescence. J Abnorm Psychol 111:471–477, 2002

Wenzel A, Holt CS: Dot probe performance in two specific phobias. Br J Clin Psychol 38:407–410, 1999

Westling BE, Öst L: Cognitive bias in panic disorder patients and changes after cognitive-behavioral treatments. Behav Res Ther 33:585–588, 1995

Williams JMG, Mathews A, MacLeod C: The emotional Stroop task and psychopathology. Psychol Bull 120:3–24, 1996

Williams M, MacLeod C, Watts F, et al: Cognitive Psychology and Emotional Disorders, 2nd Edition. London, Wiley, 1997

Wilson E, MacLeod C, Mathews A: The causal role of interpretive bias in vulnerability to anxiety. J Abnorm Psychol 115:103–111, 2006

Wilson JK, Rapee RM: The interpretation of negative social events in social phobia: changes during treatment and relationship to outcome. Behav Res Ther 43:373–389, 2005

Yiend J, Mackintosh B: The experimental modification of processing biases, in Cognition, Emotion, and Psychopathology: Theoretical, Empirical and Clinical Approaches. Edited by Yiend J. New York, Cambridge University Press, 2004, pp 190–210

Yiend J, Mackintosh B, Mathews A: Enduring consequences of experimentally induced biases in interpretation. Behav Res Ther 43:779–797, 2005

11

STRESS AND PSYCHOSOCIAL FACTORS IN ONSET OF FEAR CIRCUITRY DISORDERS

Ronald M. Rapee, Ph.D.
Richard A. Bryant, Ph.D.

Onset of Anxiety Disorders

Fear-based disorders, for the most part, appear to have their onsets in early to midadolescence or perhaps even earlier (Ost 1987). In most cases, onset is subtle and insipid and individuals cannot recall specific dates or even periods of initial onset. This is especially the case for social phobia and the specific phobias as well as for generalized anxiety disorder (GAD). The major exceptions are panic disorder, which is rare in childhood (King et al. 1993) and typically has an abrupt onset in late adolescence to early adulthood (Rapee 1985), and posttraumatic stress disorder (PTSD), which by definition can have its onset at any age. However, even for these disorders, as for the other anxiety disorders, onset of the actual disorder is often preceded by chronic symptoms and personality features that may show much in common with the disorder (Fava et al. 1988; Schmidt et al. 1997). In contrast to major depression, the anxiety disorders are also rarely episodic and most show a chronic pattern of maintenance (Keller et al. 1992; Massion et al. 2002). Thus, environmental factors important to the onset of anxiety disorders are likely to be those that are present during the early years of life. However, environmental factors in the adult years may still be of importance to the maintenance, exacerbation, or amelioration of the disorders.

Behavior Genetic Evidence

In examining the role of environmental factors in the onset of anxiety, behavior genetic data provide indications about the broad nature of environmental input. Several reviews of twin concordance in anxiety have concluded that variance in both anxious symptoms and disorder is accounted for by a combination of heritability and unique environmental influence (Eley 1999; Hettema et al. 2001). Typically, shared environmental factors account for little variance. However, data have been inconsistent with regard to whether shared environmental factors account for no appreciable variance or simply for a small but nevertheless significant amount of variance (Eley 1999; Hettema et al. 2001). In fact, one study of adult males showed that shared environmental factors accounted for significant variance in symptoms of agoraphobia and social phobia (Kendler et al. 2001).

Of greater importance is the fact that these data have been gathered in studies based on adult twin samples. Data from the relatively smaller number of child twin samples have indicated that variance in anxiety is significantly accounted for by both shared and unique environmental factors (Eley 1999; Eley and Lau 2005). In fact, in some studies, shared environmental factors account for the majority of variance in some forms of childhood anxiety (Stevenson et al. 1992; Thapar and McGuffin 1995; Topolski et al. 1997). It is unclear what these discrepant findings mean. It is possible that child and adult anxiety disorders are different problems affecting different populations. Alternately, it is possible that there are developmental differences in the expression of anxiety disorders and that different factors influence the expression of anxiety at different developmental stages.

In terms of the specificity of anxious expression, evidence from twin data has been mixed. At least one large twin study suggested that the environmental influence for anxiety and depression was distinct and that it was this unique environmental influence that distinguished anxiety from depression (Kendler et al. 1987). Distinction between anxiety disorders has been more inconsistent. Some research has suggested that a small proportion of the variance unique to several different disorders is accounted for by specific environmental components (Kendler et al. 1995, 2001). However, considerable evidence points to environmental factors that have a common influence across disorders (Kendler et al. 1995, 2001).

Family studies have shown a strong familial concordance for anxiety disorders, and in fact, some family studies have indicated a degree of specificity in the family resemblance (Fyer et al. 1995; Last et al. 1987; Noyes et al. 1987). Given the likely nonspecific genetic involvement in anxiety, such specificity would most likely reflect, primarily, environmental influence (Eley 1999; Kendler et al. 1992b). Thus, it appears that a considerable proportion of variance in symptoms of anxiety is accounted for by environmental factors. The majority of environmental variance in adult anxiety appears to be accounted for by factors that make monozygotic twins different from one another (mostly factors occurring independently to that individual). However, in childhood, variance in anxiety appears to be influenced by both unique and shared environmental factors. It is also likely that the environmental factors involved in anxiety are largely common across the disorders. However, the data are not inconsistent with the possibility that a certain proportion of the variance in each disorder is predicted by unique environmental factors. One final point to note is that gene–environment interactions have rarely been modeled in any of the studies, yet it is highly likely that any influence of environmental factors on anxiety will be moderated by genetic influence (Eley and Lau 2005).

Demographic Factors

SOCIOECONOMIC STATUS

Several studies have demonstrated that anxious adults have significant impairments in work, use higher levels of government and health benefits, have lower education, and are less likely to be married than the general population (Andrews et al. 1999; Schneier et al. 1992; Stein and Kean 2000; Steketee et al. 1987; Wittchen et al. 1999). Commonly, comparisons have not been made between anxiety disorders, and results have indicated only small and relatively inconsistent differences (Massion et al. 1993; Norton et al. 1996; Steketee et al. 1987). Whether these differences represent cause or effect is impossible to say, although most authors consider lower socioeconomic status to be a result of the life interference caused by anxiety rather than a cause. However, some evidence has suggested that parents of anxious children and adolescents score lower on measures of socioeconomic status or education (Cronk et al. 2004; Lewinsohn et al. 1997; Xue et al. 2005), indicating that such factors may be present before onset of the disorder. It is likely that these effects represent shared genetic influence, but the possibility that low socioeconomic status acts as a risk factor for anxiety cannot be excluded at this stage.

FAMILY OF ORIGIN

From studies of adults, there is little information on the structure of their early families. However, some epidemiological research has shown that anxious children and adolescents are more likely to live in single-parent homes (Kroes et al. 2002; Lewinsohn et al. 1997). This finding is certainly not specific to anxiety and is likely to characterize a range of psychopathology. Some clinical data have suggested that this may depend on the type of anxiety disorder, with separated or divorced parents being more common only for children with separation anxiety disorder and not for those with GAD or social phobia (Rapee and Szollos 2003). In fact, one study demonstrated that paternal absence accounted for significant variance in separation anxiety, even after controlling for genetic factors (Cronk et al. 2004).

There is a similar lack of information on size of family of origin from studies of anxiety in adults. However, data from samples of children generally fail to show differences in the number of siblings between anxious and nonanxious children (Kroes et al. 2002; Rapee and Szollos 2003). On the other hand, studies have shown some possible differences in position in the family, and this may indicate one of the few specific environmental factors that is unique to a particular disorder. Following observations from Zimbardo (1977) that shy people were more likely to be the firstborn in a family, some research has demonstrated support for this suggestion (Klonsky et al. 1990; Rapee and Szollos 2003). However, some smaller studies from adult populations have failed to support the association between social phobia and birth order (Rapee and Melville 1997; Steketee et al. 1987), and research from behaviorally inhibited toddlers has also failed to support this effect (Hirshfeld-Becker et al. 2004). Furthermore, some studies have shown an association between being firstborn and having adult obsessive-compulsive disorder (OCD), although later research failed to support this association (Insel et al. 1983; Steketee et al. 1987).

GENDER AND CULTURE

Data consistently show a higher level of anxiety reported by females than males. This gender difference appears to be consistent, whether assessed by symptom measures or based on disorder, and is found in both child and adult populations (Andrews et al. 1999; Kessler et al. 1994; Kleinknecht et al. 1997; Lewinsohn et al. 1997). Examination of gender balance on related temperamental constructs, such as behavioral inhibition, shyness, or approach—especially during the earlier years—has failed to indicate differences (Hirshfeld-Becker et al. 2004; Prior 1992). The difference in expression of anxiety between genders appears to be relatively consistent across anxiety disorders and is also similar in depression, although in the latter disorder there is a difference in developmental expression that is not seen in anxiety (Hankin et al. 1998). Whether the gender imbalance reflects the influence of biology or environment has not yet been determined and is widely debated. However, a number of authors have argued that an environmental determinant for gender differences in anxiety is plausible (Gavranidou and Rosner 2003; Weich et al. 2001), an argument that is supported by the lack of gender differences observed in developmentally delayed populations (Pickersgill et al. 1994) and in nonhuman species (J.M. Warren and Levy 1979).

One of the common arguments is that sex differences in the report of anxiety disorders reflect different social pressures or different social roles for males and females. Indeed, some research has shown a decrease in levels of inhibition across time for males but not for females (Kerr et al. 1994; Zhengyan et al. 2003), which has been interpreted as consistent with the push in Western societies for males to be more dominant (Kerr et al. 1994). On the other hand, other research has failed to find a link between gender-based social roles and the sex difference in neurotic disorders (Weich et al. 2001). Furthermore, one large study comparing the frequency of anxiety disorders in general practice across 15 different countries and spanning several continents failed to find significant differences in the male-to-female ratio across countries for panic disorder, although marked differences were noted for GAD (Gater et al. 1998). Thus, if environmental effects are responsible for the gender difference in panic disorder, these would have to be relatively universal environmental conditions, something that is difficult to explain. However, for GAD, there are clearly more localized effects on the expression of the disorder, a pattern that is more consistent with the influence of sociocultural factors.

There also have been suggestions that the expression of anxiety may differ between cultures; however, empirical examination has been sparse. The most strongly investigated disorder has been social anxiety disorder, which is believed to be more common in Eastern cultures that are typically collectivistic compared with Western cultures that are more strongly individualistic. Comparison of levels of symptoms between culturally diverse populations is fraught with complexity, and perhaps as a result, comparisons have been somewhat inconsistent. However, at least some studies have indicated higher scores on measures of social anxiety in Eastern countries, including Japan and Korea, than in Western countries, including Europe, North America, and Australia (Heinrichs et al. 2006; Kleinknecht et al. 1997).

Of some considerable interest are intriguing suggestions that the diagnosis of social phobia is actually less common in Eastern countries than in Western. Three surveys in Taiwan and Korea using the Diagnostic Interview Schedule found a lifetime prevalence for social phobia, based on DSM-III (American Psychiatric Association 1980) criteria, of only around 0.5% (Furmark 2002). This is considerably lower than the 2%–8% reported in studies in Western countries in which the same instrument and the same criteria were used (Furmark 2002). Of course, the data are far too scant at this stage for conclusions to be drawn, but if these data are supported, they may be consistent with the suggestion that social anxiety, as a personality style, is more common and more broadly accepted in Eastern cultures, thus resulting in less life interference and lower rates of "disorder" (Rapee and Spence 2004). Consistent with this suggestion, some studies have shown that parents in some Asian countries are considerably less distressed by their child's internalizing behaviors, relative to externalizing behaviors, whereas the reverse is true in Western countries (Weisz et al. 1987, 1988). Furthermore, in Eastern countries, childhood shyness predicts positive functioning in adolescence (Chen et al. 1999).

From a slightly different perspective, the form of anxious expression may vary across cultures. Again, most empirical comparison studies have focused on social reticence. DSM describes a disorder known as *Taijin Kyofusho* in Japanese (TK), which refers to a fear of social interactions due to concern about causing distress to another. In contrast, social phobia is characterized by a fear of negative evaluation of the self by another. Once again, comparisons across cultures are difficult; however, some research has suggested that symptoms of TK are reported more frequently in Japanese and Korean samples than in American or Australian populations (Kleinknecht et al. 1997). Certainly, clinical diagnoses of TK are rarely made in Western countries and are restricted to the occasional case study (Clarvit et al. 1996; McNally et al. 1990).

In the context of PTSD, there are intriguing differences between rates of acute stress disorder and PTSD in studies that have used comparable methodologies in different populations. For example, rates of PTSD after traumatic injury in Switzerland (Schnyder et al. 2001) are markedly lower than rates reported in Australia (Bryant and Harvey 1998; Harvey and Bryant 1998), England (J. Murray et al. 2002), or the United States (Blanchard et al. 1996). Similarly, a number of epidemiological surveys of refugee populations have found varied, and rather low, rates of PTSD (Silove 1999). These findings suggest that the prevalence and/or expression of PTSD vary markedly depending on the cultural context in which it is assessed.

A few other "culture-specific" forms of anxiety have been reported (Dobkin de Rios 1981; Guarnaccia 1993; Russell 1989; Sachdev 1990), but empirical evaluations and comparisons with Western notions of anxiety have not been systematic. It is likely that the underlying experience and influences on anxiety are a consistent human characteristic. However, the surface expression of anxiety, the subjective experience, and the ways in which anxiety interferes with daily functioning and thus becomes a disorder are likely to be at least partly influenced by cultural considerations.

Roles of Stressors

NONSPECIFIC LIFE EVENTS

Research into the onset of anxiety disorders after nonspecific stressful life events lags well behind similar research in areas such as mood disorders. This may be largely due to the chronicity of most anxiety disorders. It is difficult to consider or evaluate a role for acute life events in the case of continuing difficulties. The obvious exceptions are PTSD and panic disorder, both of which have relatively abrupt onsets. Life events are part of the definition of PTSD; hence, an association between stressors and immediate onset of this disorder is tautological and is thus not discussed further. A number of early studies have also reported large proportions of stressful life events in the lives of individuals with panic disorder in the period 1–12 months before experience of their first panic attack (de Loof et al. 1989; Manfro et al. 1996). Only a handful of these studies has included an appropriate comparison group, and results from these studies have been mixed (Pollard et al.

1989; Rapee et al. 1990; Roy-Byrne et al. 1986). However, one of the more detailed of the studies found a marked increase in stressful life events occurring in the 2 months prior to experience of the first panic attack (Faravelli 1985). Similar increased reports of stressful life events prior to onset of symptoms has been noted in the few studies of OCD (de Loof et al. 1989; McKeon et al. 1984).

Given the onset of many anxiety disorders during the early years, examination of stressful life events during childhood would appear to be warranted. Surprisingly little research of this kind has been conducted; however, a few studies have supported the suggestion that life events are associated with anxiety disorders in children and adolescents (Boer et al. 2002; Eley and Stevenson 2000; Goodyer 1990; Goodyer et al. 1990; Tiet et al. 2001). Importantly, research has also shown that the association between independent life events and symptoms of anxiety is a result of gene–environment interactions (Silberg et al. 2001). That is, the reaction to negative life events is influenced by genetic factors.

Consistent with this suggestion, life events that are shared between siblings appear to have a greater impact on the anxious child (Boer et al. 2002). Similarly, data from both child and adult studies show that it is the impact of life events that most clearly distinguishes anxious from nonclinical populations (Rapee et al. 1990; Roy-Byrne et al. 1986). Even in the area of PTSD, research has shown that some individuals are more vulnerable to the influences of trauma. For example, a recent study indexed the tendency of firefighters to catastrophize during their cadet training (i.e., prior to trauma exposure) and found that this predicted posttraumatic stress after they were subsequently exposed to traumatic events (Bryant and Guthrie 2005).

In addition to the literature reviewed, which has shown that nonspecific life events may act in the immediate term to trigger or precipitate an anxiety disorder, some research has examined the question of whether early experiences with stressors may increase an individual's vulnerability to later anxiety. Some animal research has shown that early experience with a highly controllable environment leads to greater confidence later in development (Mineka et al. 1986) and lower levels of plasma cortisol (Insel et al. 1988). However, the specificity of these observations to anxiety disorders seems unclear, and it is more likely that early experience with an uncontrollable environment increases vulnerability to any neurotic disorder (Alloy et al. 1990; Chorpita and Barlow 1998).

SPECIFIC ENVIRONMENTAL EVENTS

Apart from PTSD, differences in the association between life events and specific anxiety disorders, anxiety, or other disorders have received little attention. Some research has suggested that anxiety is associated with stressors related to threats or dangers, whereas depression is more strongly associated with losses (Eley and Stevenson 2000; Finlay-Jones and Brown 1981). Other research has suggested that, in childhood, separation anxiety disorder is more strongly associated with life events than are other anxiety disorders (Chaffin et al. 2005; Rapee and Szollos 2003; Tiet et al. 2001). Investigations of specific types of life events and their associations with specific anxiety disorders in adults have typically shown inconsistent results (Pollard et al. 1989; Rapee et al. 1990; Roy-Byrne et al. 1986). The one disorder that stands out in this respect is PTSD, in which there is a reliable dosage effect between the likelihood of PTSD development and the severity of the threat (March 1993).

PEER VICTIMIZATION

A number of studies have shown that experiences of teasing and bullying are associated with increases in anxiety as well as depression (Hawker and Boulton 2000). A few longitudinal studies have also demonstrated that the direction of relationship is at least partly from victimization to symptoms (Bond et al. 2001). Most focus has been specifically on social anxiety (Storch and Masia-Warner 2004), and it is possible that this is one of the few specific environment–disorder relationships. In the clinical literature, some retrospective reports have indicated a greater history of victimization during childhood in adults with social phobia than in those without disorder or those with other anxiety disorders (McCabe et al. 2003). However, considerably more longitudinal research, particularly examining the issue of specificity, is required before this relationship can be confirmed.

SPECIFIC LEARNING EXPERIENCES

The best example of specific environmental events leading to particular disorders comes from the conditioning literature. In brief, theoretical models have suggested that some fear reactions and phobias develop on the basis of the association between specific negative experiences and previously innocuous—although highly specific—stimuli (Bouton et al. 2001; Mineka and Zinbarg 1995; Ohman 1993; Rachman 1977). Although a wealth of animal and human laboratory data exist to support the processes of these models, most of the evidence for this assertion in human clinical conditions is based on retrospective introspection. Consequently, some theoretical papers have argued against associative accounts of phobias (Menzies and Clarke 1994, 1995), and at least some carefully collected longitudinal evidence is inconsistent with associative notions (Poulton et al. 1998, 2001). Given that a more detailed account of this issue is provided in Chapter 5 ("Continuity and Etiology of Anxiety Disorders") of this volume, the issue is not discussed further here.

Family Factors

Given the wealth of research into the roles of family factors in the development of all areas of psychopathology and the considerable controversy this issue has generated (Hudson and Rapee 2005), a brief discussion of this area in the development of anxiety disorders is warranted.

FAMILY DISRUPTION

There have been some suggestions that family disruption may characterize anxious populations, although specificity to anxiety is unlikely. An early but small study reported a greater degree of severe family disruption in people with panic disorder relative to those with GAD (Raskin et al. 1982). More detailed examination has shown that women with a range of anxiety disorders, including panic disorder, social phobia, and GAD, reported higher-than-average levels of early family adversity, including physical and sexual abuse or parental neglect (Brown and Harris 1993). Similarly, there have been some suggestions from studies with relatively large cohorts that anxiety may be associated with paternal violence and maternal separation (Fergusson and Horwood 1998; Kendler et al. 1992a).

CHILDHOOD SEXUAL ABUSE

Several studies have reported associations between a history of sexual abuse during childhood and later anxiety disorders (Burnam et al. 1988; McCauley et al. 1997), although the link with anxiety is clearly not specific, because childhood sexual abuse is associated with a range of psychopathology (Fergusson et al. 1996). Naturally, a number of confounds exist in most studies, including perceptual distortions over time; possible lack of specificity; associated features, such as violence and family disruption; and existing prior issues, such as preexisting anxiety, poor family functioning, or low socioeconomic status.

In a prospective study in which several of these factors were measured and statistically controlled, 1,433 10- to 16-year-old youths were contacted 15 months apart (Boney-McCoy and Finkelhor 1996). Even after several preexisting factors were controlled for, new cases of sexual abuse were associated with onset of PTSD. In a more recent study, 158 sexually abused children (ages 6–13 years) and their parents were interviewed to obtain lifetime-experience histories of several anxiety disorders (separation anxiety disorder, overanxious disorder, obsessions, compulsions, phobias, and PTSD), and ages of onset for each disorder were carefully assessed (Chaffin et al. 2005). Plots of annual hazard rates showed a clear association between onset of all anxiety disorders and commencement of sexual abuse. Effects were especially strong for PTSD, separation anxiety, and phobias.

Interestingly, reduction in anxiety disorders was also associated with offset of sexual abuse, which simultaneously supports the causal status of sexual abuse in the production of anxiety but also questions its role in chronic anxiety disorders. It is important to note that although the relationship between childhood sexual abuse and adult psychopathology has been noted, there is also evidence that this is not a linear relationship, that many abused children do not develop psychopathological states, and that one's parental environment appears to be a more powerful influence on adult psychopathology than childhood sexual abuse (Kendall-Tackett et al. 1993; Rind et al. 1998).

PARENT–CHILD INTERACTION

A tremendous amount of retrospective research has pointed to an association between specific styles of parenting and adult anxiety disorders (Gerlsma et al. 1990; Rapee 1997). The limitations of this research are obvious and include self-reported recollections of perceived parenting from current patients some 20–30 years after parental influence has ceased. Nevertheless, the sheer volume of the research and the apparent consistency across many of the studies indicate that some interesting factors are at work. Whether this includes a causal role for parental styles has yet to be determined.

In general, the research indicates that parental styles characterized by overprotective behaviors and, possibly, negative and critical parental attitudes are associated with anxiety. However, the specificity of these relationships is unclear, because similar relationships have been shown between these parenting styles and depression, as well as for several other disorders (Rapee 1997). More recent research has moved to the laboratory—with its attendant limitations—and has shown that parents of clinically anxious children interact with their child in a more intrusive and protective manner than do parents of nonclinical children (Hudson and Rapee 2001, 2002; Moore et al. 2004; Wood et al. 2003). Similar research has also shown that negativity is characteristic of the parent–child interactions of parents who themselves have an anxiety disorder (Whaley et al. 1999), and that overprotection is displayed by mothers of anxious children equally to their clinically anxious child and to his or her sibling (Hudson and Rapee 2002), suggesting that the parents' own anxiety may be partly responsible for these effects.

In an attempt to disentangle some of these effects, 62 mothers of children who had anxiety disorders and 60 mothers of children without disorders interacted in the preparation of a speech (Hudson et al., in press). On one occasion each mother interacted with a child with an anxiety disorder, and on another occasion each mother interacted with a child without a disorder. Mothers in both groups were more protective of anxious children who were not their own, suggesting that anxiety in a child can elicit overprotective parenting. However, mothers of anxious children were especially positive when interacting with a nonanxious child who was not their own, suggesting that warmth in the relationship may be a result of an interaction between mother and child characteristics. As mentioned earlier, very little of this work has indicated causal status of the relationship.

In examining the role of overprotection longitudinally, two studies from the same laboratory have indicated conflicting findings. In the first, 60 toddlers were followed from ages 2 to 4 years, and ratings of shyness and parenting were taken from their parents at each time point (Rubin et al. 1999). Parents' reports of their child's shyness at age 2 predicted parents' lack of encouragement of independence of their child at age 4, but the reverse was not demonstrated. However, in a later study, observational measures were used to determine toddler inhibition (ages 2 and 4) as well as parent overprotection and negativity (Rubin et al. 2002). Results showed an interaction between temperament and parenting—inhibition at age 2 predicted shyness at age 4, but only in the presence of either overprotective or negative parenting.

Importantly, with respect to nosological considerations, there have been few indications of differences between specific anxiety disorders in parent–child interactions, although some hints from retrospective studies in adults have suggested that more consistent associations may be observed in socially anxious individuals than in other forms of anxiety (Rapee 1997).

ATTACHMENT STYLES

Another literature that is highly related to the previously described studies of parent–child interaction is found in research into the construct of attachment. The attachment literature provides the advantage of well-developed and highly standardized laboratory observations of child reactions applicable very early in development (Ungerer and McMahon 2005). Unfortunately, this very early stage of application means that very few attachment studies have examined the influence of attachment style on the development of diagnosed anxiety disorders. Nevertheless, using somewhat less reliable questionnaire and retrospective measures, several studies have shown associations between insecure attachment styles and anxiety disorders in children, adolescents, and adults (Gar et al. 2005). In one of the few laboratory studies that included diagnoses, it was shown that anxiety disorders in 4- to 5-year-old children were cross-sectionally predicted by an insecure style of attachment (Shamir-Essakow et al. 2005). This relationship held even when controlling for inhibited temperament and mothers' trait anxiety. In the only long-term study, S.L. Warren et al. (1997) found that anxious/resistant attachment at 12 months of age predicted anxiety disorders at age 17 after control for infant temperament and mothers' anxiety.

MODELING AND INFORMATION TRANSMISSION

Numerous theoretical and popular perspectives have assumed that part of the development of fears and phobias comes from observation and other information about potential dangers from external sources (Muris et al. 1996; Ollendick and King 1991; Rachman 1977). More popular views assume that much of this learning comes from parental influence. However, empirical demonstration of any such relationship is currently far from conclusive and may, in fact, be impossible to establish given the likely subtlety of this type of effect. The understanding that fears can be learned at a very young age via observation is beginning to be established, but the causal nature of such a relationship is still far from certain. In one study, 15- to 20-month-old toddlers showed fearful reactions and avoidance of a toy snake or spider up to 10 minutes after their mothers reacted negatively to the same object (Gerull and Rapee 2002). A later replication demonstrated a similar effect when a stranger (the experimenter) reacted negatively to the toy snake or spider (Egliston and Rapee 2007). However, when the infant's mother had previously reacted positively to that same object, fearful reactions were prevented. Some interesting data have shown similar patterns with socially relevant information: infants have been shown to react more fearfully to a stranger after watching their mother react negatively with that person (de Rosnay et al. 2006). Infants of mothers with social phobia have also been shown to display greater increase in fear of a stranger over time than control infants, but only when their mothers displayed overt anxiety to that stranger.

Finally, a few retrospective studies have suggested an association between early observation of parental sick-role behaviors, as well as parental encouragement of sick-role behaviors, and later experience of panic attacks (Ehlers 1993; Stewart et al. 2001; Watt et al. 1998). Some suggestion of specificity was shown in all three studies, in that panic attacks were only associated with parental modeling related specifically to symptoms of arousal and not to other nonarousal symptoms.

One adoption study has been conducted of relevance to anxiety and provided data suggesting clear contribution of an environmental factor that is most likely shared (Daniels and Plomin 1985). In predicting levels of shyness in adopted infants, significant relationships were demonstrated between levels of infants' shyness and the sociability of their adoptive mothers. The mechanisms for this effect are not clear, but it is possible that either modeling from mother to infant or direct learning/habituation by the infant may be involved.

DISTAL AND PROXIMAL CAUSES

This review has highlighted the differing roles of distal and proximal causes that can contribute to a specific anxiety disorder. Whereas *distal causes* are those that are temporally distant from the onset of the anxiety disorder, *proximal causes* are those that trigger the disorder and immediately precede the disorder onset. It is important to distinguish between these two types of causes because distal causes tend to represent vulnerability factors, and proximal causes act as precipitants. Proximal causes may have a stronger relationship with the onset of some anxiety disorders (e.g., PTSD) than others (e.g., social phobia). Also, it is likely that whereas proximal causes may permit some specificity between anxiety disorders and the stressor that triggers it (e.g., PTSD), it is more probable that distal causes are associated with anxiety generally rather than a specific anxiety disorder. It is also important to recognize that diathesis-stress models posit an interaction between distal and proximal causes, in which case the vulnerability may become operational once the individual is exposed to sufficient stress.

Conclusion

It is highly unlikely that anxiety is a purely genetic condition. Hence, some influence from the environment must be assumed and is supported by behavior genetic research. The form of that environmental influence is unclear from twin studies but may differ across the developmental span, with a greater influence from shared environmental factors earlier in development and a dominant influence from individual environmental factors in the expression of adult anxiety. Twin studies are also largely consistent with a general neurotic influence, attributed to genetic factors, and thus it is logical to suggest that differentiation between anxiety disorders may be more attributable to environmental influence. Although several environmental factors are beginning to amass greater evidence, it is still far too early either to assign causality to any specific factors or to determine specific links between environmental factors and specific disorders. From a DSM perspective, it is clearly too soon to determine diagnostic criteria based on causal environmental factors.

References

Alloy LB, Kelly KA, Mineka S, et al: Comorbidity of anxiety and depressive disorders: a helplessness-hopelessness perspective, in Comorbidity of Mood and Anxiety Disorders. Edited by Maser JD, Cloninger CR. Washington, DC, American Psychiatric Press, 1990, pp 499–543

American Psychiatric Association: Diagnostic and Statistical Manual of Mental Disorders, 3rd Edition. Washington, DC, American Psychiatric Association, 1980

Andrews G, Hall W, Teesson M, et al: The Mental Health of Australians. Canberra, Australia, Commonwealth Department of Health and Aged Care, 1999

Blanchard EB, Hickling EJ, Barton KA, et al: One-year prospective follow-up of motor vehicle accident victims. Behav Res Ther 34:775–786, 1996

Boer F, Markus MT, Maingay R, et al: Negative life events of anxiety disordered children: bad fortune, vulnerability, or reporter bias? Child Psychiatry Hum Devel 32:187–199, 2002

Bond L, Carlin JB, Thomas L, et al: Does bullying cause emotional problems? A prospective study of young teenagers. BMJ 323:480–484, 2001

Boney-McCoy S, Finkelhor D: Is youth victimization related to trauma symptoms and depression after controlling for prior symptoms and family relationships? A longitudinal prospective study. J Consult Clin Psychol 64:1406–1416, 1996

Bouton ME, Mineka S, Barlow DH: A modern learning perspective on the etiology of panic disorder. Psychol Rev 108:4–32, 2001

Brown GW, Harris TO: Aetiology of anxiety and depressive disorders in an inner-city population, 1: early adversity. Psychol Med 23:143–154, 1993

Bryant RA, Guthrie RM: Maladaptive appraisals as a risk factor for posttraumatic stress: a study of trainee firefighters. Psychol Sci 16:749–752, 2005

Bryant RA, Harvey AG: Relationship of acute stress disorder and posttraumatic stress disorder following mild traumatic brain injury. Am J Psychiatry 155:625–629, 1998

Burnam MA, Stein JA, Golding JM, et al: Sexual assault and mental disorders in a community population. J Consult Clin Psychol 56:843–850, 1988

Chaffin M, Silovsky JF, Vaughn C: Temporal concordance of anxiety disorders and child sexual abuse: implications for direct versus artifactual effects of sexual abuse. J Clin Child Adolesc Psychol 34:210–222, 2005

Chen X, Rubin KH, Li B, et al: Adolescent outcomes of social functioning in Chinese children. Int J Behav Dev 23:199–223, 1999

Chorpita BF, Barlow DH: The development of anxiety: the role of control in the early environment. Psychol Bull 124:3–21, 1998

Clarvit SR, Schneier FR, Liebowitz MR: The offensive subtype of Taijin-Kyofu-Sho in New York City: the phenomenology and treatment of a social anxiety disorder. J Clin Psychiatry 57:523–527, 1996

Cronk NJ, Slutske WS, Madden PAF, et al: Risk for separation anxiety disorder among girls: paternal absence, socioeconomic disadvantage, and genetic vulnerability. J Abnorm Psychol 113:237–247, 2004

Daniels D, Plomin R: Origins of individual differences in infant shyness. Dev Psychol 21:118–121, 1985

de Loof C, Zandbergen J, Lousberg H, et al: The role of life events in the onset of panic disorder. Behav Res Ther 27:461–463, 1989

de Rosnay M, Cooper PJ, Tsigaras N, et al: Transmission of social anxiety from mother to infant: an experimental study using a social referencing paradigm. Behav Res Ther 44:1165–1175, 2006

Dobkin de Rios M: Saladerra: a culture-bound misfortune syndrome in the Peruvian Amazon. Cult Med Psychiatry 5:193–213, 1981

Egliston K-A, Rapee RM: Inhibition of fear acquisition in toddlers following positive modelling by their mothers. Behav Res Ther 45:1871–1882, 2007

Ehlers A: Somatic symptoms and panic attacks: a retrospective study of learning experiences. Behav Res Ther 31:269–278, 1993

Eley TC: Behavioral genetics as a tool for developmental psychology: anxiety and depression in children and adolescents. Clin Child Fam Psychol Rev 2:21–36, 1999

Eley TC, Lau JYF: Genetics and the family environment, in Psychopathology and the Family. Edited by Hudson JL, Rapee RM. Oxford, UK, Pergamon/Elsevier, 2005, pp 3–19

Eley TC, Stevenson J: Specific life events and chronic experiences differentially associated with depression and anxiety in young twins. J Abnorm Child Psychol 28:383–394, 2000

Faravelli C: Life events preceding the onset of panic disorder. J Affect Disord 9:103–105, 1985

Fava GA, Grandi S, Canestrari R: Prodromal symptoms in panic disorder with agoraphobia. Am J Psychiatry 145:1564–1567, 1988

Fergusson DM, Horwood LJ: Exposure to interparental violence in childhood and psychosocial adjustment in young adulthood. Child Abuse Negl 22:339–357, 1998

Fergusson DM, Horwood LJ, Lynskey MT: Childhood sexual abuse and psychiatric disorder in young adulthood, II: psychiatric outcomes of childhood sexual abuse. J Am Acad Child Adolesc Psychiatry 34:1365–1374, 1996

Finlay-Jones R, Brown GW: Types of stressful life event and the onset of anxiety and depressive disorders. Psychol Med 11:803–815, 1981

Furmark T: Social phobia: overview of community surveys. Acta Psychiatr Scand 105:84–93, 2002

Fyer AJ, Mannuzza S, Chapman TF, et al: Specificity in familial aggregation of phobic disorders. Arch Gen Psychiatry 52:564–573, 1995

Gar NS, Hudson JL, Rapee RM: Family factors and the development of anxiety disorders, in Psychopathology and the Family. Edited by Hudson JL, Rapee RM. Oxford, United Kingdom, Elsevier, 2005, pp 125–145

Gater R, Tansella M, Korten A, et al: Sex differences in the prevalence and detection of depressive and anxiety disorders in general health care settings. Arch Gen Psychiatry 55:405–413, 1998

Gavranidou M, Rosner R: The weaker sex? Gender and post-traumatic stress disorder. Depress Anxiety 17:130–139, 2003

Gerlsma C, Emmelkamp PMG, Arrindell WA: Anxiety, depression and perception of early parenting: a meta-analysis. Clin Psychol Rev 10:251–277, 1990

Gerull FC, Rapee RM: Mother knows best: effects of maternal modelling on the acquisition of fear and avoidance behaviour in toddlers. Behav Res Ther 40:279–287, 2002

Goodyer IM: Recent life events and psychiatric disorder in school age children. J Child Psychol Psychiatry 31:839–848, 1990

Goodyer IM, Wright C, Altham P: The friendships and recent life events of anxious and depressed school-age children. Br J Psychiatry 156:689–698, 1990

Guarnaccia PJ: Ataques de nervios in Puerto Rico: culture-bound syndrome or popular illness? Med Anthropol 15:157–170, 1993

Hankin BL, Abramson LY, Silva PA, et al: Development of depression from preadolescence to young adulthood: emerging gender differences in a 10-year longitudinal study. J Abnorm Psychol 107:128–140, 1998

Harvey AG, Bryant RA: Relationship of acute stress disorder and posttraumatic stress disorder following motor vehicle accidents. J Consult Clin Psychol 66:507–512, 1998

Hawker DSJ, Boulton MJ: Twenty years' research on peer victimization and psychosocial maladjustment: a meta-analytic review of cross-sectional studies. J Child Psychol Psychiatry 41:441–455, 2000

Heinrichs N, Rapee RM, Alden LA, et al: Cultural differences in perceived social norms and social anxiety. Behav Res Ther 44:1187–1197, 2006

Hettema JM, Neale MC, Kendler KS: A review and meta-analysis of the genetic epidemiology of anxiety disorders. Am J Psychiatry 158:1568–1578, 2001

Hirshfeld-Becker DR, Biederman J, Faraone SV, et al: Lack of association between behavioral inhibition and psychosocial adversity factors in children at risk for anxiety disorders. Am J Psychiatry 161:547–555, 2004

Hudson JL, Rapee RM: Parent–child interactions and anxiety disorders: an observational study. Behav Res Ther 39:1411–1427, 2001

Hudson JL, Rapee RM: Parent–child interactions in clinically anxious children and their siblings J Clin Child Adolesc Psychol 31:548–555, 2002

Hudson JL, Rapee RM (eds): Psychopathology and the Family. Oxford, UK, Pergamon/Elsevier, 2005

Hudson JL, Doyle A, Gar NS: Child and maternal influence on parenting behavior in clinically anxious children. J Clin Child Adolesc Psychol (in press)

Insel TR, Hoover C, Murphy DL: Parents of patients with obsessive-compulsive disorder. Psychol Med 13:807–811, 1983

Insel TR, Scanlan J, Champoux M, et al: Rearing paradigm in a nonhuman primate affects response to B-CCE challenge. Psychopharmacology (Berl) 96:81–86, 1988

Keller MB, Lavori PW, Wunder J, et al: Chronic course of anxiety disorders in children and adolescents. J Am Acad Child Adolesc Psychiatry 31:595–599, 1992

Kendall-Tackett KA, Williams L, Finkelhor D: Impact of sexual abuse on children: a review and synthesis of recent empirical studies. Psychol Bull 113:164–180, 1993

Kendler KS, Heath A, Martin NG, et al: Symptoms of anxiety and symptoms of depression: same genes, different environments? Arch Gen Psychiatry 44:451–457, 1987

Kendler KS, Neale MC, Kessler RC, et al: Childhood parental loss and adult psychopathology in women: a twin study perspective. Arch Gen Psychiatry 49:109–116, 1992a

Kendler KS, Neale MC, Kessler RC, et al: The genetic epidemiology of phobias in women: the interrelationship of agoraphobia, social phobia, situational phobia and simple phobia. Arch Gen Psychiatry 49:273–281, 1992b

Kendler KS, Walters EE, Neale M, et al: The structure of the genetic and environmental risk factors for six major psychiatric disorders in women: phobia, generalized anxiety disorder, panic disorder, bulimia, major depression, and alcoholism. Arch Gen Psychiatry 52:374–383, 1995

Kendler KS, Myers J, Prescott CA, et al: The genetic epidemiology of irrational fears and phobias in men. Arch Gen Psychiatry 58:257–265, 2001

Kerr M, Lambert WW, Stattin H, et al: Stability of inhibition in a Swedish longitudinal sample. Child Dev 65:138–146, 1994

Kessler RC, McGonagle KA, Zhao S, et al: Lifetime and 12-month prevalence of DSM-III-R psychiatric disorders in the United States: results from the national comorbidity survey. Arch Gen Psychiatry 5:18–19, 1994

King NJ, Gullone E, Tonge BJ, et al: Self-reports of panic attacks and manifest anxiety in adolescents. Behav Res Ther 31:111–116, 1993

Kleinknecht RA, Dinnel DL, Kleinknecht EE: Cultural factors in social anxiety: a comparison of social phobia symptoms and Taijin Kyofusho. J Anxiety Disord 11:157–177, 1997

Klonsky BG, Dutton DL, Liebel CL: Developmental antecedents of private self-consciousness, public self-consciousness and social anxiety. Genet Soc Gen Psychol Monogr 116:273–297, 1990

Kroes M, Kalff AC, Steyaert J, et al: A longitudinal community study: do psychosocial risk factors and Child Behavior Checklist scores at 5 years of age predict psychiatric diagnoses at a later age? J Am Acad Child Adolesc Psychiatry 41:955–963, 2002

Last CG, Phillips JE, Statfeld A: Childhood anxiety disorders in mothers and their children. Child Psychiatry Hum Dev 18:103–112, 1987

Lewinsohn PM, Zinbarg R, Seeley JR, et al: Lifetime comorbidity among anxiety disorders and between anxiety disorders and other mental disorders in adolescents. J Anxiety Disord 11:377–394, 1997

Manfro GG, Otto MW, McArdle ET, et al: Relationship of antecedent stressful life events to childhood and family history of anxiety and the course of panic disorder. J Affect Disord 41:135–139, 1996

March JS: The stressor criterion in DSM-IV posttraumatic stress disorder, in Posttraumatic Stress Disorder in Review: Recent Research and Future Developments. Edited by Davidson JR, Foa EB. Washington, DC, American Psychiatric Press, 1993, pp 37–54

Massion AO, Warshaw MG, Keller MB: Quality of life and psychiatric morbidity in panic disorder and generalized anxiety disorder. Am J Psychiatry 150:600–607, 1993

Massion AO, Dyck IR, Shea MT, et al: Personality disorders and time to remission in generalized anxiety disorder, social phobia, and panic disorder. Arch Gen Psychiatry 59:434–440, 2002

McCabe RE, Antony MM, Summerfelt LJ: Preliminary examination of the relationship between anxiety disorders in adults and self-reported history of teasing or bullying experiences. Cogn Behav Ther 32:187–193, 2003

McCauley J, Kern DE, Kolodner K, et al: Clinical characteristics of women with a history of childhood abuse: unhealed wounds. JAMA 277:1362–1368, 1997

McKeon J, Roa B, Mann A: Life events and personality traits in obsessive-compulsive neurosis. Br J Psychiatry 144:185–189, 1984

McNally RJ, Cassiday KL, Calamari JE: Taijin-kyofu-sho in a Black American woman: behavioral treatment of a "culture-bound" anxiety disorder. J Anxiety Disord 4:83–87, 1990

Menzies RG, Clarke JC: Retrospective studies of the origins of phobias: a review. Anxiety Stress Coping 7:305–318, 1994

Menzies RG, Clarke JC: The etiology of phobias: a nonassociative account. Clin Psychol Rev 15:23–48, 1995

Mineka S, Zinbarg R: Conditioning and ethological models of social phobia, in Social Phobia: Diagnosis, Assessment and Treatment. Edited by Heimberg RG, Liebowitz MR, Hope DA, et al. New York, Guilford, 1995, pp 134–162

Mineka S, Gunnar M, Champoux M: Control and early socioemotional development: infant rhesus monkeys reared in controllable versus uncontrollable environments. Child Dev 57:1241–1256, 1986

Moore PS, Whaley SE, Sigman M: Interactions between mothers and children: impacts of maternal and child anxiety. J Abnorm Psychol 113:471–476, 2004

Muris P, Steerneman P, Merckelbach H, et al: The role of parental fearfulness and modeling in children's fear. Behav Res Ther 34:265–268, 1996

Murray J, Ehlers A, Mayou RA: Dissociation and post-traumatic stress disorder: two prospective studies of road traffic accident survivors. Br J Psychiatry 180:363–368, 2002

Murray L, de Rosnay M, Pearson J, et al: Intergenerational transmission of social anxiety: the role of social referencing processes in infancy. Child Dev 79:1049–1064

Norton GR, McLeod L, Guertin J, et al: Panic disorder or social phobia: which is worse? Behav Res Ther 34:273–276, 1996

Noyes JR, Clarkson C, Crowe RR, et al: A family study of generalized anxiety disorder. Am J Psychiatry 144:1019–1024, 1987

Ohman A: Fear and anxiety as emotional phenomena: clinical phenomenology, evolutionary perspectives, and information processing mechanisms, in Handbook of Emotions. Edited by Lewis M, Haviland JM. New York, Guilford, 1993, pp 511–536

Ollendick TH, King NJ: Origins of childhood fears: an evaluation of Rachman's theory of fear acquisition. Behav Res Ther 29:117–123, 1991

Ost LG: Age of onset in different phobias. J Abnorm Psychol 96:223–229, 1987

Pickersgill MJ, Valentine JD, May R, et al: Fears in mental retardation, I: types of fears reported by men and women with and without mental retardation. Advances in Behaviour Research and Therapy 16:277–296, 1994

Pollard CA, Pollard HJ, Corn KJ: Panic onset and major events in the lives of agoraphobics: a test of contiguity. J Abnorm Psychol 98:318–321, 1989

Poulton R, Davies S, Menzies RG, et al: Evidence for a non-associative model of the acquisition of a fear of heights. Behav Res Ther 36:537–544, 1998

Poulton R, Milne BJ, Craske MG, et al: A longitudinal study of the etiology of separation anxiety. Behav Res Ther 39:1395–1410, 2001

Prior M: Childhood temperament. J Child Psychol Psychiatry 33:249–279, 1992

Rachman S: The conditioning theory of fear acquisition: a critical examination. Behav Res Ther 15:375–387, 1977

Rapee R: Distinctions between panic disorder and generalised anxiety disorder: clinical presentation. Aust N Z J Psychiatry 19:227–232, 1985

Rapee R: Potential role of childrearing practices in the development of anxiety and depression. Clin Psychol Rev 17:47–67, 1997

Rapee RM, Melville LF: Retrospective recall of family factors in social phobia and panic disorder. Depress Anxiety 5:7–11, 1997

Rapee RM, Spence SH: The etiology of social phobia: empirical evidence and an initial model. Clin Psychol Rev 24:737–767, 2004

Rapee RM, Szollos AA: Developmental antecedents of clinical anxiety in childhood. Behav Change 19:146–157, 2003

Rapee R, Litwin EM, Barlow DH: Impact of life events on subjects with panic disorder and on comparison subjects. Am J Psychiatry 147:640–644, 1990

Raskin M, Peeke HVS, Dickman W, et al: Panic and generalized anxiety disorders. Arch Gen Psychiatry 39:687–689, 1982

Rind B, Tromovitch P, Bauserman R: A meta-analytic examination of assumed properties of child sexual abuse using college samples. Psychol Bull 124:22–53, 1998

Roy-Byrne PP, Geraci M, Uhde TW: Life events and the onset of panic disorder. Am J Psychiatry 143:1424–1427, 1986

Rubin KH, Nelson LJ, Hastings P, et al: The transaction between parents' perceptions of their children's shyness and their parenting styles. Int J Behav Dev 23:937–957, 1999

Rubin KH, Burgess KB, Hastings PD: Stability and social-behavioral consequences of toddlers' inhibited temperament and parenting behaviors. Child Dev 73:483–495, 2002

Russell JG: Anxiety disorders in Japan: a review of the Japanese literature on Shinkeishitsu and Taijinkyofusho. Cult Med Psychiatry 13:391–403, 1989

Sachdev PS: Whakama: Culturally determined behaviour in the New Zealand Maori. Psychol Med 20:433–444, 1990

Schmidt NB, Lerew DR, Jackson RJ: The role of anxiety sensitivity in the pathogenesis of panic: prospective evaluation of spontaneous panic attacks during acute stress. J Abnorm Psychol 106:355–364, 1997

Schnyder U, Moergeli H, Klaghofer R, et al: Incidence and prediction of posttraumatic stress disorder symptoms in severely injured accident victims. Am J Psychiatry 158:594–599, 2001

Schneier FR, Johnson J, Hornig CD, et al: Social phobia: comorbidity and morbidity in an epidemiologic sample. Arch Gen Psychiatry 49:282–288, 1992

Shamir-Essakow G, Ungerer JA, Rapee RM: Attachment, behavioral inhibition, and anxiety in preschool children. J Abnorm Child Psychol 33:131–143, 2005

Silberg J, Rutter M, Neale M, et al: Genetic moderation of environmental risk for depression and anxiety in adolescent girls. Br J Psychiatry 179:116–121, 2001

Silove DM: The psychosocial effects of torture, mass human rights violations, and refugee trauma: toward an integrated conceptual framework. J Nerv Ment Dis 187:200–207, 1999

Stein MB, Kean YM: Disability and quality of life in social phobia: epidemiologic findings. Am J Psychiatry 157:1606–1613, 2000

Steketee G, Grayson JB, Foa EB: A comparison of characteristics of obsessive-compulsive disorder and other anxiety disorders. J Anxiety Disord 1:325–335, 1987

Stevenson J, Batten N, Cherner M: Fears and fearfulness in children and adolescents: a genetic analysis of twin data. J Child Psychol Psychiatry 33:977–985, 1992

Stewart SH, Taylor S, Jang KL, et al: Causal modeling of relations among learning history, anxiety sensitivity, and panic attacks. Behav Res Ther 39:443–456, 2001

Storch EA, Masia-Warner C: The relationship of peer victimization to social anxiety and loneliness in adolescent females. J Adolesc 27:351–362, 2004

Thapar A, McGuffin P: Are anxiety symptoms in childhood heritable? J Child Psychol Psychiatry 36:439–447, 1995

Tiet QQ, Bird HR, Hoven CW, et al: Relationship between specific adverse life events and psychiatric disorders. J Abnorm Child Psychol 2:153–164, 2001

Topolski TD, Hewitt JK, Eaves L, et al: Genetic and environmental influences on child reports of manifest anxiety and symptoms of separation anxiety and overanxious disorders: a community-based twin study. Behav Genet 27:15–28, 1997

Ungerer JA, McMahon C: Attachment and psychopathology: a lifespan perspective, in Psychopathology and the Family. Edited by Hudson JL, Rapee RM. Oxford, United Kingdom, Elsevier, 2005, pp 35–52

Warren JM, Levy SJ: Fearfulness in female and male cats. Anim Learn Behav 7:521–524, 1979

Warren SL, Huston L, Egeland B, et al: Child and adolescent anxiety disorders and early attachment. J Am Acad Child Adolesc Psychiatry 36:637–644, 1997

Watt MC, Stewart SH, Cox BJ: A retrospective study of the learning history origins of anxiety sensitivity. Behav Res Ther 36:505–525, 1998

Weich S, Sloggett A, Lewis G: Social roles and the gender difference in rates of the common mental disorders in Britain: a 7-year population-based cohort study. Psychol Med 31:1055–1064, 2001

Weisz JR, Suwanlert S, Chaiyasit W, et al: Over- and undercontrolled referral problems among children and adolescents from Thailand and the United States: the Wat and Wai of cultural differences. J Consult Clin Psychol 55:719–726, 1987

Weisz JR, Suwanlert S, Chaiyasit W, et al: Thai and American perspectives on over- and undercontrolled child behavior problems: exploring the threshold model among parents, teachers, and psychologists. J Consult Clin Psychol 56:601–609, 1988

Whaley SE, Pinto A, Sigman M: Characterizing interactions between anxious mothers and their children. J Consult Clin Psychol 67:826–836, 1999

Wittchen HU, Stein MB, Kessler RC: Social fears and social phobia in a community sample of adolescents and young adults: prevalence, risk factors and co-morbidity. Psychol Med 29:309–323, 1999

Wood JJ, McLeod BD, Sigman M, et al: Parenting and childhood anxiety: theory, empirical findings, and future directions. J Child Psychol Psychiatry 44:134–151, 2003

Xue Y, Leventhal T, Brooks-Gunn J, et al: Neighborhood residence and mental health problems of 5- to 11-year-olds. Arch Gen Psychiatry 62:554–563, 2005

Zhengyan W, Huichang C, Xinyin C: The stability of children's behavioral inhibition: a longitudinal study from two to four years of age. Acta Psychologica Sinica 35:93–100, 2003

Zimbardo PG: Shyness: What It Is and What to Do About It. Sydney, Australia, Addison-Wesley, 1977

12

NEUROIMAGING AND NEUROANATOMY OF STRESS-INDUCED AND FEAR CIRCUITRY DISORDERS

Scott L. Rauch, M.D.
Wayne C. Drevets, M.D.

Phenomenology of Stress-Induced and Fear Circuitry Disorders

Other chapters in this volume provide a more detailed account of the clinical factors that weigh in favor of specific definitions of diagnoses, as well as their grouping within broader diagnostic categories. One premise of this enterprise has been that the current grouping of conditions as "anxiety disorders" is suboptimal. Specifically, it has been proposed that a subset of the current diagnostic entities within the anxiety disorders be reconstituted beneath the rubric of "stress-induced and fear circuitry disorders," based on etiological and pathophysiological considerations, whereas other anxiety disorder diagnoses might be repositioned in association with conditions already outside the anxiety disorder category.

The tentatively proposed scheme includes the following conditions among the stress-induced and fear circuitry disorders: posttraumatic stress disorder (PTSD), panic disorder, specific phobia, and social anxiety disorder (SocAD; also called *social phobia*). Other diagnostic entities, including acute stress disorder and agoraphobia, are not a focus of this section, although their respective links to PTSD and panic disorder make it likely that they will ultimately be included under the same rubric. In contrast, several other conditions have been intentionally and explicitly excluded—for example, generalized anxiety disorder (which might be better conceptualized as associated with major affective disorders) and obsessive-compulsive disorder (OCD, which might be better conceptualized as part of a group of "obsessive-compulsive spectrum disorders," including body dysmorphic disorder, trichotillomania, and Tourette disorder). Consequently, issues of specificity are especially germane, if support is to be found for the proposed scheme, in terms of excluding these entities previously included in the anxiety disorder category. In this context, we wish to note that the goals and benefits of grouping diagnoses within categories are somewhat less clear than are the goals and benefits of having specific diagnoses and operational diagnostic criteria that define them.

Anxiety and fear are normal human emotional states, and as is the case with a broader array of stress responses, these presumably serve adaptive functions. In contrast, anxiety disorders, as currently conceptualized, represent one category of psychiatric syndromes that is characterized by maladaptive anxiety symptoms that cause distress and impair function (American Psychiatric Association 2000).

POSTTRAUMATIC STRESS DISORDER

PTSD is one of few psychiatric conditions for which the etiology is nominally defined. In PTSD, individuals evolve a constellation of symptoms in the aftermath of a severe emotionally traumatic event. The cardinal features of PTSD include reexperiencing phenomena (e.g., flashbacks that can occur spontaneously or in response to reminders of the traumatic event); avoidance (e.g., avoiding situations that remind the individual of the traumatic event); and hyperarousal (e.g., exaggerated startle response). Given the phenomenology of PTSD, the classical fear conditioning and extinction learning paradigms (discussed later) are considered to afford valuable models for developing hypotheses about this disorder's pathophysiology.

PANIC DISORDER

Panic disorder is characterized by recurrent panic episodes, typically occurring spontaneously and without overt precipitants. Panic attacks entail a rapid escalation to extreme anxiety accompanied by physical symptoms, such as tachypnea, palpitations, sweating, and dizziness, as well as emotional and cognitive symptoms, such as the feeling that something catastrophic is about to happen or that immediate escape is necessary. Individuals with panic disorder often develop avoidance of places or situations (i.e., contexts) where they believe panic attacks are more likely to occur (including where such attacks have occurred in the past) or where escape may be difficult (e.g., crowded or confined places). In its most extreme form, this avoidance manifests as agoraphobia. Notably, panic attacks are far more common than panic disorder; consequently, we submit that the focus in modeling the pathogenesis of this disorder might be directed toward the progression from panic attack to panic disorder as opposed to the historical focus on the underpinnings of panic attacks per se. It is also relevant that heightened anxiety sensitivity (e.g., heightened awareness of interoceptive stimuli such as one's own heartbeat) is a common characteristic of individuals with panic disorder.

PHOBIAS

Phobias are characterized by exaggerated anxiety responses to relatively innocuous stimuli or situations. Such phobic responses include both the psychic experience of anxiety and peripheral manifestations of anxiety (e.g., changes in heart rate) as well as the tendency to avoid the feared object or situation.

Specific Phobias

Specific phobias entail phobic responses to any of various particular stimuli or situations (e.g., small animals, enclosed spaces).

Social Phobia

SocAD entails phobic responses specifically to social situations. Although there is some appeal to models based on learned fear for these disorders (as for PTSD), in fact, existing data about phobias do not provide support for the hypothesis that these are fundamentally learned phenomena from initial traumatic exposures to the feared object/situation. To the contrary, current evidence suggests that there may be a strong familial component to phobias, perhaps based on inherited aspects of temperament (Kendler et al. 2001; Rosenbaum et al. 1991).

Bridging From Phenomenology to Neurocircuitry

Neurocircuitry models of these conditions have been constructed by the following means: a) identifying the functional domains that appear to be abnormal on the basis of the phenomenology of the disorders; b) establishing the mediating anatomy of the associated normal functions; c) testing for the presence of abnormalities in the nodes of those circuits in individuals with the disorders (vs. control groups); and finally, d) demonstrating associations between such abnormalities and the clinical features of the disorders in question (e.g., documenting correlations between the magnitude of a brain abnormality and the severity or course of the disorder).

With respect to the four disorders in question, we selected several functional domains to illustrate these concepts: 1) persistent or indelible learning about threat-related stimuli, 2) exaggerated fear responses, 3) impaired extinction capacity, 4) deficient ability to suppress attention/response to disorder-relevant stimuli, 5) excessive contextual conditioning and/or inability to appreciate safe contexts, 6) exaggerated interoceptive/anxiety sensitivity, and 7) perceptual hypersensitivity to threat-related stimuli. The neural circuits supporting these functional domains are discussed with respect to their neurophysiological and neuroanatomical correlates in anxiety disorders. In contrast, the endocrine and neurotransmitter systems that are known to modulate these neural circuits, and which also have been implicated in the neurobiology of stress and anxiety disorders, are not reviewed here because of space constraints, but they are reviewed elsewhere (see Charney and Drevets 2002).

In general, two lines of research have been most influential in shaping neurocircuitry models of these disorders. First, animal studies using variants of the classical fear conditioning paradigm and human neuroimaging studies in healthy subjects have helped to establish the neurocircuitry that mediates normal functions related to the domains listed earlier. In parallel, through a variety of imaging modalities and paradigms, neuroimaging studies of subjects with anxiety disorders have begun to provide convergent evidence regarding the neural substrates of these disorders.

Neurocircuitry of Relevant Functional Domains: Animal Research

Given that the literature on animal research relevant to fear circuitry and stress is vast, here we focus on classical fear-conditioning paradigms as influential and pertinent examples (for reviews, see Charney and Drevets 2002; Davis 1998; LeDoux 1996; Rauch et al. 2006). Briefly, an animal (e.g., a rat) is exposed to a series of inherently innocuous sensory stimuli (tones) in a conditioning procedure, such that one (or more) of these stimuli is paired with an inherently aversive stimulus (e.g., a shock, called the unconditioned stimulus [UCS]), whereas other stimuli are presented without shock and come to be associated with relative safety. These conditioned stimuli (CS) are termed the CS+ (predictive of the aversive UCS) and the CS− (predictive of no UCS). Following conditioning, exposure to the CS+ alone induces a constellation of physiological responses that can be conceptualized as preparatory for an anticipated aversive event and that bear resemblance to fear or anxiety; these include elevations in autonomic tone, increased startle, and freezing in rodents. The conditioning phase may be followed by an extinction learning phase, during which the animal is given an opportunity to modify the learned association; a series of CS+ presentations are given without delivery of an accompanying UCS, indicating that the CS+ no longer signals shock. Finally, after a delay (e.g., the following day) the response to the CS+ is tested as an index of extinction retention over time. Interestingly, if the initial fear conditioning occurs in one context (e.g., a chamber of identifiable features; Cx+) and the extinction training occurs in a different context (e.g., a different chamber; Cx–), testing the following day reveals differential extinction retention versus renewal that is context dependent. Specifically, extinction learning is recalled in the Cx– (the extinction/safe context), whereas the conditioned fear response is typically significantly greater in the Cx+ (the conditioned/dangerous context). The context-gated return of the fear response following extinction is called *renewal*.

More generally, other paradigms can be used to demonstrate fear conditioning to contexts as well as to specific cues. As noted earlier, this basic paradigm has relevance to the phenomenology of anxiety disorders, because individuals with such disorders conceivably may show exaggerated learned-fear responses, failure to extinguish learned-fear associations, failure to retain such extinction learning, or failure to appreciate safe contexts. Notably, the extant behavioral therapies for anxiety disorders are based on principles of extinction. Consequently, the capacity for extinction learning, retention, and generalization across contexts may underpin effective behavior therapy, and interventions that enhance or fortify these processes could improve the response to such therapies.

The extensive and elegant animal research in this field has largely mapped the neurocircuitry responsible for the various elemental functions. In simple terms, by means of a fast track through the thalamus, the amygdala plays a central role in rapidly (and automatically) processing sensory stimuli in the service of assessing their threat value. The amygdala also plays a role in forming conditioned fear associations and in mediating (via its descending projections) the fear response (e.g., increased autonomic tone). Amygdala function is modulated by top-down influences from various cortical structures. In particular, although extinction learning per se may largely also depend on structures intrinsic to the amygdala as well as medial prefrontal cortex (mPFC; Morgan et al. 1993), the capacity to retain and recall extinction information in rodents is purportedly mediated in part by a region of the ventromedial prefrontal cortex (vmPFC) called the infralimbic cortex (Milad and Quirk 2002). Likewise, the hippocampus plays a critical role in contextual conditioning and hence in the capacity to distinguish between safe and dangerous contexts (Bouton 2004; Corcoran and Maren 2004).

Theorists have extrapolated from these data in animals to pose hypotheses regarding dysfunction in the homologous structures in humans with anxiety disorders (Rauch et al. 2006). Specifically, it has been hypothesized that individuals with anxiety disorders exhibit intrinsically exaggerated amygdala hyperresponsivity and/or deficient top-down modulation of the amygdala response due to deficiencies in function within mPFC and/or the hippocampus (Rauch et al. 2006). Behavioral data consistent with these hypotheses have been reported for some anxiety disorders within the context of fear conditioning and extinction studies. For example, PTSD samples have been shown to acquire de novo conditioned responses more readily and extinguish them more slowly than control samples (Orr et al. 2000; Peri et al. 2000). As is reviewed later, the extant neuroimaging data also are compatible with such hypotheses in that they show exaggerated amygdala responses and impaired function and/or abnormal structure in the mPFC and hippocampus.

The capacity to test such hypotheses directly has generally required two types of human neuroimaging studies. First, a large body of research has focused on investigating normal mediating anatomy of relevant functions and developing sensitive probes of functional response in brain regions of interest. In tandem, a substantial series of studies have been performed in subjects with anxiety disorders, typically in comparison with control groups.

A general limitation of both approaches has been that the relatively low resolution of state-of-the-art in vivo human neuroimaging techniques has precluded anatomically precise comparisons with the data available from parallel studies conducted in experimental animals. For example, although the amygdaloid complex is composed of multiple nuclei for which discrete functions have been demonstrated during fear conditioning, fear expression, anticipatory anxiety, and other relevant emotional behaviors, neuroimaging studies have been thus far unable to resolve these specific nuclei and thus have treated this nuclear complex as though it were functionally monolithic. As neuroimaging technology continues to evolve, therefore, the incremental improvements in spatial resolution and sensitivity will enable increasingly sophisticated comparisons with the animal literature and progressively refined hypotheses regarding the pathophysiology of anxiety disorders.

Human Neuroimaging Techniques

Although a comprehensive explanation and discussion of modern neuroimaging methods is beyond the scope of this chapter (see Dougherty and Rauch 2001; Raichle et al. 1987), here we briefly outline the various methods employed in the neuroimaging studies that we subsequently review later.

STRUCTURAL NEUROIMAGING TECHNIQUES

Morphometric magnetic resonance imaging (MRI) involves automated or semi-automated segmentation of brain structures of interest, enabling investigators to measure indices of size or features of shape from high resolution structural MRI data. Relatively new methods in this field include techniques for parcellating cortical subterritories and automated procedures for measuring cortical thickness (Caviness et al. 1996; Fischl and Dale 2000; Rauch et al. 2003b). Other emerging methods include voxel-based morphometry, which is an entirely automated method for identifying voxels where structural differences can be inferred from signal intensity differences on structural MRI scans analyzed in voxelwise fashion (e.g., Yamasue et al. 2003), and diffusion tensor imaging, which enables investigation of white matter tract orientation (Taylor et al. 2004). In addition to supporting tests of between-group differences in regional size, shape, and structural composition, significant associations have been reported between such structural imaging indices and a variety of clinical and behavioral measures (Bremner et al. 1995).

FUNCTIONAL NEUROIMAGING TECHNIQUES AND PARADIGMS

Various experimental paradigms have been employed, in conjunction with functional neuroimaging modalities, in efforts to delineate the neurophysiological correlates of normal brain functions as well as the pathophysiological correlates of psychiatric disorders. Commonly applied methods include positron emission tomography (PET), with tracers that measure blood flow (e.g., oxygen-15-labeled water) or glucose metabolism (i.e., fluorine-18-labeled fluorodeoxyglucose [FDG]); single photon emission tomography (SPECT), with tracers that measure correlates of blood flow (e.g., technetium-99-labeled hexamethyl propylene amine oxime); and functional magnetic resonance imaging (fMRI) to measure blood oxygenation level–dependent signal changes. Each of these techniques yields maps that reflect regional brain activity. Although some controversy remains regarding the optimal interpretation of functional imaging measures, current knowledge indicates that these indices predominantly reflect metabolic activity within neuronal terminal fields, rather than in cell bodies, so that the tightly coupled cerebral blood flow and glucose metabolic signals within a region reflect an integration of the synaptic activity or local field potential within that region, as opposed to the neuronal firing rates of local cell bodies per se (Magistretti and Pellerin 1999; Raichle et al. 1987).

Such brain activity profiles are sensitive to the state of the subject at the time of tracer distribution or image acquisition. Thus, functional imaging paradigms can be categorized on the basis of the type of state manipulations employed by the investigators, and the principal statistical comparisons can be applied. In *neutral state* paradigms, subjects are studied during a nominal "resting" state or while performing a nonspecific continuous task. Thus, hypotheses regarding between-group differences in regional brain activity are tested without particular attention to momentary state variables. In *symptom provocation* paradigms, subjects are scanned during a symptomatic state (after having their symptoms intentionally induced) as well as during control conditions. Within-group comparisons can be made to test hypotheses regarding the mediating anatomy of the symptomatic state, and group-by-condition interactions can be sought to distinguish responses in patients versus control groups. Behavioral and/or pharmacological challenges can be used to induce symptoms. In some cases when symptomatic states occur spontaneously, experiments are designed to capture these events without the need for provocation or induction per se.

In *cognitive-behavioral activation* paradigms, subjects are studied while performing specially designed cognitive-behavioral tasks. This approach is intended to increase sensitivity by employing tasks that specifically activate brain systems of interest. In healthy subjects, within-group analyses are used to establish the normal mediating anatomy for functional domains of interest. Subsequently, group-by-condition interactions are sought to test the functional responsivity or integrity of specific brain systems in patients versus control subjects.

Any of these three paradigm types can also be employed in the context of a longitudinal design. For example, in treatment studies, subjects are scanned both before and after a treatment trial. Then, within-group comparisons are made to test hypotheses regarding changes in brain activity profiles associated with symptomatic improvement. Alternatively, correlation analyses can be performed to identify pretreatment brain activity characteristics that predict subsequent treatment response.

Imaging studies of neurochemistry have employed PET and SPECT methods in conjunction with radiolabeled high-affinity ligands. In this way, the regional receptor binding potential (modeled as density × affinity) can be characterized in vivo (i.e., receptor characterization studies). Other approaches include the use of magnetic resonance spectroscopy (MRS) to measure the regional relative concentration of select "MRS-visible" compounds. For instance, MRS can be used to measure the compound *N*-acetyl aspartate (NAA), which is a purported marker of healthy neuronal density.

Neurocircuitry of Functional Domains Relevant to Anxiety Disorders: Human Imaging Research

NEUROIMAGING STUDIES OF FEAR CONDITIONING AND EXTINCTION

Neuroimaging studies have been conducted to investigate the mediating anatomy of conditioned fear acquisition, extinction, and extinction retention. Consistent with animal research (e.g., LeDoux 1996), several neuroimaging experiments of fear conditioning in healthy humans have likewise implicated the amygdala. Such studies have found significant correlation between PET–regional cerebral blood flow (rCBF) changes in right amygdala and electrodermal activity changes (Fredrikson et al. 1995a; Furmark et al. 1997) as well as interregional correlations between amygdala and thalamus (Morris et al. 1997). Using PET and backward masking techniques, Morris et al. (1998) found bilateral activation in amygdala; right amygdala activation was found in the condition where subjects were aware, whereas left amygdala activation was found in the condition where subjects were unaware of the emotionally expressive face stimuli. Several fMRI studies have also demonstrated amygdala activation during fear conditioning (Cheng et al. 2003; LaBar et al. 1998; Morris and Dolan 2004). Knight et al. (2004) also found amygdala involvement during contingency changes in fear conditioning/extinction. Finally, an fMRI paradigm has been developed in which an aversive air puff (UCS) is used to engage the amygdala during conditioning in pediatric subjects (Pine et al. 2001).

An fMRI study found involvement of the vmPFC during the recall of extinction in humans (Phelps et al. 2004). Activation of the amygdala and vmPFC, specifically a region of the pregenual anterior cingulate cortex (pACC), was observed as participants acquired conditioned fear, extinguished conditioned fear in the same session, and recalled this extinction learning 24 hours later. Consistent with previous studies (LaBar et al. 1998), activation of the amygdala in response to a CS+ compared with a CS− was correlated with the strength of the conditioned response during acquisition. Amygdala activation correlated with extinction success in the same session, although in this case a greater response to a CS−, compared with the CS+, indicated greater extinction, suggesting the amygdala may also play a role in early extinction training (Knight et al. 2004; Myers and Davis 2002). During the recall of extinction after a 24-hour delay, activation of the vmPFC predicted extinction success and was correlated with amygdala activation (Gottfried and Dolan 2004), consistent with animal models indicating that the infralimbic cortex may act to inhibit the amygdala response during the recall of extinction (Milad and Quirk 2002). Most recently, employing a similar extinction retention design (Milad et al. 2005a), Milad et al. (2005b) showed that cortical thickness at a specific locus within medial orbitofrontal cortex was directly correlated with the magnitude of extinction recall. Of note, this locus was mapped to within one resolution unit (~1 cm) of the peak voxel in the Phelps et al. (2004) fMRI study of extinction recall. Taken together, these data implicate vmPFC (and perhaps specifically medial orbitofrontal cortex) as the human homologue of infralimbic cortex in rodents with respect to extinction retention function.

Recent studies in humans have demonstrated context dependency of extinction retention using peripheral physiological endpoints, such as skin conductance (Milad et al. 2005a; Vansteenwegen et al. 2005). In addition, damage to the hippocampus in humans leads to an impairment in contextually mediated reinstatement of an extinguished fear (LaBar and Phelps 2005), consistent with animal models (Bouton 2004). Thus, these findings provide a foundation for developing analogous paradigms for use in conjunction with functional imaging.

However, hippocampal activation has yet to be demonstrated in association with fear conditioning/extinction-related context effects by human neuroimaging methods. Neuroimaging research on context effects faces a unique challenge due to the fact that the imaging suite environment represents a powerful fixed context in its own right. Consequently, it is difficult to effectively manipulate context within an experimental imaging session. One approach to meet this challenge involves the use of virtual reality to achieve or simulate meaningful context manipulations during neuroimaging acquisition (Maguire et al. 1998; Milad et al. 2005a).

These relatively recently developed neuroimaging paradigms not only implicate the amygdala and vmPFC in human fear conditioning/extinction processes but also provide tools for future investigation of the neural substrates of potential abnormalities of these functions across the anxiety disorders. To date, however, other cognitive activation paradigms have been more extensively developed to probe relevant brain regions of interest and applied to the study of anxiety disorders.

COGNITIVE ACTIVATION PROBES OF AMYGDALA FUNCTION

Paradigms designed to probe amygdala function have principally involved viewing face stimuli or other emotionally valenced pictorial stimuli. An initial series of functional imaging studies showed that passive viewing of human face stimuli produces reliable amygdala activation (Breiter et al. 1996a; Morris et al. 1996) and that amygdala responses appear to be greatest with fearful faces as opposed to neutral, happy, or angry faces (Whalen et al. 2001). Hence, such paradigms represent tools for potentially assessing amygdala responses to a particular class of socially relevant threat-related stimuli that are not disorder specific. Interestingly, whereas overtly presented face stimuli recruit a broad array of other brain areas in addition to the amygdala (e.g., frontal cortical territories), when face stimuli are instead presented beneath the level of awareness (e.g., by using a backward masking technique), isolated amygdala activation is observed (Morris et al. 1998; Whalen et al. 1998a). Consequently, such masked-faces paradigms provide a potential tool for exploring automatic amygdala responses relatively dissociated from the top-down influences of frontal cortex. Furthermore, a series of studies have shown that the repeated presentation of face stimuli can be used to demonstrate habituation of amygdala responses (Phillips et al. 2001; Wright et al. 2001). Such paradigms provide a potential tool for characterizing habituation profiles within the amygdala. Of note, these studies, together with the large extant literature on neuroimaging and face stimuli, indicate that humans exhibit differential responses within the right and left amygdala. The right amygdala appears to show a more temporally dynamic pattern of response, whereas the left amygdala appears to exhibit a more temporally stable response, with a more robust difference in response based on the emotional valence of the stimuli.

Other paradigms that involve viewing pictures have indicated robust and reliable amygdala activation in response to emotionally valenced versus neutral stimuli (Irwin et al. 1996; Lane et al. 1997). In particular, the International Affective Picture System (Lang 1993) and various sets of emotionally expressive face pictures (Ekman and Friesen 1976) have provided well-characterized and validated sets of visual stimuli for constructing such paradigms to assess amygdala responses on the basis of emotional valence or arousal.

INTEROCEPTIVE FUNCTION AND THE INSULAR CORTEX

A number of human functional imaging studies have implicated the insular cortex in the mediating anatomy of interoceptive function and, specifically, sensitivity to one's own heartbeat (Critchley et al. 2004). In a complementary line of neuroimaging research, investigators have shown that viewing the facial emotion of disgust, as well as viewing disgusting pictures or generating internal images of disgust, likewise is associated with insular cortical activation (Fitzgerald et al. 2004; Phillips et al. 1997; Wright et al. 2004). Thus, such paradigms have been established for probing insular responses in the context of interoceptive sensitivity.

COGNITIVE ACTIVATION PROBES OF ANTERIOR CINGULATE CORTEX

Numerous paradigms have been shown to activate various subterritories of the anterior cingulate cortex (ACC; Bush et al. 1998). For example, a battery of various Stroop-type tasks has been developed for studying ACC function in anxiety disorders. The rationale for using such interference tasks has been that the function of the ACC most germane to anxiety disorders is the capacity to suppress attention/response to a particular information stream in favor of attention/response to another stream. In anxiety disorders, there is a well-established deficit in suppressing attention to disorder-relevant information in favor of non-disorder-relevant information (McNally 1998). Indeed, a series of fMRI studies has shown that a pACC is activated during the emotional counting Stroop task, where attention/response to emotional information must be suppressed in favor of nonemotional information (Whalen et al. 1998b). In contrast, a more dorsal subterritory is activated when attention/response to nonemotional information must be suppressed (Bush et al. 1998). This neurocognitive probe has now been applied to demonstrate deficiencies in pACC recruitment in subjects with anxiety disorders (Shin et al. 2001).

COGNITIVE ACTIVATION PROBES OF HIPPOCAMPUS

The roles of hippocampus in explicit learning and memory and contextual conditioning have been well established (Bouton 2004; LeDoux 1996; Schacter and Wagner 1999). Therefore, to date, investigators have used explicit learning and memory paradigms (e.g., encoding/recalling word lists) in conjunction with neuroimaging as robust probes of hippocampal function. In contrast, human neuroimaging studies of contextual conditioning have yet to be published.

Neuroimaging Studies of the Anatomical Correlates of Anxiety Disorders

POSTTRAUMATIC STRESS DISORDER

Amygdalocentric Model

We previously presented a neurocircuitry model of PTSD that emphasizes the role of the amygdala and its interactions with the hippocampus and mPFC (Rauch et al. 1998a). Briefly, this model hypothesizes hyperresponsivity within the amygdala to threat-related stimuli, with inadequate top-down governance over the amygdala by the mPFC and the hippocampus. Amygdala hyperresponsivity mediates symptoms of hyperarousal and explains the indelible quality of the emotional memory for the traumatic event; dysfunction involving the pACC underlies deficits in suppressing attention/response to trauma-related stimuli; deficient vmPFC influence underlies deficits in extinction retention; and decreased hippocampal function underlies deficits in identifying safe contexts as well as accompanying explicit memory difficulties (Bremner et al. 1995). This model represents a final common pathophysiological pathway. Consequently, the pathogenesis of PTSD can be conceptualized as a fear-conditioning process that is superimposed over some diathesis, which could entail any combination of premorbid intrinsic amygdala hyperresponsivity, pACC/vmPFC deficiency, hippocampal deficiency, or exaggerated susceptibility to stress. Furthermore, chronic PTSD might involve progressive deterioration of function (and structure) within these stress-modulating systems.

Functional Imaging Findings

An initial PET symptom-provocation study of PTSD (Rauch et al. 1996) used a script-driven imagery method for inducing symptoms. For the provoked versus control conditions, increased rCBF was found within right orbitofrontal, anterior insular, anterior temporal, and visual cortices as well as in the pACC and the right amygdala. Decreases in rCBF were observed within the left inferior frontal (Broca's area) and left middle temporal cortices. Interpretations of this initial study, with regard to the pathophysiology of PTSD, were limited by the absence of a comparison group. A series of subsequent functional imaging studies were conducted in which comparisons were made between subjects with PTSD and trauma-exposed subjects without PTSD for contrasts between provoked versus control conditions and to test hypotheses about the pathophysiology of PTSD. Convergent results suggested that when exposed to reminders of traumatic events (vs. control conditions), subjects with PTSD (vs. subjects without PTSD) exhibit greater hemodynamic responses within the amygdala (Hendler et al. 2003; Liberzon et al. 1999; Pissiotta et al. 2002; Protopopescu et al. 2005a; Shin et al. 1997), attenuated responses within the mPFC (Bremner et al. 1999a, 1999b; Lanius et al. 2001;

Lindauer et al. 2004a; Shin et al. 1999), and exaggerated deactivation (seen as reductions in hemodynamic activity) within other heteromodal frontal cortical regions (Shin et al. 1997, 1999). These findings from symptom-provocation studies were interpreted as providing support for the amygdalocentric neurocircuitry model of PTSD. However, replication across this full complement of experiments has been far from perfect, possibly because the small sample sizes of subsequent studies increased the risk of type II error, inconsistencies existed in the experimental paradigms across studies, and biological and clinical heterogeneity likely existed across subject samples meeting the entrance criteria for PTSD (Lanius et al. 2001).

As further tests of this model, cognitive activation studies were used to measure the functional integrity at each node of the circuit: pACC, amygdala, and hippocampus. Using fMRI to measure hemodynamic responses of the amygdala to fearful faces that had been "masked" by a neutral face, such that subjects were only explicitly aware of having seen the neutral face (Whalen et al. 1998a), Rauch et al. (2000) found that, in comparison to trauma-exposed subjects without PTSD, subjects with PTSD exhibited exaggerated responses to the masked fearful face in the right dorsal amygdala. Across individual subjects, the blood oxygenation level–dependent response within the amygdala to masked-fearful versus masked-happy faces correlated with an index of PTSD symptom severity (i.e., Clinician-Administered PTSD Scale score) but did not correlate with an index of depression severity (i.e., Beck Depression Inventory score). Furthermore, an assessment of the main effect of condition across all subjects replicated the finding that this contrast illustrates recruitment of the amygdala in the absence of frontal cortical activation. Independent replication also has been reported, showing a correlation between PTSD symptom severity and right amygdala responses to masked fearful versus happy faces (Armony et al. 2005). Thus, these findings represent additional evidence of hyperresponsivity of the amygdala to threat-related stimuli in PTSD, even when relatively dissociated from the top-down influences of the prefrontal cortex.

Using an fMRI–emotional counting Stroop paradigm, Shin et al. (2001) found that, in comparison with trauma-exposed subjects without PTSD, PTSD subjects exhibited attenuated recruitment of pACC in the context of a task that requires suppression of attention and response to trauma-related information in favor of general negative information. This finding, which has now been replicated in an independent cohort (Bremner et al. 2004), indicates deficient function of pACC in PTSD in this context.

Moreover, a recent fMRI study of PTSD versus control subjects, using overtly presented emotional face stimuli, found exaggerated amygdala responses as well as diminished mPFC responses to fear versus happy faces (Shin et al. 2005). An inverse relationship was found whereby greater amygdala activation was associated with lesser mPFC activation. This represents one of several studies that have provided data regarding interregional correlations, specifically with regard to potential mPFC–amygdala interactions (e.g., Gilboa et al. 2004; Shin et al. 2004b). Furthermore, an initial PET study using a fear-conditioning and extinction paradigm found that PTSD subjects versus control subjects exhibited exaggerated amygdala responses during fear conditioning and diminished ACC activation during extinction learning (Bremner et al. 2005).

PET studies have utilized explicit learning paradigms as probes of hippocampal function in PTSD. Bremner and colleagues reported relatively diminished activation of the hippocampus during performance of a verbal paired associates task in abuse survivors with PTSD (Bremner et al. 2003a) as well as during encoding of a narrative paragraph (Bremner et al. 2003b). Likewise, using a word stem completion task, Shin et al. (2004a) found diminished recruitment of the hippocampus in firefighters with PTSD relative to firefighters without PTSD. These results thus add support for the model of hippocampal dysfunction in PTSD.

Complementary Neuroimaging Findings: Structure and Chemistry

To date, morphometric MRI studies of PTSD have focused on subtle between-group differences with respect to hippocampal volume. The possibility of reduced hippocampal and mPFC volume and function is scientifically appealing, given that studies in animals have shown that pyramidal neuron dendritic trees atrophy within the hippocampus and the mPFC during repeated stress because of interactions between the increased glutamatergic transmission within these regions and the elevated systemic glucocorticoid secretion that accompany stress (McEwen 2005; Sapolsky et al. 1990). In contrast, the dendritic arborization *increases* within some amygdala nuclei during some types of stress (Vyas et al. 2002, 2003). The findings from these animal models of repeated stress suggest hypotheses regarding the neurobiological mechanisms that may account for both the heightened physiological responsiveness to emotional stimuli seen within the amygdala and the reduced volumes and/or physiological responses to emotional stimuli seen within the hippocampus and mPFC structures (such as the pACC) in PTSD as well as in some other anxiety disorders (discussed later) (Drevets and Price 2005).

An initial series of four studies showed smaller hippocampal volumes in adult subjects with PTSD versus healthy control subjects (Bremner et al. 1995, 1997; Gurvits et al. 1996; Stein et al. 1997) and/or trauma-exposed subjects without PTSD (Gurvits et al. 1996). In some instances, these findings remained after alcohol abuse or years of education were controlled for (Bremner et al. 1995; Gurvits et al. 1996). These investigators also found that measures of hippocampal volume correlated with measures of verbal memory (Bremner et al. 1995) or dissociative symptoms (Stein et al. 1997), as well as indices of trauma exposure and PTSD symptom severity (Gurvits et al. 1996). In addition, MRS studies found significantly reduced levels of NAA, a putative neuronal viability marker, in the hippocampus in PTSD versus control subjects (Mohanakrishnan Menon et al. 2003; Schuff et al. 2001), and some subsequent research has further replicated the finding of hippocampal volumetric reductions in PTSD (Bremner et al. 2003b; Lindauer et al. 2004b; Shin et al. 2004a).

However, several subsequent MRI studies failed to show hippocampal volume differences when assessing children and adolescents with PTSD (Carrion et al. 2001; DeBellis et al. 1999), and two longitudinal studies failed to find reductions in hippocampal volumes over 6-month to 2-year follow-up periods (Bonne et al. 2001; DeBellis et al. 2001). A unique monozygotic twin study, employing a twin design with discordance for trauma exposure, yielded findings suggesting that reduced hippocampal volume may represent a risk factor for developing PTSD if the individual is exposed to trauma (Gilbertson et al. 2002). One study of adult burn patients indicated smaller hippocampal volume associated with traumatic exposure compared with hippocampal volume in PTSD (Winter and Irle 2004). Consequently, although initial MRI and MRS findings provided support for the hypothesis that PTSD is associated with reduced hippocampal size, which in turn is associated with cognitive deficits and PTSD symptoms, subsequent results have complicated the picture with regard to the relationship between hippocampal volume and PTSD. Of note, a recent study indicated that chronic treatment with paroxetine was associated with improvement of PTSD symptom severity and declarative memory and increased hippocampal volume, although this finding awaits replication (Vermetten et al. 2003).

An initial cortical parcellation study (Rauch et al. 2003b) found that Vietnam War nurses with PTSD, versus those without PTSD, exhibited selectively reduced volumes in pACC and subcallosal cortex. These findings of pACC structural abnormalities are convergent with voxel-based morphometric findings in two subsequent reports (Corbo et al. 2005; Yamasue et al. 2003). These structural neuroimaging findings implicating pACC resonate with a recent MRS study (DeBellis et al. 2000) in which maltreated children exhibited reduced NAA in a comparable region of ACC.

SPECT/iomazenil findings of frontal cortical benzodiazepine-binding abnormalities in PTSD (Bremner et al. 2000a) were not replicated in a second study (Fujita et al. 2004).

Summary

Taken together, imaging data support the current neurocircuitry model of PTSD that emphasizes the functional relationship between a triad of brain structures: the amygdala, mPFC, and hippocampus. When exposed to reminders of traumatic events, subjects appear to recruit anterior paralimbic regions and the amygdala while exhibiting decreased activity within other heteromodal cortical areas. In comparison with control subjects, patients with PTSD exhibit pACC activation of diminished magnitude, but exaggerated activation, within other limbic (amygdala) and paralimbic regions (including the insula), along with exaggerated neurophysiological deactivations within widespread areas associated with higher cognitive functions. Cognitive activation experiments designed to probe the functional integrity within the nodes of this circuitry have indicated hyperresponsivity within the amygdala to threat-related stimuli and during fear conditioning, diminished pACC activation during emotional Stroop tasks, and diminished activation of the hippocampus during various explicit encoding and retrieval tasks. To date, structural imaging studies have yielded replicable findings implicating reduced volumes in pACC and hippocampus, without evidence of volumetric abnormality involving the amygdala. Reduced hippocampal volume may represent a risk factor for developing PTSD. In parallel, MRS studies have found reduced NAA in ACC and hippocampus.

PANIC DISORDER

Neuroanatomical Models

Although neurocircuitry models of panic disorder resemble those of PTSD (Gorman et al. 2000), theories of panic disorder have emphasized a wide range of disparate elements (Coplan and Lydiard 1998), including dysregulated ascending noradrenergic and/or serotonergic systems, aberrant responsivity to CO_2 at the level of brain stem (i.e., "false suffocation alarm"), and global cerebral abnormalities in lactate metabolism, as well as abnormalities in the interactions between hippocampus, parahippocampal cortex, and amygdala (Klein 1993). Whereas the behavioral sequelae of panic attacks (e.g., agoraphobic avoidance) putatively can be explained by learning theory and fear conditioning, a satisfactory model of panic disorder must also explain the occurrence of spontaneous panic episodes.

One possibility is that a core physiological (i.e., normal) anxiety response, mediated by the anxiety/fear circuitry, is recruited spontaneously as an aberrant event due to homeostatic deficits. This possibility is exemplified by the suffocation alarm model (Klein 1993) and by theories regarding fundamental monoaminergic dysregulation (reviewed in Charney and Drevets 2002). Another possibility is that panic attacks evolve in the context of what should be minor anxiety episodes, but because of failures in the systems responsible for limiting such normal responses, the anxiety response becomes excessive to an extent that is maladaptive. Similar to the aforementioned model of PTSD, hippocampal or other temporal cortical deficits might underlie such a mechanism in the case of panic disorder (McNaughton 1997).

Finally, it is conceivable that panic episodes described as spontaneous (i.e., without identifiable precipitants) may reflect anxiety responses to stimuli that are not processed at the conscious (i.e., explicit) level but instead recruit anxiety circuitry without awareness (i.e., implicitly). This concept is compatible with evidence that the amygdala can be recruited into action in the absence of explicit awareness that a threat-related stimulus has been presented (Whalen et al. 1998a). According to this model, panic disorder might be characterized by fundamental amygdala hyperresponsivity to subtle environmental cues, triggering full-scale, threat-related responses in the absence of conscious awareness. Furthermore, the absence of explicit awareness may be attributable to dysfunction, involving the hippocampus or parahippocampal regions, which allows abnormal escalation in response to contextual stimuli that would not be recognized as inherently threatening.

Functional Imaging Findings

In an initial PET neutral-state study, Reiman et al. (1986) found that, in comparison with control subjects, a subset of panic disorder patients who were vulnerable to lactate-induced panic exhibited lower left:right ratios of parahippocampal rCBF while resting with eyes closed. In a resting-state SPECT study, DeCristofaro et al. (1993) found that, in comparison with control subjects, panic disorder subjects exhibited elevated rCBF in left occipital cortex and reduced rCBF in the hippocampal area bilaterally. In a resting-state PET-FDG study, panic disorder subjects exhibited a lower left:right hippocampal ratio of regional cerebral metabolic rate for glucose (rCMRglu) compared with control subjects (Nordahl et al. 1990). In contrast, another PET-FDG study found that panic disorder subjects exhibited elevated rCMRglu in the left hippocampus and parahippocampal area, but reduced rCMRglu in the right superior temporal regions, compared with control subjects (Bisaga et al. 1998).

One fMRI study of symptom provocation using script-driven imagery in panic disorder versus control subjects found exaggerated activation in inferior frontal, cingulate, and orbitofrontal cortex, as well as hippocampus, in the panic disorder group (Bystritsky et al. 2001). Four symptom-provocation studies of panic disorder that employed pharmacological challenges have been published. Stewart et al. (1988) used SPECT and ^{133}Xe inhalation to measure cerebral blood flow in superficial cortical areas during lactate-induced panic; in comparison with normal control subjects and panic disorder subjects who did not experience lactate-induced panic attacks, the subjects who did experience lactate-induced panic attacks displayed global cortical decreases in cerebral blood flow, possibly reflecting the effects of hyperventilation on cerebrovascular function. Woods et al. (1988) employed SPECT and yohimbine infusions and found that panic disorder subjects experienced increased anxiety and exhibited decreased rCBF in bilateral frontal cortex compared with control subjects. In a PET study, Reiman et al. (1989) showed that, in comparison with normal subjects and panic disorder subjects who did not experience lactate-induced panic, panic disorder subjects who did have lactate-induced panic episodes exhibited rCBF increases in bilateral temporopolar cortex and bilateral insular cortex/claustrum/putamen and the midbrain in the vicinity of the periaqueductal gray. The temporopolar findings were subsequently shown to predominantly reflect the cerebral blood flow changes in the extracranial musculature (Benkelfat et al. 1995; Drevets et al. 1992a). Using PET and pentagastrin challenge to induce panic attacks in panic disorder subjects, versus control subjects, Boshuisen et al. (2002) found decreases in anterior insula and inferior frontal cortex, as well as exaggerated activation in parahippocampal gyrus, superior temporal cortex, and ACC.

In a fifth report, a spontaneous panic attack was captured in a single case; the PET data showed decreased rCBF in right orbitofrontal cortex, subcallosal cortex, ACC, and anterior temporal cortex during the acute event (Fischer et al. 1998).

In a study of medicated panic disorder subjects, Nordahl et al. (1998) used PET-FDG methods to assess regional glucose metabolism in imipramine-treated subjects with panic disorder and reported a rightward shift in asymmetry within hippocampus and posterior inferior frontal cortex, similar to that which they had observed in nontreated patients with panic disorder (Nordahl et al. 1990). Furthermore, in comparison with the untreated group, the imipramine-treated group exhibited metabolic decreases in posterior orbitofrontal cortex. Unpublished data from fMRI cognitive-activation studies of panic disorder subjects versus healthy control subjects indicate exaggerated right amygdala responses to masked fearful versus happy faces and deficient pACC activation during the emotional counting Stroop (Whalen PJ, Rauch SL, Shin LM, et al., unpublished data, 2003). These findings precisely mirror the results in PTSD reported by the same laboratory (Rauch et al. 2000; Shin et al. 2001).

Complementary Neuroimaging Findings: Structure and Chemistry

Morphometric MRI studies of panic disorder patients, versus control subjects, have found abnormalities in the temporal lobe, including overall smaller left temporal lobe volume (Uchida et al. 2003); smaller temporal cortical volumes bilaterally, with no differences in hippocampal volume (Vythilingam et al. 2000); and less gray matter density in parahippocampal cortex (Massana et al. 2003a). A single study found smaller amygdalar volumes bilaterally (Massana et al. 2003b).

With respect to neurochemical abnormalities in panic disorder, in a series of MRS studies, Dager et al. (1995, 1999) demonstrated that, in comparison with healthy control subjects, panic disorder subjects show a significantly greater rise in brain lactate in response to the same level of hyperventilation and exhibit a significantly greater brain lactate level during lactate infusion. These data are consistent with reduced clearance, rather than higher production, of lactate in panic disorder. Moreover, the broad distribution of this phenomenon suggests a global or widespread abnormality in cerebrovascular function in panic disorder.

Although receptor characterization studies focusing on benzodiazepine binding have yielded inconsistent results, they have repeatedly implicated prefrontal and temporal cortical regions of abnormality. In a SPECT-iomazenil study, in comparison with control subjects, panic disorder subjects exhibited a greater left:right ratio in benzodiazepine receptor uptake, especially in prefrontal cortex (Kuikka et al. 1995). In an analogous SPECT-iomazenil study of panic disorder subjects versus healthy control subjects, Bremner et al. (2000b) found reduced distribution volume in left hippocampus and precuneus in those with panic disorder; subjects who experienced a panic attack during tracer uptake exhibited reduced distribution in prefrontal cortex. In a PET study, using carbon-11-labeled flumazenil, in comparison with a control group, the panic disorder group exhibited a global reduction in benzodiazepine binding that was most pronounced in right orbitofrontal and right insular cortex (Malizia et al. 1998). Whereas these three initial experiments may have been confounded by prior treatment, Brandt et al. (1998), using SPECT-iomazenil, found that medication-naïve panic disorder subjects, compared with healthy control subjects, exhibited significantly elevated benzodiazepine receptor binding within right supraorbital frontal cortex as well as a trend toward elevated binding in the right temporal cortex. Most recently, Neumeister et al. (2004a), using PET and fluoride-18-labeled FCWAY, found that in comparison with normal control subjects, panic disorder subjects exhibited diminished 5-HT$_{1A}$ binding within ACC, posterior cingulate cortex (PCC), and raphe. This abnormality extended to panic disorder subjects both with and without comorbid depression and to subjects with and without prior exposure to antidepressant drugs.

Summary

Taken together, the neuroimaging data on panic disorder suggest abnormalities in hippocampal/parahippocampal activity at rest; during a symptomatic state patients exhibit activation of insular and motor striatal regions as well as reduced activity in widespread cortical regions, including prefrontal cortex. Unpublished data suggest striking similarities to PTSD in terms of amygdala hyperresponsivity to general threat-related stimuli and deficient pACC recruitment to panic-related words. Morphometric studies have most consistently implicated abnormalities involving parahippocampal/temporal cortex. MRS studies of brain lactate implicate a global phenomenon consistent with an exaggerated hemodynamic response to hypocapnea. Such differences underscore the problems with using frankly symptom-provoking paradigms (such as fear conditioning) to study panic disorder with fMRI or cerebral blood flow–based methods.

Similarly, receptor-binding studies suggest widespread abnormalities in the γ-aminobutyric acid (GABA)/benzodiazepine system, which also appear to be most pronounced in prefrontal, paralimbic, and temporal cortices. Likewise, 5-HT$_{1A}$ abnormalities have now also been demonstrated within the raphe and its projection fields in paralimbic cortex (ACC and PCC). Consistent with prevailing neurobiological models of panic disorder, fundamental abnormalities in monoaminergic neurotransmitter systems originating in the brain stem may underlie the abnormalities of metabolism, hemodynamics, and chemistry found in widespread territories of cortex. Moreover, these abnormalities conceivably may mediate the increased risk for having initial panic attacks. Furthermore, regional abnormalities within the temporal lobes provide support for theories regarding dysfunctional influence over the amygdala via temporal cortex and/or the hippocampus in panic disorder. These latter aspects may mediate the liability for developing the disorder following initial panic attacks.

SPECIFIC PHOBIAS

Neuroanatomical Models of Phobias

Phobias may represent the product of dysregulated systems specific to assessing potentially threatening stimuli or situations that are of particular ethological significance. For example, it has been hypothesized that if humans evolved a neural network specifically designed to assess threat from small animals, this network might represent the neural substrates for the pathophysiology underlying phobias. Until recently, neurocircuitry models of phobias reflected extrapolations from animal research, with limited human data to draw on (Fyer 1998). However, neuroimaging data from human subjects are accruing and beginning to provide an empirical basis for neurocircuitry models of specific phobia. Specifically, although the amygdala had been the theoretical focus because of its critical role in mediating conditioned and innate fear, the human imaging data more directly have implicated anterior paralimbic regions and sensory cortical regions known to interact with the amygdala.

Functional Imaging Findings

Initial studies of specific phobia principally employed PET symptom-provocation paradigms. Although the first PET study (Mountz et al. 1989), using older data analytic methods, found no significant changes in rCBF, a subsequent series of studies yielded convergent results. During exposure to videotapes of phobic stimuli, versus control videotapes, subjects with snake phobia (Wik et al. 1993) exhibited increases in rCBF within secondary visual cortex and rCBF decreases within the prefrontal, posterior cingulate, and anterior temporopolar cortices and the hippocampus. These findings were replicated in an analogous study of subjects with spider phobia (Fredrikson et al. 1993, 1995b). A PET study involving subjects with a variety of small animal phobias and in vivo exposure to phobia-related and control stimuli found different results (Rauch et al. 1995), with the difference attributable to the fact that rCBF measures were obtained while subjects had their eyes closed, whereas previous studies were performed with subjects' eyes open. This study found significant rCBF increases within multiple anterior paralimbic territories, left somatosensory cortex, and left thalamus. Dominant-sided somatosensory cortical activation was interpreted in the context of subjects' reports that they engaged in tactile imagery, worrying that the phobic stimulus would come in bodily contact with them. This was conceptualized as analogous to visual cortical activation in the other specific phobia studies in which exposures to phobic stimuli were mediated via the visual sensory modality. In this context, it is interesting to note that the amygdala is known to project to sensory areas and is believed to facilitate responsivity in those areas when the amygdala is activated, such as in response to threatening stimuli in the environment (Amaral et al. 1992).

More recently, fMRI studies have found medial temporal (amygdala, hippocampus, and parahippocampal gyrus) and anterior paralimbic activation that is greater in subjects with animal phobias versus comparison subjects in response to phobia-relevant, versus control, pictures (Dilger et al. 2003; Veltman et al. 2004) but no group differences in amygdala responses to emotionally expressive face stimuli (Wright et al. 2003). Moreover, another fMRI study found greater prefrontal cortex, insular cortex, and PCC activation in response to phobia-related, versus control, words in subjects with animal phobias compared with control subjects (Straube et al. 2004b). In a treatment study of subjects with spider phobia using fMRI and films of spiders versus control scenes, Paquette et al. (2003) found activation in right dorsolateral prefrontal cortex (~Brodmann area 10), parahippocampal gyrus, and bilateral visual association cortex. After successful cognitive-behavioral therapy, the activations in the frontal and parahippocampal regions were no longer evident.

Complementary Neuroimaging Findings: Structure and Chemistry

One structural MRI study of subjects with animal phobias found increased cortical thickness in pACC as well as insular cortex and PCC (Rauch et al. 2004).

Summary

Imaging findings in specific phobia suggest activation of anterior paralimbic regions (including insular cortex) and sensory cortex, corresponding to stimulus inflow associated with a symptomatic state. Such results are consistent with a hypersensitive system for assessment of, or response to, specific threat-related cues—a system in which the amygdala likely plays a central role. The available fMRI data suggest amygdala hyperresponsivity in specific phobia that is selective to phobia-relevant stimuli. Future studies that assess the pACC function during emotional Stroop tasks and obtain morphometric measures of cortical volume in the pACC, hippocampus, amygdala, anterior paralimbic regions, and sensory cortices may prove particularly informative in elucidating the anatomical correlates of specific phobia.

SOCIAL PHOBIA (SOCIAL ANXIETY DISORDER)

Neuroanatomical Models

As in specific phobia, models of SocAD consider increased sensitivity to the potential threat value of a specific class of stimuli—in this case, socially relevant stimuli. Although leading possibilities in this regard include enhanced sensitivity to or learning about social threat, it is also conceivable that heightened responses to novel social stimuli (Schwartz et al. 2003), as well as decreased reward value of neutral/positive social stimuli (Stein 1998), play a role in the disorder. Consequently, research paradigms in this area have focused on responses to social stimuli (e.g., faces) varied for valence, arousal, and novelty, as well as the context of conditioning protocols. Thus, the brain regions considered in the neurocircuitry of SocAD include the amygdala; sensory association cortices regions; anterior paralimbic areas, including mPFC and insular cortex; and ventral striatum.

Functional Imaging Findings

Although no significant differences in rCBF were identified between subjects with SocAD and healthy control subjects in the resting state in a SPECT study (Stein and Leslie 1996), subsequent studies performed using activation paradigms in conjunction with PET and fMRI yielded more informative results. Symptom provocation studies employing public-speaking challenges found exaggerated activation within the amygdala in SocAD subjects versus healthy control subjects (Lorberbaum et al. 2004; Tillfors et al. 2001). Studies utilizing cognitive activation paradigms also implicated exaggerated amygdala responses in SocAD in response to face stimuli. Birbaumer et al. (1998) used fMRI to study SocAD subjects versus healthy control subjects while they were exposed to slides of neutral human faces or aversive odors. In comparison with the control group, the SocAD group exhibited hyperresponsivity within the amygdala that was specific to the human face stimuli. More recently, two studies contrasting responses to socially threatening (i.e., angry and/or contemptuous) faces found exaggerated amygdala activation in SocAD versus control groups (Stein et al. 2002; Straube et al. 2004a).

Finally, Schneider et al. (1999) used fMRI to study SocAD subjects, versus healthy control subjects, in the context of a classical conditioning paradigm; neutral-face stimuli were the CS, and odors (negative odor, odorless air) served as the UCS. In response to the CS associated with the negative odor, the SocAD group displayed signal increases within amygdala and hippocampus, whereas healthy comparison subjects displayed signal decreases in these same regions.

Complementary Neuroimaging Findings: Structure and Chemistry

Potts et al. (1994) used morphometric MRI to examine volumetric measures of total cerebrum, caudate, putamen, and thalamus in SocAD subjects and healthy control subjects. No significant between-group differences were found in any of these regional brain volumes. Thus, further morphometric brain imaging studies of SocAD are needed to study regions in which morphometric abnormalities were identified in other anxiety disorders. Tiihonen et al. (1997) used SPECT and [123I]-labeled beta-CIT to measure the density of dopamine reuptake sites in 11 SocAD subjects and 28 healthy comparison subjects. These investigators found significantly reduced striatal dopamine reuptake binding-site density in the SocAD group. This finding awaits replication.

Summary

Studies of SocAD indicate exaggerated responsivity of medial temporal lobe structures to human face stimuli as well as an aberrant pattern of activity within medial temporal lobe structures during aversive conditioning with human face stimuli. In particular, amygdala hyperresponsivity has been demonstrated in response to in vivo social challenges as well as exposure to socially threatening faces. This is consistent with a hypersensitive system for the assessment or assignment of threat to human faces as a neural substrate for the underpinnings of social anxiety in SocAD. Moreover, the preliminary finding of dopamine receptor abnormalities in SocAD is compatible with theories of dysregulated reward as a factor in social deficits (Stein 1998).

Commonalities and Specificity Across Disorders

In general, the imaging data gathered thus far suggest some commonalities among four anxiety disorders—PTSD, panic disorder, specific phobia, and SocAD—as currently defined. PTSD and panic disorder appear to share amygdala hyperresponsivity to disorder-specific, as well as general, threat-related stimuli. This stands in contrast to the phobias, specific phobia and SocAD, in which amygdala hyperresponsivity appears to be limited to disorder-specific stimuli. In a recent review (Fredrikson and Furmark 2003) that compared data from several separate studies of patients with PTSD, SocAD, and specific phobia, significant positive correlations were found between *right amygdala* responses and the severity of symptoms for each of these disorders. Together with convergent data from other laboratories and unpublished data on panic disorder, these findings implicate hyperresponsivity of the right amygdala as a common substrate across the proposed stress-induced and fear circuitry disorders.

With respect to hippocampal involvement, the data are strongest for PTSD and panic disorder, but with different profiles. In PTSD, the hippocampus appears volumetrically small, with increased resting activity and deficient capacity for activation in the context of explicit learning paradigms. In contrast, in panic disorder, temporal lobe volumetric abnormalities have been principally found in extrahippocampal regions, and most resting activity findings suggest a rightward shift in laterality of function. The hippocampus has been rarely implicated in SocAD or specific phobia.

Finally, with respect to frontal cortical involvement, again, PTSD and panic disorder appear to share profiles of deficient recruitment of pACC. In contrast, in specific phobia pACC size (thickness) is reportedly increased—as opposed to the decreases in volume reported for PTSD—and evidence of dysfunction in frontal cortex is lacking. For SocAD, the data are inconsistent, with at least some suggestion of diminished frontal cortical recruitment in pACC. Interestingly, increased anterior insular activation has been found, incidentally, across all four of these disorders, suggesting that future studies utilizing specific probes of insular response in the context of interoceptive function are warranted.

These profiles of similarities and differences among PTSD, panic disorder, specific phobia, and SocAD are arguably in keeping with the notion that the diseases are distinct from one another, while sharing sufficient similarities in terms of implicated circuitry, to merit inclusion in one disease category. However, such a contention must consider the relative specificity of these findings balanced against the profiles of other disorders that have been excluded from this proposed category of diseases.

As for other anxiety disorders, there are abundant neuroimaging data implicating different neurocircuitry in OCD; numerous convergent studies indicate involvement of orbitofrontal-striatal circuitry and, to date, there are few studies implicating amygdala hyperresponsivity (e.g., Breiter et al. 1996b). In particular, we know of no published evidence of amygdala hyperresponsivity to general negative stimuli, and at least one OCD study has shown *decreased* amygdala responses to face stimuli (Cannistraro et al. 2004). Likewise, OCD is distinguished from the stress-induced and fear circuitry disorders because there is no indication of deficient function nor reduced volume in pACC or hippocampus. Instead, OCD has been associated with altered activity in the orbitofrontal cortex, dorsal ACC, basal ganglia (especially the caudate), and hippocampus (Insel 1992; Rauch et al. 1994, 1997, 1998b, 2007; Saxena et al. 1998).

With respect to generalized anxiety disorder, there are insufficient neuroimaging data to comment on evidence for or against amygdala, pACC, hippocampal, or insular involvement.

The literature on major depressive disorder (MDD) also suggests a central role for the amygdala. Prevailing neurocircuitry models of MDD involve exaggerated activity within a ventral compartment, including the amygdala and ventral prefrontal regions, and deficient activity within a dorsal compartment, including anterolateral and dorsal prefrontal cortical regions, striatum, and hippocampus (Drevets 2000). The amygdala has been found to be hyperactive in resting-state studies of patients with MDD (e.g., Drevets et al. 1992b), and there is some suggestion that this finding is left-lateralized (i.e., the severity of depressive symptoms is correlated with *left amygdala* activity). The hyperactivity within this region is attenuated with successful treatment (Drevets et al. 2002).

Beyond neutral-state studies, using an emotional faces paradigm, Sheline et al. (2001) found that, in comparison with healthy control subjects, subjects with MDD exhibited exaggerated left amygdala responses to masked-fearful faces. Moreover, they found that the magnitude of left amygdala activation correlated with an index of depression severity rather than anxiety severity and that this abnormal activation profile returned toward normal with successful antidepressant medication treatment. Likewise, Fu et al. (2004), in an fMRI study of MDD, demonstrated exaggerated activation in the left amygdala in response to SocAD faces, with return toward normal after antidepressant treatment.

Within the subgenual portion of the ACC, the resting cerebral blood flow and metabolism are reduced in depressive subjects, relative to control subjects, but this reduction in activity appeared to be largely accounted for by a reduction in cortex volume in this region (Drevets et al. 1997; Öngur et al. 1998). Moreover, metabolic activity is increased in this region during the depressed phase, relative to the remitted phase of MDD, as shown both by longitudinal studies demonstrating that metabolism decreases in the subgenual ACC during successful antidepressant drug treatment (Drevets et al. 2002; Mayberg et al. 1999) and by studies in remitted MDD cases showing that activity in this region increases during the depressive relapse induced by tryptophan depletion (Neumeister et al. 2004b). Potentially consistent with these findings regarding the mood state–dependence of subgenual ACC activity in MDD, this region, together with the anterior insula, exhibits elevated activity during induced states of transient sadness in healthy humans (George et al. 1995; Mayberg et al. 1999). In contrast, cognitive activation studies have indicated an attenuated capacity for patients with mood disorder to successfully recruit dorsal ACC (George et al. 1997).

Most germane to comparisons with the stress-induced and fear circuitry disorders, studies of MDD also have identified abnormalities in the pACC, which include elevated resting state metabolic activity (Drevets et al. 1992b), increased serotonin turnover (Agren and Reibring 1994), and histopathological changes (reviewed in Drevets and Price 2005). In addition, pretreatment resting glucose metabolism within pACC has been found to predict subsequent response to antidepressant medication (Mayberg et al. 1997).

Critical Considerations: Past, Present, and Future

SENSITIVITY, SPECIFICITY, AND REPLICATION

Although we have tried to portray the neuroimaging literature pertinent to stress-induced and fear circuitry disorders, we want to emphasize that despite convergence and replication across studies in several instances, nonreplication is also a frequent occurrence. We noted cases of replication, and there are many instances in which a finding has been ostensibly reproduced across a total of two or more studies conducted by two or more laboratories. However, in general, it is rare to find instances in which there are more than two positive studies without at least one-third of the total number of studies yielding negative findings. Moreover, in positive studies, when data are extracted from them and presented for individual subjects, substantial overlap exists between the individual values for the diagnostic group in question and those for the healthy control subjects. For instance, even with thresholds assigned post hoc, it is very rare to find any neuroimaging index in these studies that distinguishes one of these disorders from healthy control subjects at greater than 90% sensitivity and specificity.

Several factors likely contribute to this modest profile of sensitivity, specificity, and reproducibility. Most fundamentally, the tautological reliance on clinical diagnoses as the gold standard can undermine progress toward a pathophysiology-based nomenclature. In other words, if 20% of a sample diagnosed with panic disorder fails to exhibit a neuroimaging marker, this may reflect either the insensitivity of the marker or the imprecision of the diagnosis for identifying people with a common neurobiological substrate. If we aspire to a pathophysiology-based diagnostic scheme, until such time as we have well-established pathophysiology-based, gold standard diagnostic criteria for psychiatric diseases, we may need to identify alternative gold standards—such as treatment response or long-term course—that do not unduly bias us toward retaining the syndrome-based diagnostic scheme of the present. Second, most studies to date have employed pilot probes. We will need to refine and optimize the neuroimaging measures and paradigms that we employ, in an iterative fashion, to enhance sensitivity, specificity, and reliability. Third, most neuroimaging studies are underpowered because the number of subjects studied does not take into account the very stringent statistical criteria used, based on correction for multiple comparisons. Therefore, reproducibility, sensitivity, and specificity must be established in studies that are adequately powered (e.g., larger numbers of subjects per group), which will prove challenging given the pressures of cost and scientific precedent.

Although the issue of reliability has been well studied with respect to structural neuroimaging measures (yielding quite high reliability in general), it has been poorly studied with respect to functional neuroimaging in psychiatry. This is an especially vexing challenge in functional neuroimaging studies of mood and anxiety disorders in which the circuitry of interest (e.g., the limbic system) may be particularly sensitive to novelty/experience effects and the measures are known to be exquisitely sensitive to state variables. Consequently, it is problematic to repeat the same protocol and expect equivalent results across test and retest. Studies formally investigating this issue are long overdue and only beginning to make their way into the peer-reviewed literature (e.g., Johnstone et al. 2005). Ultimately, demonstrating reliability will be essential for the credibility of functional neuroimaging find-

DEVELOPMENTAL PERSPECTIVE AND MARKERS OF RISK VERSUS DISEASE

Although there are other chapters in this volume devoted to the developmental perspective (see Chapter 5, "Continuity and Etiology of Anxiety Disorders," and Chapter 9, "Serotonin, Sensitive Periods, and Anxiety"), we think that the importance of the issue warrants coverage here as well. Developmental neuroimaging studies are essential for several reasons, among them the capacity to study new-onset disease to minimize confounds of chronicity and treatment as well as the potential for identifying the neural underpinnings of risk and predictors of disease onset. Markers of risk are critical for developing strategies for prevention and early intervention.

However, recognizing that neuroimaging markers for risk likely exist also raises the challenge of distinguishing risk markers from markers of disease per se. To illustrate this point, we refer to the example of behavioral inhibition to the unfamiliar as a temperament. Behavioral inhibition to the unfamiliar has been identified as a behavioral phenotype in childhood, characterized by withdrawal/avoidance and reactivity to novel stimuli, that appears to confer risk for the development of later SocAD and perhaps other anxiety disorders (Rosenbaum et al. 1991). It has recently been associated with neuroimaging findings of exaggerated amygdala responses to novel versus neutral faces (Schwartz et al. 2003). This finding underscores the potential liability in cross-sectional studies of adults with and without a given disorder, with respect to interpreting between-group differences. Although investigators may be inclined to attribute such differences to the pathophysiology of disease, such experiments cannot rule out that the observed differences only represent markers of risk. To rule out such confounding influences, investigators must study comparison groups of subjects who have the risk factor but not the full disease.

Furthermore, acknowledging the developmental perspective leads to the consideration of normal versus pathophysiological trajectories over time with respect to brain structure and function. Any brain-based criteria for disease must account for age, in addition to sex, medication effects, and a host of other pertinent temporal variables, such as stage of hormonal cycle for women, and diurnal variations for both sexes (Goldstein et al. 2005; Protopopescu et al. 2005b; Reiman et al. 1996).

Mapping the Agenda for Future Research

In this section we propose 10 key landmarks around which to map the future research agenda with respect to neuroimaging and neurocircuitry of the stress-induced and fear circuitry disorders.

CONDUCTING TRANSLATIONAL RESEARCH

As noted, animal studies have been critical to defining the neurocircuitry of fear conditioning. Such work in animals will continue to be an essential complement to human neuroimaging studies. For instance, animal studies can delineate the relevant neural circuits at greater spatial and temporal resolution and enable the manipulation of the circuitry (e.g., via lesions) not possible in humans.

DEFINING NEW GOLD STANDARDS

We envision innovative human study designs whereby neuroimaging profiles represent independent variables that provide an alternative method for defining group designation for subjects. In the transition from a syndrome-based to a pathophysiology-based nomenclature, interim gold standards such as clinical course and treatment response will be necessary to search for, and find, biological markers that outperform current diagnostic criteria.

OPTIMIZING IMAGING TECHNIQUES

The discipline of psychiatric neuroimaging remains a relatively immature field, in that the basic methods as well as the specific paradigms are destined to evolve substantially over the next 10–25 years. It is premature to rely heavily on the techniques of yesterday or today. Rather, we should equally invest in optimizing existing methods and developing the new applications of tomorrow. We submit that certain very-large-scale studies should await further refinement of the tools available as well as refinement in the hypotheses to be tested.

ASSESSING AND ESTABLISHING RELIABILITY

As neuroimaging methods are developed and applied, it is essential that formal tests of their reliability be conducted. As noted, in the case of functional measures made in conjunction with activation paradigms, this may not be an entirely straightforward enterprise. Therefore, research aimed at developing temporally stable paradigms for measuring limbic system function would be of great value, as would studies that characterize the reliability of popular probes.

REPLICATING AND EXTENDING FINDINGS, WITH ATTENTION TO POWER AND SUBJECT CHARACTERISTICS

Reproducibility is the hallmark of valid science. A premium should be placed on studies that seek to replicate key findings and resolve discrepant findings, particularly by meeting power demands via studies of sufficient subject number. Future research also should seek to extend initial findings, even when previously replicated, by investigating the generalizability of these findings in studies of samples that represent the total population with respect to age, sex, and ethnicity. Likewise, extension studies can seek to address issues of confounding comorbidity and medication effects as well as potential subtypes within a given disorder.

CONDUCTING FOLLOW-UP STUDIES TO ADDRESS ISSUES OF LATERALITY AND INTERREGIONAL EFFECTS

In many instances, initial positive findings warrant follow-up studies to refine the interpretations of the results with respect to anatomical designations. For example, it will be important to conduct such follow-up investigations to formally test for laterality effects, to interrogate precise subdivisions or discrete subnuclei within larger structures, and to conduct tests of interregional interactions. Beyond two-region interactions, progressively sophisticated models must consider interactions across multinodal networks that reflect the inherent organization of brain circuits.

PERFORMING DEVELOPMENTAL/LONGITUDINAL STUDIES

Longitudinal and developmental studies are critical for identifying markers of risk and distinguishing them from markers of disease. Such study designs will also be essential for comparing neuroimaging markers with current diagnostic designations in the prediction of outcome.

CONDUCTING NEUROIMAGING STUDIES OF TREATMENT EFFECTS

Pragmatically, neuroimaging studies that leverage clinical trials provide the most direct opportunities for clinical application. Such studies promise to provide useful information regarding predictors of treatment response as well as quantitative indices of treatment effects on brain structure and physiology

INCORPORATING MULTIMODAL IMAGING

Formal integration of data across imaging modalities has great potential for enhancing the sensitivity and specificity of findings. For instance, combining data acquired using diffusion tensor imaging and functional imaging techniques promises to enable the integration of structural and functional connectivity data. Also, magnetoencephalography or electroencephalography could be integrated with fMRI to delineate network dynamics—an approach that would capitalize on the complementary strengths of these imaging modalities in temporal resolution and spatial resolution, respectively.

COMBINING NEUROIMAGING WITH GENETICS

Studies that combine imaging with genetics may have the greatest impact on advancing our understanding of the interplay between nature, nurture, risk, and disease. Already, pioneering efforts in this field have yielded insights regarding the relatively large amount of variance in brain structural and functional measures that is explained by genotypic information (Hariri et al. 2006; Pezawas et al. 2005).

Conclusion

The convergence of physiological and anatomical data, obtained from basic studies in experimental animals, with the systems neuroscience data, obtained from human neuroimaging studies, has contributed to the development of tentative neurocircuitry models of anxiety disorders. In particular, human neuroimaging studies of PTSD, panic disorder, specific phobia, and SocAD—versus control groups—have provided support for amygdalocentric models of disease, with varying involvement of mPFC subterritories and hippocampus. Interestingly, anterior insular involvement may be another universal feature of these conditions. Thus, commonalities and differences in brain imaging profiles for these four syndromes offer support for maintaining these as distinct diagnoses, categorized together as "stress-induced and fear circuitry disorders." Although this line of inquiry appears quite promising, the reliability, sensitivity, and specificity of the extant human neuroimaging findings have been limited. Further research is needed to refine methods, establish reliability, replicate published results, and extend findings to larger and more representative samples. Moreover, innovative study designs are needed to disentangle neural substrates of risk, compensatory processes, and epiphenomena from fundamental substrates of pathophysiology. In this context, developmental studies are warranted. At present such data are very limited and suggest lack of specificity as well as discontinuities with respect to current diagnostic designations. In addition to a critical review of the relevant human neuroimaging data, we have provided suggestions regarding key considerations for the future research agenda in this domain.

References

Agren H, Reibring L: PET studies of presynaptic monoamine metabolism in depressed patients and healthy volunteers. Pharmacopsychiatry 27:2–6, 1994

Amaral DG, Price JL, Pitkanen A, et al: Anatomical organization of the primate amygdaloid complex, in The Amygdala: Neurobiological Aspects of Emotion, Memory and Mental Dysfunction. Edited by Aggleton JP. New York, Wiley-Liss, 1992, pp 1–66

American Psychiatric Association: Diagnostic and Statistical Manual of Mental Disorders, 4th Edition, Text Revision. Washington, DC, American Psychiatric Association, 2000

Armony JL, Corbo V, Clement MH, et al: Amygdala response in patients with acute PTSD to masked and unmasked emotional facial expressions. Am J Psychiatry 162:1961–1963, 2005

Benkelfat C, Bradwejn J, Meyer E, et al: Functional neuroanatomy of CCK4-induced anxiety in normal healthy volunteers. Am J Psychiatry 152:1180–1184, 1995

Birbaumer N, Grodd W, Oliver D, et al: fMRI reveals amygdala activation to human faces in social phobics. Neuroreport 9:1223–1226, 1998

Bisaga A, Katz JL, Antonini A, et al: Cerebral glucose metabolism in women with panic disorder. Am J Psychiatry 155:1178–1183, 1998

Bonne O, Brandes D, Gilboa A et al: Longitudinal MRI study of hippocampal volume in trauma survivors with PTSD. Am J Psychiatry 158:1248–1251, 2001

Boshuisen ML, Ter Horst GJ, Paans AM, et al: rCBF differences between panic disorder patients and control subjects during anticipatory anxiety and rest. Biol Psychiatry 52:126–135, 2002

Bouton ME: Context and behavioral processes in extinction. Learn Mem 11:485–494, 2004

Brandt CA, Meller J, Keweloh L, et al: Increased benzodiazepine receptor density in the prefrontal cortex in patients with panic disorder. J Neural Transm 105:1325–1333, 1998

Breiter HC, Etcoff NL, Whalen PJ, et al: Response and habituation of the human amygdala during visual processing of facial expression. Neuron 17:875–887, 1996a

Breiter HC, Rauch SL, Kwong KK, et al: Functional magnetic resonance imaging of symptom provocation in obsessive compulsive disorder. Arch Gen Psychiatry 53:595–606, 1996b

Bremner JD, Randall P, Scott TM, et al: MRI-based measurement of hippocampal volume in patients with combat-related posttraumatic stress disorder. Am J Psychiatry 152:973–981, 1995

Bremner JD, Randall P, Vermetten E, et al: Magnetic resonance imaging-based measurement of hippocampal volume in posttraumatic stress disorder related to childhood physical and sexual abuse: a preliminary report. Biol Psychiatry 41:23–32, 1997

Bremner JD, Narayan M, Staib LH, et al: Neural correlates of memories of childhood sexual abuse in women with and without posttraumatic stress disorder. Am J Psychiatry 156:1787–1795, 1999a

Bremner JD, Staib LH, Kaloupek D et al: Neural correlates of exposure to traumatic pictures and sound in Vietnam combat veterans with and without posttraumatic stress disorder: a positron emission tomography study. Biol Psychiatry 45:806–816, 1999b

Bremner JD, Innis RB, Southwick SM, et al: Decreased benzodiazepine receptor binding in prefrontal cortex in combat-related posttraumatic stress disorder. Am J Psychiatry 157:1120–1126, 2000a

Bremner JD, Innis RB, White T, et al: SPECT [I-123]iomazenil measurement of the benzodiazepine receptor in panic disorder. Biol Psychiatry 47:96–106, 2000b

Bremner JD, Vythilingam M, Vermetten E, et al: MRI and PET study of deficits in hippocampal structure and function in women with childhood sexual abuse and posttraumatic stress disorder. Am J Psychiatry 160:924–932, 2003a

Bremner JD, Vythilingam M, Vermetten E et al: Neural correlates of declarative memory for emotionally valenced words in women with posttraumatic stress disorder related to early childhood sexual abuse. Biol Psychiatry 53:879–889, 2003b

Bremner JD, Vermetten E, Vythilingam M, et al: Neural correlates of the classic color and emotional Stroop in women with abuse-related posttraumatic stress disorder. Biol Psychiatry 55:612–620, 2004

Bremner JD, Vermetten E, Schmahl C, et al: Positron emission tomographic imaging of neural correlates of a fear acquisition and extinction paradigm in women with childhood sexual-abuse-related post-traumatic stress disorder. Psychol Med 35:791–806, 2005

Bush G, Whalen PJ, Rosen BR, et al: The Counting Stroop: an interference task specialized for functional neuroimaging—validation study with functional MRI. Hum Brain Mapp 6:270–282, 1998

Bystritsky A, Pontillo D, Powers M, et al: Functional MRI changes during panic anticipation and imagery exposure. Neuroreport 12:3953–3957, 2001

Cannistraro PA, Wright CI, Wedig MM, et al: Amygdala responses to human faces in obsessive-compulsive disorder. Biol Psychiatry 56:916–920, 2004

Carrion VG, Weems CF, Eliez S, et al: Attenuation of frontal asymmetry in pediatric posttraumatic stress disorder. Biol Psychiatry 50:943–951, 2001

Caviness VS Jr, Kennedy DN, Richelme C, et al: The human brain age 7–11 years: a volumetric analysis based upon magnetic resonance images. Cereb Cortex 6:726–736, 1996

Charney DS, Drevets WC: The neurobiological basis of anxiety disorders, in Psychopharmacology: The Fifth Generation of Progress. Edited by Davis K, Charney DS, Coyle J, et al. Baltimore, MD, Lippincott Williams & Wilkins, 2002, pp 901–930

Cheng DT, Knight DC, Smith CN, et al: Functional MRI of human amygdala activity during pavlovian fear conditioning: stimulus processing versus response expression. Behav Neurosci 117:3–10, 2003

Coplan JD, Lydiard RB: Brain circuits in panic disorder. Biol Psychiatry 44:1264–1276, 1998

Corbo V, Clement MH, Armony JL, et al: Size versus shape differences: contrasting voxel-based and volumetric analyses of the anterior cingulate cortex in individuals with acute posttraumatic stress disorder. Biol Psychiatry 58:119–124, 2005

Corcoran KA, Maren S: Factors regulating the effects of hippocampal inactivation on renewal of conditional fear after extinction. Learn Mem 11:598–603, 2004

Critchley HD, Wiens S, Rotshtein P, et al: Neural systems supporting interoceptive awareness. Nat Neurosci 7:189–195, 2004

Dager SR, Strauss WL, Marro KI, et al: Proton magnetic resonance spectroscopy investigation of hyperventilation in subjects with panic disorder and comparison subjects. Am J Psychiatry 152:666–672, 1995

Dager SR, Friedman SD, Heide A, et al: Two-dimensional proton echo-planar spectroscopic imaging of brain metabolic changes during lactate-induced panic. Arch Gen Psychiatry 56:70–77, 1999

Davis M: Are different parts of the extended amygdala involved in fear versus anxiety? Biol Psychiatry 44:1239–1247, 1998

DeBellis MD, Keshavan MS, Clark DB, et al: Developmental traumatology, part II: brain development. Biol Psychiatry 45:1271–1284, 1999

DeBellis MD, Keshavan MS, Spencer S, et al: N-Acetylaspartate concentration in the anterior cingulate of maltreated children and adolescents with PTSD. Am J Psychiatry 157:1175–1177, 2000

DeBellis MD, Hall J, Boring AM, et al: A pilot longitudinal study of hippocampal volumes in pediatric maltreatment-related posttraumatic stress disorder. Biol Psychiatry 50:305–309, 2001

De Cristofaro MT, Sessarego A, Pupi A, et al: Brain perfusion abnormalities in drug-naive, lactate-sensitive panic patients: a SPECT study. Biol Psychiatry 33:505–512, 1993

Dilger S, Straube T, Mentzel HJ, et al: Brain activation to phobia-related pictures in spider phobic humans: an event-related functional magnetic resonance imaging study. Neurosci Lett 348:29–32, 2003

Dougherty DD, Rauch SL (eds): Psychiatric Neuroimaging Research: Contemporary Strategies. Washington, DC, American Psychiatric Publishing, 2001

Drevets WC: Neuroimaging studies of mood disorders. Biol Psychiatry 48:813–829, 2000

Drevets WC, Price JL: Neuroimaging and neuropathological studies of mood disorders, in Biology of Depression: From Novel Insights to Therapeutic Strategies, Vol 1. Edited by Licinio J, Wong ML. Weinheim, Germany, Wiley-VCH Verlag, 2005, pp 427–466

Drevets WC, Videen TO, MacLeod AK, et al: PET images of blood flow changes during anxiety: a correction. Science 256:1696, 1992a

Drevets WC, Videen TO, Price JL, et al: A functional anatomical study of unipolar depression. J Neurosci 12:3628–3641, 1992b

Drevets WC, Price JL, Simpson JR, et al: Subgenual prefrontal cortex abnormalities in mood disorders. Nature 386:824–827, 1997

Drevets WC, Frank E, Price JC: Serotonin type-1A receptor imaging in depression. Nucl Med Biol 27:499–507, 2000

Drevets WC, Bogers W, Raichle ME: Functional anatomical correlates of antidepressant drug treatment assessed using PET measures of regional glucose metabolism. Eur Neuropsychopharmacol 12:527–544, 2002

Ekman P, Friesen WV: Pictures of Facial Affect. Palo Alto, CA, Consulting Psychologists Press, 1976

Fischer H, Andersson JL, Furmark T, et al: Brain correlates of an unexpected panic attack: a human positron emission tomographic study. Neurosci Lett 251:137–140, 1998

Fischl B, Dale AM: Measuring the thickness of the human cerebral cortex from magnetic resonance images. Proc Natl Acad Sci U S A 97:11050–11055, 2000

Fitzgerald DA, Posse S, Moore GJ, et al: Neural correlates of internally generated disgust via autobiographical recall: a functional magnetic resonance imaging investigation. Neurosci Lett 370:91–96, 2004

Fredrikson M, Furmark T: Amygdaloid regional cerebral blood flow and subjective fear during symptom provocation in anxiety disorders. Ann N Y Acad Sci 985:341–347, 2003

Fredrikson M, Wik G, Greitz T, et al: Regional cerebral blood flow during experimental fear. Psychophysiology 30:126–130, 1993

Fredrikson M, Wik G, Annas P, et al: Functional neuroanatomy of visually elicited simple phobic fear: additional data and theoretical analysis. Psychophysiology 32:43–48, 1995a

Fredrikson M, Wik G, Fischer H, et al: Affective and attentive neural networks in humans: a PET study of pavlovian conditioning. Neuroreport 7:97–101, 1995b

Fu CH, Williams SC, Cleare AJ, et al: Attenuation of the neural response to sad faces in major depression by antidepressant treatment: a prospective, event-related functional magnetic resonance imaging study. Arch Gen Psychiatry 61:877–889, 2004

Fujita M, Southwick SM, Denucci CC, et al: Central type benzodiazepine receptors in Gulf War veterans with posttraumatic stress disorder. Biol Psychiatry 56:95–100, 2004

Furmark T, Fischer H, Wik G, et al: The amygdala and individual differences in fear conditioning. Neuroreport 8:3957–3960, 1997

Fyer AJ: Current approaches to etiology and pathophysiology of specific phobia. Biol Psychiatry 44:1295–1304, 1998

George MS, Ketter TA, Parekh PI, et al: Brain activity during transient sadness and happiness in healthy women. Am J Psychiatry 15:341–351, 1995

George MS, Ketter TA, Parekh PI, et al: Blunted left cingulate activation in mood disorder subjects during a response interference task (the Stroop). J Neuropsychiatry Clin Neurosci 9:55–63, 1997

Gilbertson MW, Shenton ME, Ciszewski A, et al: Smaller hippocampal volume predicts pathologic vulnerability to psychological trauma. Nat Neurosci 5:1242–1247, 2002

Gilboa A, Shalev AY, Laor L, et al: Functional connectivity of the prefrontal cortex and the amygdala in posttraumatic stress disorder. Biol Psychiatry 55:263–272, 2004

Goldstein JM, Jerram M, Poldrack R, et al: Hormonal cycle modulates arousal circuitry in women using functional magnetic resonance imaging. J Neurosci 25:9309–9316, 2005

Gorman JM, Kent JM, Sullivan GM, et al: Neuroanatomical hypothesis of panic disorder, revised. Am J Psychiatry 157:493–505, 2000

Gottfried JA, Dolan RJ: Human orbitofrontal cortex mediates extinction learning while accessing conditioned representations of value. Nat Neurosci 7:1144–1152, 2004

Gurvits TV, Shenton ME, Hokama H, et al: Magnetic resonance imaging study of hippocampal volume in chronic, combat-related posttraumatic stress disorder. Biol Psychiatry 40:1091–1099, 1996

Hariri AR, Drabant EM, Weinberger DR: Imaging genetics: perspectives from studies of genetically driven variation in serotonin function and corticolimbic affective processing. Biol Psychiatry 59:888–897, 2006

Hendler T, Rotshtein P, Yeshurun Y, et al: Sensing the invisible: differential sensitivity of visual cortex and amygdala to traumatic context. Neuroimage 19:587–600, 2003

Insel TR: Toward a neuroanatomy of obsessive-compulsive disorder. Arch Gen Psychiatry 49:739–744, 1992

Irwin W, Davidson RJ, Lowe MJ, et al: Human amygdala activation detected with echo-planar functional magnetic resonance imaging. Neuroreport 7:1765–1769, 1996

Johnstone T, Somerville LH, Alexander AL, et al: Stability of amygdala BOLD response to fearful faces over multiple scan sessions. Neuroimage 25:1112–1123, 2005

Kendler KS, Myers J, Prescott CA, et al: The genetic epidemiology of irrational fears and phobias in men. Arch Gen Psychiatry 58:257–267, 2001

Klein DF: False suffocation alarms, spontaneous panics, and related conditions. Arch Gen Psychiatry 50:306–317, 1993

Knight DC, Smith CN, Cheng DT, et al: Amygdala and hippocampal activity during acquisition and extinction of human fear conditioning. Cogn Affect Behav Neurosci 4:317–325, 2004

Kuikka JT, Pitkanen A, Lepola U, et al: Abnormal regional benzodiazepine receptor uptake in the prefrontal cortex in patients with panic disorder. Nucl Med Commun 16:273–280, 1995

LaBar KS, Phelps EA: Reinstatement of conditioned fear in humans is context dependent and impaired in amnesia. Behav Neurosci 119:677–686, 2005

LaBar KS, Gatenby C, Gore JC, et al: Human amygdala activation during conditioned fear acquisition and extinction: a mixed-trial fMRI study. Neuron 20:937–945, 1998

Lane RD, Reiman EM, Bradley MM, et al: Neuroanatomical correlates of pleasant and unpleasant emotion. Neuropsychologia 35:1437–1444, 1997

Lang PJ: Looking at pictures: affective, facial, visceral and behavioral reactions. Psychophysiology 30:261–273, 1993

Lanius RA, Williamson PC, Densmore M, et al: Neural correlates of traumatic memories in posttraumatic stress disorder: a functional MRI investigation. Am J Psychiatry 158:1920–1922, 2001

LeDoux JE: The Emotional Brain. New York, Simon and Schuster, 1996

Liberzon I, Taylor SF, Amdur R, et al: Brain activation in PTSD in response to trauma-related stimuli. Biol Psychiatry 45:817–826, 1999

Lindauer RJ, Booij J, Habraken JB, et al: Cerebral blood flow changes during script-driven imagery in police officers with posttraumatic stress disorder. Biol Psychiatry 56:853–861, 2004a

Lindauer RJ, Vlieger EJ, Jalink M, et al: Smaller hippocampal volume in Dutch police officers with posttraumatic stress disorder. Biol Psychiatry 56:356–363, 2004b

Lorberbaum JP, Kose S, Johnson MR, et al: Neural correlates of speech anticipatory anxiety in generalized social phobia. Neuroreport 15:2701–2705, 2004

Magistretti PJ, Pellerin L: Cellular mechanisms of brain imaging metabolism and their relevance to functional brain imaging. Philos Trans R Soc Lond B Biol Sci 354:1155–1163, 1999

Maguire EA, Burgess N, Donnett JG, et al: Knowing where and getting there: a human navigation network. Science 280:921–924, 1998

Malizia AL, Cunningham VJ, Bell CJ, et al: Decreased brain GABA(A)-benzodiazepine receptor binding in panic disorder: preliminary results from a quantitative PET study. Arch Gen Psychiatry 55:715–720, 1998

Massana G, Serra-Grabulosa JM, Salgado-Pineda P, et al: Amygdalar atrophy in panic disorder patients detected by volumetric magnetic resonance imaging. Neuroimage 19:80–90, 2003a

Massana G, Serra-Grabulosa JM, Salgado-Pineda P et al: Parahippocampal gray matter density in panic disorder: a voxel-based morphometric study. Am J Psychiatry 160:566–568, 2003b

Mayberg HS, Brannan SK, Mahurin RK, et al: Cingulate function in depression: a potential predictor of treatment response. Neuroreport 8:1057–1061, 1997

Mayberg HS, Liotti M, Brannan SK, et al: Reciprocal limbic-cortical function and negative mood: converging PET findings in depression and normal sadness. Am J Psychiatry 156: 675–682, 1999

McEwen BS: Glucocorticoids, depression, and mood disorders: structural remodeling in the brain. Metabolism 54(suppl):20–23, 2005

McNally RJ: Experimental approaches to cognitive abnormality in posttraumatic stress disorder. Behav Res Ther 32:119–122, 1998

McNaughton N: Cognitive dysfunction resulting from hippocampal hyperactivity: a possible cause of anxiety disorder? Pharmacol Biochem Behav 56:603–611, 1997

Milad MR, Quirk GJ: Neurons in medial prefrontal cortex signal memory for fear extinction. Nature 420:70–74, 2002

Milad MR, Orr SP, Pitman RK, et al: Context modulation of memory for fear extinction in humans. Psychophysiology 42:456–464, 2005a

Milad MR, Quinn BT, Pitman RK, et al: Thickness of ventromedial prefrontal cortex in humans is correlated with extinction memory. Proc Natl Acad Sci U S A 102:10706–10711, 2005b

Mohanakrishnan Menon P, Nasrallah HA, Lyons JA, et al: Single-voxel proton MR spectroscopy of right versus left hippocampi in PTSD. Psychiatry Res 123:101–108, 2003

Morgan MA, Romanski LM, LeDoux JE: Extinction of emotional learning: contribution of medial prefrontal cortex. Neurosci Lett 163:109–113, 1993

Morris JS, Dolan RJ: Dissociable amygdala and orbitofrontal responses during reversal fear conditioning. Neuroimage 22:372–380, 2004

Morris JS, Frith CD, Perrett DI, et al: A differential neural response in the human amygdala to fearful and happy facial expressions. Nature 383:812–815, 1996

Morris JS, Friston KJ, Dolan RJ: Neural responses to salient visual stimuli. Proc Biol Sci 264:769–775, 1997

Morris JS, Öhman A, Dolan RJ: Conscious and unconscious emotional learning in the human amygdala. Nature 393: 467–470, 1998

Mountz JM, Modell JG, Wilson MW, et al: Positron emission tomographic evaluation of cerebral blood flow during state anxiety in simple phobia. Arch Gen Psychiatry 46:501–504, 1989

Myers KM, Davis M: Behavioral and neural analysis of extinction. Neuron 36:567–584, 2002

Neumeister A, Bain E, Nugent AC, et al: Reduced serotonin type 1A receptor binding in panic disorder. J Neurosci 24:589–591, 2004a

Neumeister A, Nugent AC, Waldeck T, et al: Behavioral and neural responses to tryptophan depletion in unmedicated remitted patients with major depressive disorder and controls. Arch Gen Psychiatry 61:765–773, 2004b

Nordahl TE, Semple WE, Gross M, et al: Cerebral glucose metabolic differences in patients with panic disorder. Neuropsychopharmacology 3:261–272, 1990

Nordahl TE, Stein MB, Benkelfat C, et al: Regional cerebral metabolic asymmetries replicated in an independent group of patients with panic disorders. Biol Psychiatry 44:998–1006, 1998

Öngür D, Drevets WC, Price JL: Glial reduction in the subgenual prefrontal cortex in mood disorders. Proc Natl Acad Sci U S A 95:13290–13295, 1998

Orr SP, Metzger LJ, Lasko NB, et al: De novo conditioning in trauma-exposed individuals with and without posttraumatic stress disorder. J Abnorm Psychol 109:290–298, 2000

Paquette V, Levesque J, Mensour B, et al: "Change the mind and you change the brain": effects of cognitive-behavioral therapy on the neural correlates of spider phobia. Neuroimage 18:401–409, 2003

Peri T, Ben-Shakhar G, Orr SP, et al: Psychophysiologic assessment of aversive conditioning in posttraumatic stress disorder. Biol Psychiatry 47:512–519, 2000

Pezawas L, Meyer-Lindenberg A, Drabant EM, et al: 5-HTTLPR polymorphism impacts human cingulate-amygdala interactions: a genetic susceptibility mechanism for depression. Nat Neurosci 8:828–834, 2005

Phelps EA, Delgado MR, Nearing KI, et al: Extinction learning in humans: role of the amygdala and vmPFC. Neuron 43:897–905, 2004

Phillips ML, Young AW, Senior C, et al: A specific neural substrate for perceiving facial expressions of disgust. Nature 389:495–498, 1997

Phillips ML, Medford N, Young AW, et al: Time courses of left and right amygdalar responses to fearful facial expressions. Hum Brain Mapp 12:193–202, 2001

Pine DS, Fyer A, Grun J, et al: Methods for developmental studies of fear conditioning circuitry. Biol Psychiatry 50:225–228, 2001

Pissiota A, Frans O, Fernandez M, et al: Neurofunctional correlates of posttraumatic stress disorder: a PET symptom provocation study. Eur Arch Psychiatry Clin Neurosci 252:68–75, 2002

Potts NL, Davidson JR, Krishnan KR, et al: Magnetic resonance imaging in social phobia. Psychiatry Res 52:35–42, 1994

Protopopescu X, Pan H, Altemus M, et al: Orbitofrontal cortex activity related to emotional processing changes across the menstrual cycle. Proc Natl Acad Sci U S A 102:16060–16065, 2005a

Protopopescu X, Pan H, Tuescher O, et al: Differential time courses and specificity of amygdala activity in posttraumatic stress disorder subjects and normal control subjects. Biol Psychiatry 57:464–473, 2005b

Raichle ME: Circulatory and metabolic correlates of brain function in normal humans, in Handbook of Physiology: The Nervous System, V. Edited by Brookhart JM, Mountcastle VB. Baltimore, MD, American Physiological Society, 1987, pp 643–674

Rauch SL: Neuroimaging and the neurobiology of anxiety disorders, in Handbook of Affective Sciences. Edited by Davidson RJ, Scherer K, Goldsmith HH. New York, Oxford University Press, 2003, pp 963–975

Rauch SL, Jenike MA, Alpert NM, et al: Regional cerebral blood flow measured during symptom provocation in obsessive-compulsive disorder using ^{15}O-labeled CO_2 and positron emission tomography. Arch Gen Psychiatry 51:62–70, 1994

Rauch SL, Savage CR, Alpert NM, et al: A positron emission tomographic study of simple phobic symptom provocation. Arch Gen Psychiatry 52:20–28, 1995

Rauch SL, van der Kolk BA, Fisler RE, et al: A symptom provocation study of posttraumatic stress disorder using positron emission tomography and script-driven imagery. Arch Gen Psychiatry 53:380–387, 1996

Rauch SL, Savage CR, Alpert NM: Probing striatal function in obsessive-compulsive disorder: a PET study of implicit sequence learning. J Neuropsychiatry Clin Neurosci 9:568–573, 1997

Rauch SL, Shin LM, Whalen PJ, et al: Neuroimaging and the neuroanatomy of PTSD. CNS Spectr 3(suppl):30–41, 1998a

Rauch SL, Whalen PJ, Dougherty DD, et al: Neurobiological models of obsessive compulsive disorders, in Obsessive-Compulsive Disorders: Practical Management. Edited by Jenike MA, Baer L, Minichiello WE. Boston, MA, Mosby, 1998b, pp 222–253

Rauch SL, Whalen PJ, Shin LM, et al: Exaggerated amygdala responses to masked facial stimuli in posttraumatic stress disorder: a functional MRI study. Biol Psychiatry 47:769–776, 2000

Rauch SL, Shin LM, Segal E, et al: Selectively reduced regional cortical volumes in posttraumatic stress disorder. Neuroreport 14:913–916, 2003a

Rauch SL, Shin LM, Wright CI: Neuroimaging studies of amygdala function in anxiety disorders. Ann N Y Acad Sci 985:389–410, 2003b

Rauch SL, Wright CI, Martis B, et al: A magnetic resonance imaging study of cortical thickness in animal phobia. Biol Psychiatry 55:946–952, 2004

Rauch SL, Shin LM, Phelps EA: Neurocircuitry models of posttraumatic stress disorder and extinction: human neuroimaging research past, present and future. Biol Psychiatry 60:376–382, 2006

Rauch SL, Wedig MM, Wright CI, et al: A functional magnetic resonance imaging study of regional brain activation during implicit sequence learning in obsessive compulsive disorder. Biol Psychiatry 61:330–336, 2007

Reiman EM, Raichle ME, Robins E, et al: The application of positron emission tomography to the study of panic disorder. Am J Psychiatry 143:469–477, 1986

Reiman EM, Raichle ME, Robins E, et al: Neuroanatomical correlates of a lactate-induced anxiety attack. Arch Gen Psychiatry 46:493–500, 1989

Reiman EM, Armstrong SM, Matt KS, et al: The application of positron emission tomography to the study of the normal menstrual cycle. Hum Reprod 11:2799–2805, 1996

Rosenbaum JF, Biederman J, Hirshfeld DR, et al: Further evidence of an association between behavioral inhibition and anxiety disorders: results from a family study of children from a nonclinical sample. J Psychiatr Res 25:49–65, 1991

Sapolsky RM, Uno H, Rebert CS, et al: Hippocampal damage associated with prolonged glucocorticoid exposure in primates. J Neurosci 10:2897–2902, 1990

Saxena S, Brody AL, Schwartz JM, et al: Neuroimaging and frontal-subcortical circuitry in obsessive-compulsive disorder. Br J Psychiatry 173(suppl):26–37, 1998

Schacter DL, Wagner AD: Medial temporal lobe activations in fMRI and PET studies of episodic encoding and retrieval. Hippocampus 9:7–24, 1999

Schneider F, Weiss U, Kessler C, et al: Subcortical correlates of differential classical conditioning of aversive emotional reactions in social phobia. Biol Psychiatry 45:863–871, 1999

Schuff N, Neylan TC, Lenoci MA, et al: Decreased hippocampal N-acetyl aspartate in the absence of atrophy in posttraumatic stress disorder. Biol Psychiatry 50:952–959, 2001

Schwartz CE, Wright CI, Shin LM, et al: Inhibited and uninhibited infants "grown up": adult amygdalar response to novelty. Science 300:1952–1953, 2003

Sheline YI, Barch DM, Donnelly JM, et al: Increased amygdala response to masked emotional faces in depressed subjects resolves with antidepressant treatment: an fMRI study. Biol Psychiatry 50:651–658, 2001

Shin LM, Kosslyn SM, McNally RJ, et al: Visual imagery and perception in posttraumatic stress disorder: a positron emission tomographic investigation. Arch Gen Psychiatry 54:233–241, 1997

Shin LM, McNally RJ, Kosslyn SM, et al: Regional cerebral blood flow during script-driven imagery in childhood sexual abuse-related posttraumatic stress disorder: a PET investigation. Am J Psychiatry 156:575–584, 1999

Shin LM, Whalen PJ, McInerney SC, et al: An fMRI study of anterior cingulate function in posttraumatic stress disorder. Biol Psychiatry 50: 932–942, 2001

Shin LM, Orr SP, Carson MA, et al: Regional cerebral blood flow in amygdala and medial prefrontal cortex during traumatic imagery in male and female Vietnam veterans with PTSD. Arch Gen Psychiatry 61:168–176, 2004a

Shin LM, Shin PS, Heckers S, et al: Explicit memory and hippocampal function in posttraumatic stress disorder. Hippocampus 14:292–300, 2004b

Shin LM, Wright CI, Cannistraro PA, et al: A functional magnetic resonance imaging study of amygdala and medial prefrontal cortex responses to overtly presented fearful faces in posttraumatic stress disorder. Arch Gen Psychiatry 62:273–281, 2005

Stein MB: Neurobiological perspectives on social phobia: from affiliation to zoology. Biol Psychiatry 44:1277–1285, 1998

Stein MB, Leslie WD: A brain SPECT study of generalized social phobia. Biol Psychiatry 39:825–828, 1996

Stein MB, Koverola C, Hanna C, et al: Hippocampal volume in women victimized by childhood sexual abuse. Psychol Med 27:951–960, 1997

Stein MB, Goldin PR, Sareen J, et al: Increased amygdala activation to angry and contemptuous faces in generalized social phobia. Arch Gen Psychiatry 59:1027–1034, 2002

Stewart RS, Devous MD Sr, Rush AJ, et al: Cerebral blood flow changes during sodium-lactate-induced panic attacks. Am J Psychiatry 145:442–449, 1988

Straube T, Kolassa IT, Glauer M, et al: Effect of task conditions on brain responses to threatening faces in social phobics: an event-related functional magnetic resonance imaging study. Biol Psychiatry 56:921–930, 2004a

Straube T, Mentzel HJ, Glauer M, et al: Brain activation to phobia-related words in phobic subjects. Neurosci Lett 372:204–208, 2004b

Taylor WD, Hsu E, Krishnan KR, et al: Diffusion tensor imaging: background, potential, and utility in psychiatric research. Biol Psychiatry 55:201–207, 2004

Tiihonen J, Kuikka J, Bergstrom K, et al: Dopamine reuptake site densities in patients with social phobia. Am J Psychiatry 154:239–242, 1997

Tillfors M, Furmark T, Marteinsdottir I, et al: Cerebral blood flow in subjects with social phobia during stressful speaking tasks: a PET study. Am J Psychiatry 158:1220–1226, 2001

Uchida RR, Del-Ben CM, Santos AC, et al: Decreased left temporal lobe volume of panic patients measured by magnetic resonance imaging. Braz J Med Biol Res 36:925–929, 2003

Vansteenwegen D, Hermans D, Vervliet B, et al: Return of fear in a human differential conditioning paradigm caused by a return to the original acquisition context. Behav Res Ther 43:323–336, 2005

Veltman DJ, Tuinebreijer WE, Winkelman D, et al: Neurophysiological correlates of habituation during exposure in spider phobia. Psychiatry Res 132:149–158, 2004

Vermetten E, Vythilingam M, Southwick SM, et al: Long-term treatment with paroxetine increases verbal declarative memory and hippocampal volume in posttraumatic stress disorder. Biol Psychiatry 54:693–702, 2003

Vyas A, Mitra R, Shankaranarayana Rao BS, et al: Chronic stress induces contrasting patterns of dendritic remodeling in hippocampal and amygdaloid neurons. J Neurosci 22:6810–6818, 2002

Vyas A, Bernal S, Chattarji S: Effects of chronic stress on dendritic arborization in the central and extended amygdala. Brain Res 965:290–294, 2003

Vythilingam M, Anderson ER, Goddard A, et al: Temporal lobe volume in panic disorder: a quantitative magnetic resonance imaging study. Psychiatry Res 99:75–82, 2000

Whalen PJ, Bush G, McNally RJ, et al: The Emotional Counting Stroop paradigm: an fMRI probe of the anterior cingulate affective division. Biol Psychiatry 44:1219–1228, 1998a

Whalen PJ, Rauch SL, Etcoff NL, et al: Masked presentations of emotional facial expressions modulate amygdala activity without explicit knowledge. J Neurosci 18:411–418, 1998b

Whalen PJ, Shin LM, McInerney SC, et al: A functional MRI study of human amygdala responses to facial expressions of fear vs. anger. Emotion 1:70–83, 2001

Wik G, Fredrikson M, Ericson K, et al: A functional cerebral response to frightening visual stimulation. Psychiatry Res 50:15–24, 1993

Winter H, Irle E: Hippocampal volume in adult burn patients with and without posttraumatic stress disorder. Am J Psychiatry 161:2194–2200, 2004

Woods SW, Koster K, Krystal JK, et al: Yohimbine alters regional cerebral blood flow in panic disorder. Lancet 2:678, 1988

Wright CI, Fischer H, Whalen PJ, et al: Differential habituation in the prefrontal cortex and amygdala to repeatedly presented emotional facial stimuli. Neuroreport 12:379–383, 2001

Wright CI, Martis B, McMullin K, et al: Amygdala and insular responses to emotionally valenced human faces in small animal specific phobia. Biol Psychiatry 54:1067–1076, 2003

Wright P, He G, Shapira NA, et al: Disgust and the insula: fMRI responses to pictures of mutilation and contamination. Neuroreport 15:2347–2351, 2004

Yamasue H, Kasai K, Iwanami A, et al: Voxel-based analysis of MRI reveals anterior cingulate gray-matter volume reduction in posttraumatic stress disorder due to terrorism. Proc Natl Acad Sci U S A 100:9039–9043, 2003

13

ROLE OF NEUROCHEMICAL AND NEUROENDOCRINE MARKERS OF FEAR IN CLASSIFICATION OF ANXIETY DISORDERS

Rachel Yehuda, Ph.D.

Representative Neurochemical and Neuroendocrine Findings

Although a comprehensive review of the literature is not undertaken here, Table 13–1 provides a summary of representative findings that are consistent with the majority of published reports. Within the four anxiety disorders—panic disorder, PTSD, GAD, and phobic disorder—there is no uniformity of results with respect to a single major ambient neurotransmitter/hormone level, nor is there uniformity of responses to neurochemical or neuroendocrine provocations. Each of these disorders appears to have a distinct biological signature.

Generally, panic disorder and PTSD are more similar to each other in showing analogous responses to cholecystokinin, catecholaminergic (e.g., yohimbine), and serotonergic (e.g., *meta*-chlorophenylpiperazine [mCPP]) provocations, whereas subjects with GAD and phobias do not differ from control subjects. Yet panic disorder and PTSD differ on neuroendocrine baseline and challenge measures. With respect to corticotropin-releasing factor (CRF), the majority of studies do not find

TABLE 13–1. Directional differences in biological findings among anxiety disorders

	Panic	PTSD	GAD	Phobia
Neurochemical provocation				
Cholecystokinin	↑ (Kennedy et al. 1999)	↑ (Kellner et al. 2000)	↔ (Katzman et al. 2004)	↔ (Katzman et al. 2004)
Catecholamine	↑ (Charney et al. 1984)	↑ (Southwick et al. 1993, 1997)	↔ (Charney et al. 1984)	↔ (Charney et al. 1984)
Serotonin	↑ (Charney et al. 1987; Kahn et al. 1991)	↑ (Southwick et al. 1997)	↔ (Charney et al. 1987)	↔ (Charney et al. 1987)
Lactate/CO_2	↑ (Peskind et al. 1998; Tancer et al. 1994–1995)	↑ (Jensen et al. 1997)	↔ (Perna et al. 1999)	↔ (Perna et al. 1999; Tancer et al. 1994–1995)
Neuroendocrine baseline				
CRF concentration	↔ (Fossey et al. 1996; Tharmalingam et al. 2006)	↑ (Bremner et al. 1997; Yehuda 2002)	↔ (Fossey et al. 1996)	↔ (Fossey et al. 1996)
Cortisol concentration	↑ (Uhde et al. 1988, 1994)	↓ (Hoen-Saric et al. 1991; Yehuda 2002; Yehuda et al. 1996)	↔ (Rosenbaum et al. 1983)	↔ (Condren et al. 2002; Furlan et al. 2001; Potts et al. 1991)
Neuroendocrine challenge				
DST	↑ (Carson et al. 1988; Kathol et al. 1988; Uhde et al. 1994)	↓ (Yehuda 2002; Yehuda et al. 2004)	↔ (Avery et al. 1985)	↔ (Avery et al. 1985; Uhde et al. 1994)

Note.   ↑=increased response of dependent variable; ↓=decreased response of dependent variable; ↔=no significant difference compared with normal control; CRF=corticotropin-releasing factor; DST=dexamethasone suppression test; GAD=generalized anxiety disorder; PTSD=posttraumatic stress disorder.

evidence for increased CRF in any of the anxiety disorders, other than PTSD. With respect to ambient cortisol levels, generally, PTSD has been associated with normal to low cortisol levels, whereas the other three anxiety disorders have been associated with normal—and in rare circumstances, increased—cortisol levels. Cortisol responses on the dexamethasone suppression test are generally in the direction of hypersuppression in PTSD, increased suppression in panic disorder, and unaltered suppression in GAD and phobias. Although this review is far from complete and does not take into consideration disparate observations within a diagnostic category, it does illustrate an essential feature of the literature: namely, that there is no particular neurochemical or neuroendocrine pattern of findings that allows the anxiety disorders to be subsumed into one category.

There are interesting observations supporting the idea that biological alterations in these conditions are also different from those associated with normative responses of fear. For example, although eliciting fear in laboratory animals is accompanied by increased cortisol levels, neither provoked nor spontaneous panic attacks are associated with increased cortisol levels. Persons with GAD and social phobia do not show any neurochemical or neuroendocrine alterations, compared with control subjects, but they do seem to show increased neuroendocrine responses to induced stressors in the laboratory.

In contrast to neurochemical and neuroendocrine findings in the anxiety disorders, neuroimaging data have provided consistent evidence implicating the amygdala, hypothalamus, and other brain regions involved in fear responses (see Chapter 12, "Neuroimaging and Neuroanatomy of Stress-Induced and Fear Circuitry Disorders"). These data have been more uniform in suggesting linkages within and between different anxiety disorders, similar to findings that would be anticipated on the basis of animal studies of fear. That both structural and functional changes in these regions are present in patients with anxiety disorders raises several questions, ranging from the utility of neurochemical and neuroendocrine data in the anxiety disorders to the conceptual problem of resolving discrepancies between information obtained from neuroimaging studies and information from investigations using these more peripheral measures.

Why Anxiety Disorders May Not Be Similar From a Neurochemical/Neuroendocrine Perspective

There are several sources that contribute to disparate findings, all of which have implications for whether anxiety disorders are manifestations of fear-related responses. The first concerns methodological error: that differences in how studies are conducted account for the lack of uniformity in the findings. The lack of cohesive findings may be a result of the way the clinical syndromes are currently defined. For example, classification by current diagnostic criteria, rather than specific behavioral domains, may reduce the power of these measures to map to underlying pathophysiology. Alternatively, the concept of fear responses on which hypotheses are based may be flawed or incomplete. To the extent that preclinical paradigms do not offer a complete conceptual model of anxiety disorders, there may not be a good match between biological alterations observed in those models and those seen in patients with anxiety disorders. Moreover, it may be that the disorders that are thought to be expressions of fear are actually expressions of a different affect.

Methodological Problems

Historically, neurochemical and neuroendocrine studies have relied on peripheral measures that have been criticized for not necessarily reflecting brain processes. Such measures may, it is argued, be too far "downstream" from measures that would actually be informative or may be subject to competing regulatory influences and therefore not able to accurately portray the central processes articulated in basic science studies. However, these criticisms only apply to understanding why peripheral markers show discrepant findings from central measures obtained with neuroimaging techniques. The criticisms do not explain why the different anxiety disorders show different patterns from one another. Nor do they provide a compelling explanation for why findings such as low cortisol levels in persons with PTSD and failure of cortisol levels to increase during induced or spontaneous panic attacks are very different from findings of cortisol levels obtained from animals and healthy volunteers who are exposed to laboratory provocations designed to induce fear.

Study design is a source of variation that may explain differences among the anxiety disorders. It is not always clear what the appropriate comparison groups are for anxiety disorders. It is particularly problematic to study "healthy" comparison subjects if the biological alteration of interest is related to risk or genetics, because such subjects may have the same diathesis for anxiety disorders without the precipitating stressor. Thus, if some disorders are more likely to be based on genetic diatheses or subject to environmental modification of neurochemical/neuroendocrine systems, these disorders may be different from one another on these measures. Furthermore, to the extent that biological measures of fear exist on a normal continuum, examination of baseline measures may not be sufficiently distinct to yield diagnostic differences.

What is not considered here are the methodological confounds that potentially account for lack of reproducibility of biological findings within a particular diagnostic grouping. Although such issues are important, they are not relevant to the larger observation of directional differences in markers across anxiety disorders—especially those observed within the context of a single design. Certainly, neurochemical and neuroendocrine studies are informative to the extent that investigators are careful to use adequate sample numbers and minimize contributions of individual differences. However, because of the extent that biological measures are affected by individual differences, such measures might be poor biomarkers.

In this context it is important to make a distinction between an unreliable marker and an uninformative one. The former might actually be more problematic with respect to diagnostic classification. If the goal is to utilize biological measures to make decisions with respect to DSM-V classifications, based on fear-related pathophysiology, the measures must provide meaningful and valid information about biological aspects of fear.

Definitional Problems in DSM-IV

The impetus for determining whether to reclassify panic disorder, PTSD, GAD, and phobias is based on the clinical similarities and overlapping symptoms of these disorders. This is the rationale for attempting to delineate a common underlying biological basis. It therefore becomes important to consider the possibility that discrepant findings between, and sometimes within, anxiety disorders could be a result of failure to appropriately capture the salient clinical features that represent the correlates of the biological measures. Thus, rather than being associated with presence or absence of a specific constellation of symptoms as required by the DSM-IV (American Psychiatric Association 1994, 2000) formulation, biological measures in anxiety disorders may be related to symptom severity, level of disability, or behavioral dimensions. To the extent that specific correlates of fear markers and clinical indices in anxiety disorders could be related, this might enhance the ability of these peripheral markers to justify a link between anxiety disorders based on fear. Such relationships may or may not create an argument for reconceptualizing diagnostic criteria for specific anxiety disorders.

Anxiety disorders are often comorbid with mood, personality, and substance abuse disorders. These comorbid conditions may complicate the use of biological measures to justify diagnostic groupings but do not provide evidence that disparate conditions are not linked. Importantly, the attribution that the failure of neurochemical and neuroendocrine markers to classify anxiety disorders—based on fear and stress—is related to diagnostic criteria or clinical heterogeneity of samples constitutes an affirmation of our faith in the capacity of both the biological measures and the underlying conceptions to inform classification.

Conceptual Foundations

Clinical reality is the conceptual foundation of psychiatric research. Thus, although specific issues regarding presence or absence of diagnostic criteria could be debated, it is not in question that such conditions exist and cause impairment. In attempting to focus on the similarities across the anxiety disorders, it is possible that the salient features that make these conditions so impairing are not based on the obvious signs of fear and stress that they seem to have in common. One reason for the mismatch between neurochemical/neuroendocrine data and the fear literature might be a result of false attribution of the fundamental clinical problem to fear responses simply because these aspects are present.

For example, PTSD occurs after exposure to an event that elicited extreme fear. However, because many persons who experience fear do not experience PTSD, experiencing fear does not sufficiently explain the development of this disorder. It is also arguable whether persons who have chronic PTSD continue to experience fear. Certainly, PTSD patients are extremely physiologically and psychologically distressed by reminders of their traumatic events. They avoid reminders of these events and show an increased vigilance, presumably in an attempt to maintain their safety. Yet, interestingly, neither fear nor anticipatory anxiety is a criterion for PTSD.

With GAD, many of the same psychological and physiological symptoms are present as in PTSD, but an event has not actually happened. Rather, the symptoms appear to result from excessive worrying and anticipation of an event that has not happened. It is not clear whether the anticipatory worry is analogous to a realized fear from an event that has occurred. In contrast, patients with panic disorder experience real heart-pounding fear but presumably do not do so in response to a particular stimulus. Thus, although the reaction is clearly one that looks like fear, in the absence of a environmental event that is interpreted as fearful it is not clear whether such a response would be neurochemically or endocrinologically analogous to fear in the presence of a stimulus. With phobias, the fear evoked by a specific stimulus is thought to be irrational. However, it is not clear whether the critical and impairing factor is the response of fear or the irrationality of the fear.

These distinctions suggest that although anxiety disorders may seem on the surface to resemble manifestations of stress and fear, the underlying pathological components of the disorders may lie in the fact that the fear response deviates from how it might manifest in the absence of disorder. That is, in PTSD, the alteration may be the inability to mobilize biological systems necessary for recovering from fear or stress. In GAD, the alteration may involve a failure to mobilize yet other biological systems necessary for providing corrective information or comforting or calming thoughts. If this were the case, then biological measures that represent deviations from those expected in response to fear would actually be more informative than those related to fear.

Role of Environment

One of the central problems in using nonclinical models of stress and fear as a basis for identifying biological systems involved in the pathophysiology of anxiety disorders is that in the experimental situation, there is usually a clearly defined event that is the precipitant of the fear reactions. As discussed earlier, with the exception of PTSD, the fear-like responses occurring in patients are thought to occur even in the absence of an event. In PTSD, the occurrence of an event that precipitates the disorder does not provide a sufficient explanation for why the fear response does not abate with time.

There are several problems to contend with in considering the extent to which experimental studies of fear and anxiety can be helpful in studies of the biology of anxiety disorders. The first is identifying the extent to which symptoms in anxiety disorders actually represent a response to an event or anticipation of a precipitating environmental event. The second is determining whether the symptoms of anxiety disorders are representations of normative responses to fear or are qualitatively different, particularly to the extent where they do not seem to be the product of an environmental event that is interpreted as fearful. A third and challenging problem, related to the second, is considering the extent to which the symptoms of anxiety disorders are similar to manifestations of anxiety that occur in the absence of disorder.

Reconceptualizing the Role of Fear and Stress in Anxiety Disorders From Existing Data

The previous discussion highlights that there are both similarities and differences across the anxiety disorders. It is reasonable to postulate that biological alterations that reflect the features these disorders share in common would be similar. For example, it may be that exaggerated activation of the amygdala in response to provocation is a consequence of experiencing anxiety, regardless of whether the anxiety is anticipatory or based on interpretations of threat in the environment. In addition, neurochemical and neuroendocrine alterations may reflect different types of processes that relate to differences between disorders.

There are several issues. With respect to biological measures common to the anxiety disorders, there is probably a good case for deemphasizing the role of stress in PTSD and reemphasizing it in other disorders, particularly if the biological measure is associated with responding to stress or provocation. Thus, the organizing framework for the anxiety disorders would center around presence of a precipitating event and the necessity for persistent reactions, either because events are re-created or because of the fear that they will be. In PTSD, an environmental event may have occurred but may not be relevant to the pathophysiological features of the disorder. Similarly, the other anxiety disorders could reflect—as they largely do—anticipation, rather than realization, of events.

Anxiety disorders could also be reconceptualized in terms of abnormal expressions of stress and fear, as suggested earlier. If this were to occur, the emphasis of biological research would shift from trying to find similarities with normal fear, experienced in appropriate contexts, to delineating the biological processes that differentiate responses in disorders. Such a reconceptualization would potentially support a reclassification based on disorders representing abnormal manifestations of fear responses. In such cases, observed biological *differences*—not similarities—between fear responses as they occur in anxiety disorders and those described in the preclinical or normal human literature would constitute important targets for drug development. Neurochemical and neuroendocrine studies would then potentially be relevant to pathophysiology, whereas imaging findings would be reflections of physiology—that is, to the extent that the physiology expresses the normal circuitry of fear in the brain, it may not be a reflection of the interesting pathological processes that explain, provoke, and sustain fear in patients with anxiety disorders.

Clinical Implications

The question of whether anxiety disorders reflect processes associated with fear responses is important with respect to nosology and treatment. It is essential to understand the extent to which anxiety disorders represent overreactions due to a failure of biological mechanisms associated with suppressing or containing fear reactions. All persons are subjected to fearful and stressful situations at times, but few individuals develop chronic psychiatric disturbances as a result. It is important that we do not consider events, even those that result in fear responses, as pathogens and, moreover, that the expected fear and stress responses to such events are not conceptualized as pathology.

Current treatment of anxiety disorders suggests that we are not concerned with reversing the biological consequences of fearful events or fear responses. These are neither the proximal causes of psychopathology nor the targets of psychopharmacological interventions. Although biological alterations associated with fear may be present in persons who are expressing stress, such alterations may not be the problem or the solution in anxiety disorders and probably ought to not then be the basis for a reconceptualization of these disorders as relating to fear. To date, treatments focus on reducing symptoms, usually by modifying neurotransmitter and neuroendocrine systems. Such an approach seems warranted but leaves questions unanswered with respect to pathophysiology that can hopefully be examined by combining neuroimaging and neurochemical/neuroendocrine biological strategies.

References

American Psychiatric Association: Diagnostic and Statistical Manual of Mental Disorders, 4th Edition. Washington, DC, American Psychiatric Association, 1994

American Psychiatric Association: Diagnostic and Statistical Manual of Mental Disorders, 4th Edition, Text Revision. Washington, DC, American Psychiatric Association, 2000

Avery DH, Osgood TB, Ishiki DM, et al: The DST in psychiatric outpatients with generalized anxiety disorder, panic disorder, or primary affective disorder. Am J Psychiatry 142:844–848, 1985

Bremner JD, Licinio J, Darnell A, et al: Elevated CSF corticotropin-releasing factor concentrations in posttraumatic stress disorder. Am J Psychiatry 154:624–629, 1997

Carson SW, Halbreich U, Yeh CM: Altered plasma dexamethasone and cortisol suppressibility in patients with panic disorders. Biol Psychiatry 24:56–62, 1988

Charney DS, Heninger GR, Breier A: Noradrenergic function in panic anxiety: effects of yohimbine in healthy subjects and patients with agoraphobia and panic disorder. Arch Gen Psychiatry 41:751–763, 1984

Charney DS, Woods SW, Goodman WK: Serotonin function in anxiety, II: effects of the serotonin agonist MCPP in panic disorder patients and healthy subjects. Psychopharmacology (Berl) 92:14–24, 1987

Condren RM, O'Neill A, Ryan MC, et al: HPA axis response to a psychological stressor in generalised social phobia. Psychoneuroendocrinology 27:693–703, 2002

Fossey MD, Lydiard RB, Ballenger JC: Cerebrospinal fluid corticotropin-releasing factor concentrations in patients with anxiety disorders and normal comparison subjects. Biol Psychiatry 39:703–707, 1996

Furlan PM, DeMartinis N, Schweizer E, et al: Abnormal salivary cortisol levels in social phobic patients in response to acute psychological but not physical stress. Biol Psychiatry 50:254–259, 2001

Hoen-Saric R, McLeod DR, Lee YB, et al: Cortisol levels in generalized anxiety disorder. Psychiatry Res 38:313–315, 1991

Jensen CF, Keller TW, Peskind ER, et al: Behavioral and neuroendocrine responses to sodium lactate infusion in subjects with posttraumatic stress disorder. Am J Psychiatry 154:266–268, 1997

Kahn RS, Wetzler S, Asnis GM, et al: Pituitary hormone responses to meta-chlorophenylpiperazine in panic disorder and healthy control subjects. Psychiatry Res 37:25–34, 1991

Kathol RG, Noyes R, Lopez A: Similarities in hypothalamic-pituitary-adrenal axis activity between patients with panic disorder and those experiencing external stress. Psychiatr Clin North Am 11:335–348, 1988

Katzman MA, Koszycki D, Bradwejn J: Effects of CCK-tetrapeptide in patients with social phobia and obsessive-compulsive disorder. Depress Anxiety 20:51–58, 2004

Kellner M, Wiedemann K, Yassouridis A, et al: Behavioral and endocrine response to cholecystokinin tetrapeptide in patients with posttraumatic stress disorder. Biol Psychiatry 47:107–111, 2000

Kennedy JL, Bradwejn J, Koszycki D, et al: Investigation of cholecystokinin system genes in panic disorder. Mol Psychiatry 4:284–285, 1999

Perna G, Bussi R, Allevi L, et al: Sensitivity to 35% carbon dioxide in patients with generalized anxiety disorder. J Clin Psychiatry 60:379–384, 1999

Peskind ER, Jensen CF, Pascualy M, et al: Sodium lactate and hypertonic sodium chloride induce equivalent panic incidence, panic symptoms, and hypernatremia in panic disorder. Biol Psychiatry 44:1007–1016, 1998

Potts NL, Davidson JR, Krishnan KR, et al: Levels of urinary free cortisol in social phobia. J Clin Psychiatry 52(suppl):41–42, 1991

Rosenbaum AH, Schatzberg AF, Jost FA, et al: Urinary free cortisol levels in anxiety. Psychosomatics 24:835–837, 1983

Southwick SM, Krystal JH, Morgan CA, et al: Abnormal noradrenergic function in posttraumatic stress disorder. Arch Gen Psychiatry 50:266–274, 1993

Southwick SM, Krystal JH, Bremner JD, et al: Noradrenergic and serotonergic function in posttraumatic stress disorder. Arch Gen Psychiatry 54:749–758, 1997

Tancer ME, Stein MB, Uhde TW: Lactic acid response to caffeine in panic disorder: comparison with social phobics and normal controls. Anxiety 1:138–140, 1994–1995

Tharmalingam S, King N, De Luca V, et al: Lack of association between the corticotrophin-releasing hormone receptor 2 gene and panic disorder. Psychiatr Genet 16:93–97, 2006

Uhde TW, Joffe RT, Jimerson DC, et al: Normal urinary free cortisol and plasma MHPG in panic disorder: clinical and theoretical implications. Biol Psychiatry 23:575–585, 1988

Uhde TW, Tancer ME, Gelernter CS, et al: Normal urinary free cortisol and postdexamethasone cortisol in social phobia: comparison to normal volunteers. J Affect Disord 30:155–161, 1994

Yehuda R: Current status of cortisol findings in post-traumatic stress disorder. Psychiatr Clin North Am 25:341–368, 2002

Yehuda R, Teicher MH, Trestman RL, et al: Cortisol regulation in posttraumatic stress disorder and major depression: a chronobiological analysis. Biol Psychiatry 40:79–88, 1996

Yehuda R, Halligan SL, Golier JA, et al: Effects of trauma exposure on the cortisol response to dexamethasone administration in PTSD and major depressive disorder. Psychoneuroendocrinology 29:389–404, 2004

14

ANXIETY AND SUBSTANCE ABUSE

Implications for Pathophysiology and DSM-V

Edward V. Nunes, M.D.
Carlos Blanco, M.D., Ph.D.

The challenge facing the field of psychiatry as it moves toward the development of DSM-V is in updating the nosology so it remains most clinically useful while pursuing the long-term goal of developing a nosology based primarily on pathophysiology, thereby moving psychiatric nosology closer to the classification of disorders in the rest of medicine. Why is it important to address substance use disorders in the development of the nosology of the DSM-V anxiety disorders?

The high degree of co-occurrence between anxiety disorders and substance use disorders is well known from studies of both clinical and large community samples. Attention to this relationship has been somewhat overshadowed by the prevalence and high co-occurrence of *mood* disorders among substance-dependent patients. However, the strengths of association with substance use disorders are as strong, if not stronger, for the anxiety disorders as for the mood disorders, particularly so for those anxiety disorders falling on the spectrum of fear and fear-related conditions, including panic disorder, phobias, and posttraumatic stress disorder (PTSD).

In a simplified conceptualization, three basic etiological relationships may exist between anxiety disorders and substance abuse (see also Figure 14–1):

1. An anxiety disorder may function as an etiological risk factor contributing to the development of a substance use disorder.

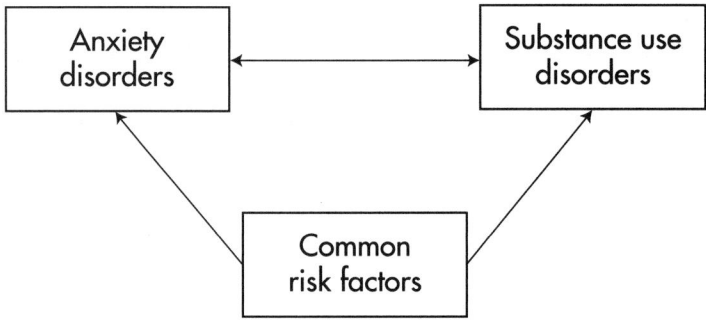

FIGURE 14–1. Potential etiological relationships between anxiety disorders and substance use disorders.

2. Conversely, substance use or abuse may contribute etiologically to the development of anxiety disorders.
3. Both anxiety and substance-use disorders may share common risk factors.

In this chapter, we review evidence from the literature on epidemiology, treatment, and neurobiology to assess the evidence supporting each of these possible relationships. Understanding the potentially shared neurobiology of these disorders should help to push forward the goal of a pathophysiologically based nosology. At the same time, the data will have practical implications for anxiety disorders in the DSM-V.

Epidemiology of Anxiety and Substance Abuse

Anxiety symptoms are very common among substance-dependent patients. In rethinking the nosology of anxiety and substance use disorders, it is well to remember the relative lack of clarity that prevailed prior to the advent of neo-Kraepelian diagnostic criteria in the form of the Feighner, Research Diagnostic, DSM-III, and DSM-IV criteria (American Psychiatric Association 1980, 1994; Feighner et al. 1972). Syndromes often were defined on the basis of internal states that were difficult to observe or objectify or upon etiological presumptions. The field was also divided as to the meaning of psychiatric symptoms, such as anxiety, among substance-dependent patients. Some practitioners, particularly those with a background in psychiatry, tended to see symptoms of drug or alcohol abuse as symptomatic of underlying personality, mood, or anxiety disorders, a tendency that led to a therapeutic focus on treating psychopathology and a relative neglect of the substance use disorders, often to the detriment of patients. Other clinicians, often those involved in the treatment of substance use disorders, tended to view psychological symptoms, such as anxiety or depression, as predominantly byproducts of the substance use disorder, leading to the view that the treatment efforts should focus exclusively on the latter, again to the detriment of patients, whose significant psychopathology often went untreated (Nunes and Levin 2004).

The new diagnostic criteria, based on clinical phenomenology, led to a generation of epidemiological studies in both clinical and large community samples. These studies provide the groundwork for a more balanced understanding of psychiatric and substance use disorders and their comorbidity, an understanding that stands as an important accomplishment of current nosology.

A large number of studies have now been published documenting the lifetime and current prevalence of mood and anxiety disorders among various clinical samples of substance-dependent patients (for review, see Hasin et al. 2004). Studies of alcohol-dependent, cocaine-dependent, or opioid-dependent patients (the latter mainly drawn from methadone maintenance programs) show lifetime prevalences in the range of 5%–15% for panic disorder, 5%–20% for generalized anxiety disorder (GAD), and 10%–30% for PTSD. In comparison, these clinically based studies have yielded lifetime prevalences between 10% and 60% for major depressive disorder. Follow-up studies among clinical samples have tended to suggest that such psychopathology is associated with worse clinical outcome, although these follow-up studies have focused more on mood disorders than on anxiety disorders. Furthermore, several studies suggest that the presence of anxiety disorders is associated with greater illness severity or poor outcome of substance use disorders (Burns et al. 2005; Kushner et al. 2005; Schneider et al. 2001). These studies establish anxiety disorders as a highly frequent, clinically significant problem among substance-dependent patients.

At least three large community-based diagnostic surveys have confirmed and quantified the co-occurrence of anxiety and substance use disorders. These surveys include the Epidemiologic Catchment Area (ECA) study, the National Comorbidity Survey (NCS), and the National Epidemiologic Survey of Alcohol and Related Conditions (NESARC) (Angst 1996; Grant et al. 2004a, 2004b; Kessler et al. 1995, 1997a, 1997b; Magee et al. 1996; Regier et al. 1990). Odds ratios that quantify the association between substance use disorders and varying anxiety disorders in the fear conditioning spectrum are displayed in Table 14–1, along with data on depressive disorders, bipolar disorder, and antisocial personality, for comparison. As can be seen in the table, the findings are relatively consistent across these national surveys, suggesting odds ratios of association of 2 or greater, similar to the odds ratios for major depression and dysthymia. Strengths of association tend to be greater between drug dependence disorders and substance use disorders, although the associations are still significant for alcohol use disorders. These national surveys have shown that both substance use and anxiety disorders are common in the general population and that their co-occurrence is greater than would be expected by chance alone.

TABLE 14–1. Odds ratios from three community surveys for co-occurrence of substance dependence disorders with anxiety and other psychiatric disorders

	ECA[a]		NCS[a]				NESARC[b]	
			Men	Women	Men	Women		
Psychiatric disorder classification	Alcohol dependence	Other drug dependence	Alcohol dependence	Alcohol dependence	Other drug dependence	Other drug dependence	Alcohol dependence	Other drug dependence
Anxiety disorders								
Any anxiety disorder	1.8	2.4	2.22	3.08			2.6	6.2
Panic disorder	3.3	4.4	2.27	2.98				
Panic disorder with agoraphobia	1.6[c]	2.2[c]					3.6	10.5
Panic disorder without agoraphobia							3.4	7.6
Social phobia	1.6[c]	2.2[c]	2.41	2.62	2.56[e]	2.56[e]	2.5	5.4
Simple phobia	1.6[c]	2.2[c]	3.11	2.63	2.47[e]	2.47[e]	2.2	3.8
Posttraumatic stress disorder			3.2	3.6	2.97[f]	4.46[f]		
Generalized anxiety disorder			3.86	3.01			3.1	10.4
Other psychiatric disorders								
Antisocial personality disorder	14.7	15.6	8.34	17.01			7.1	18.5
Any affective disorder	2.2	4.4	3.16	4.36			4.1	12.5
Bipolar disorder	4.6	8.3	12.03[d]	5.30[d]			5.7[d]	13.9[d]

TABLE 14–1. Odds ratios from three community surveys for co-occurrence of substance dependence disorders with anxiety and other psychiatric disorders *(continued)*

	ECA[a]		NCS[a]				NESARC[b]	
	Alcohol	Other drug	Men	Women	Men	Women	Alcohol	Other drug
Psychiatric disorder classification	dependence	dependence	Alcohol dependence		Other drug dependence		dependence	dependence
Other psychiatric disorders *(continued)*								
Major depressive disorder	1.6	3.7	2.95	4.05	2.0[e]	2.0[e]	3.7	9.0
Dysthymia	2.3	3.6	3.81	3.63	1.33[e]	1.33[e]	2.8	11.3

Note. ECA=Epidemiologic Catchment Area (Regier et al. 1990); NCS=National Comorbidity Survey (Angst 1996; Kessler et al. 1995, 1997a, 1997b; Magee et al. 1996); NESARC=National Epidemiologic Survey on Alcohol and Related Conditions (Grant et al. 2004a, 2004b).
[a]Lifetime odds ratios of co-occurrence of disorders reported.
[b]12-month odds ratios of co-occurrence of disorders reported.
[c]Panic disorder with agoraphobia, social phobia, and simple phobia reported as a group.
[d]Mania (bipolar I).
[e]Odds ratios reported for men and women combined.
[f]Drug abuse or dependence.

Taken together, these studies of clinical and community samples suggest that among substance-dependent individuals, anxiety disorders are prevalent and likely to be etiologically related to substance dependence. This focuses attention on understanding the underlying pathophysiological relationships that may link these common disorders. Furthermore, the association of anxiety disorders with poor prognosis among substance-dependent patients suggests that patients with both sets of disorders may be a clinically meaningful subgroup and suggests the hypothesis that identification and treatment of anxiety disorders in substance-dependent patients should improve outcome of both anxiety and substance use disorder.

Longitudinal Studies

One way to examine the possible relationships between anxiety and substance use disorders is by examining longitudinal studies that document the relative onsets and offsets of these disorders in relation to each other. Both substance use disorders and anxiety disorders can be viewed from a developmental perspective. Substance use disorders usually have their onset in adolescence, with precursors that include childhood externalizing disorders. Similarly, anxiety disorders often have precursors in childhood, including separation anxiety, social anxiety, and anxious temperament.

Among several longitudinal studies that have followed subjects from childhood and adolescence to adulthood and that have sought to understand risk factors for the development of substance use disorders, early externalizing disorders (i.e., conduct disorder; other disruptive disorders, such as attention-deficit disorder; and temperamental features related to these disorders) and neuropsychological deficits have been identified as precursors of substance dependence.

At the same time, there is some evidence for early onset anxiety as a risk factor for the subsequent development of substance use disorders. For example, the Woodlawn study followed a large cohort of children from a Chicago neighborhood from age 7 years into adulthood. Specific childhood temperaments measured at age 7—while children were in second grade—were associated with the development of subsequent substance use disorders during adolescence and adulthood (Kellam et al. 1982). This association was found in children with angry, aggressive temperament; hyperactive, impulsive temperament; inattentive temperament; and anxious temperament. In particular, the combination of aggressive and shy temperament has been identified as increasing risk for adolescent and adult substance problems, whereas shyness alone appears in some instances to be protective (Crum et al. 2006; Ensminger et al. 2002; Juon et al. 2002). Identification of these associations led to the development of preventive interventions that focused on improved behavioral management techniques for teachers or parents that, in part, target shyness (Furr-Holden et al. 2004).

Studies have also shown that early onset of nicotine (Breslau et al. 1993) or marijuana use (Brook et al. 2002; Fergusson et al. 2002; Patton et al. 2002) increases the risk for the later development of depressive or anxiety disorders. Data such as these raise the possibility that drug exposure alters brain development during adolescence in such a way as to increase susceptibility to psychopathology, including mood or anxiety disorders. It is also possible that common risk factors (genetic or environmental, e.g., stress) drive the emergence of substance use and other psychopathology, and in the presence of these risk factors substance abuse and other externalizing problems may tend to appear sooner in development. However, animal models suggest that the mechanism of early exposure to substances, resulting in relatively permanent alterations in brain functioning, needs to be taken seriously. Such studies have focused on early drug exposure and functioning of brain reward systems (Malanga and Kosofsky 2003). Analogous studies that examine early drug exposure and the development of brain systems involved in anxiety and fear conditioning are needed. The possibility of relatively permanent brain changes due to early substance exposure certainly highlights the importance of improving preventive interventions in an effort to prevent or delay the onset of nicotine, alcohol, and other drug use during adolescence.

Role of Stress and Trauma

Among potential common or shared risk factors between anxiety disorders and substance use disorders, abuse, trauma, and stress are the most salient. Evidence clearly suggests that early childhood abuse and neglect are risk factors for most forms of psychopathology, including, most prominently, substance use disorders and anxiety disorders. Histories of significant trauma and PTSD are common among substance-dependent patients in treatment, perhaps reflecting a role for stressful life events in the development of anxiety and substance use disorders. In addition, impulsive or risk-taking behavior, in the context of substance intoxication, may increase risk for trauma or for placement of these individuals in stressful circumstances.

Treatment

Although most studies on the treatment of co-occurring psychopathology and substance use disorders have focused on depressive disorders (Nunes and Levin 2004), some studies on the treatment of co-occurring anxiety and substance use disorders have begun to emerge.

For example, studies have examined the effectiveness of buspirone, a nonsedating anxiolytic, for the treatment of alcohol dependence. Several of these studies were negative. The largest and best designed study (Kranzler et al. 1994) included alcohol-dependent patients who were recently detoxified and abstinent on an inpatient unit and who continued to have elevated scores on an anxiety scale. In these patients, buspirone was found to be superior to placebo in terms of both retention in treatment and drinking outcome over a 12-week trial. The tricyclic antidepressant imipramine was found to be effective in assisting patients with GAD in tapering off of long-term benzodiazepines (Rickels et al. 2000), and nonsignificant trends toward a beneficial effect for buspirone were observed in the same study. A small placebo-controlled trial found trends in favor of buspirone in methadone-maintained opioid-dependent patients with anxiety symptoms (McRae et al. 2004).

Manual-guided cognitive-behavioral therapies (CBTs) that target specific combinations of anxiety and substance use disorders, including PTSD (Hien et al. 2004; Najavits et al. 1998) and social anxiety (Brady et al. 2001), have been developed. Clinicians and researchers have been more hesitant to implement exposure therapy due to concerns that discomfort aroused by exposure procedures could increase risk of dropout from treatment, although one pilot study suggested the outcome was good among cocaine-dependent patients who were retained in treatment (Brady et al. 2001). A small pilot trial found paroxetine superior to placebo in alcohol-dependent patients with social anxiety (Randall et al. 2001). A recent placebo-controlled trial of sertraline for the treatment of co-occurring alcohol dependence and PTSD showed that sertraline-treated patients with early onset PTSD and less severe alcohol dependence had better drinking outcomes on sertraline than on placebo (Brady et al. 2005). Conversely, among patients with severe early-onset alcohol dependence and later-onset PTSD, drinking outcome was worse in the sertraline group compared with the placebo group. This study speaks to the multiple possible relationships between anxiety and substance use disorders and potential subtypes, with treatment implications. Another study found that among alcohol-dependent patients with agoraphobia or social phobia, treatment with combined CBT and a selective serotonin reuptake inhibitor, in addition to a relapse-prevention–oriented psychosocial intervention, improved the outcome of anxiety symptoms but not of drinking, compared with relapse prevention alone (Schade et al. 2005). In summary, these studies examining the treatment of anxiety disorders among substance-dependent patients suggest that targeting the anxiety symptoms with specific treatments is often helpful in improving the outcome of either anxiety or substance use disorders, or both.

A variety of studies have shown that offering treatment for alcohol or drug use disorders improves psychiatric symptoms (O'Leary et al. 2000; for a review, see Nunes and Raby 2005). This finding supports a role for substance abuse in causing or exacerbating mood and anxiety symptoms. The intoxication and withdrawal syndromes of various substances, which are delineated in DSM-IV and DSM-IV-TR (American Psychiatric Association 2000), include mood and anxiety symptoms. Such symptoms would be expected to improve relatively rapidly with the achievement of reduced substance use or with abstinence during treatment of a substance use disorder. Thus, it seems clear that anxiety symptoms that have been observed among substance users may often be attributed to intoxication or withdrawal. Consideration of these findings is important for clinical management and for development and refinement of diagnostic criteria.

Neurobiology of Stress, Social Anxiety, and Addiction

The role of trauma and abuse in the etiology of anxiety and substance use disorders has been corroborated in preclinical and clinical neurobiological models. The field of addictions research benefits from the availability of animal models with face validity in terms of modeling the clinical phenomena, including drug self-administration—which models addictive potential and dependence—and place conditioning and drug reinstatement after a period of abstinence, which parallel the clinical phenomena of drug seeking and relapse, respectively. Animal studies with these models have found consistently that stress increases drug self-administration and prompts the reinstatement of previously extinguished drug-seeking behavior, thereby suggesting a role of stress in the fundamental pathophysiology of drug dependence. One explanation for the stress–addiction link is the self-medication model, which holds that individuals seek out substances to reduce dysphoric states associated with stress. An alternative, the sensation-seeking hypothesis, grows from findings that activation of the hypothalamic-pituitary-adrenal (HPA) axis increases sensitivity of the brain reward system to drugs and promotes the acquisition of drug self-administration in animal models. Drugs may then be taken, in part, to induce activation of the HPA axis, resulting in a desirable state of arousal. Furthermore, during abstinence, arousal of the HPA axis by stress may promote reinstatement of drug-taking by functioning as an internal cue (Goeders 2003).

Although stress, in the animal model, often is delivered through simple mechanical means, such as uncontrollable foot shocks, social stress also has been examined in such models. For example, social isolation has been shown to increase alcohol intake in rats, and socially dominant individuals self-administer less alcohol than subordinates (Wolffgramm and Heyne 1991). Similarly, in primates it was shown that in group-housed monkeys, subordinate monkeys were susceptible to cocaine self-administration, whereas dominant monkeys were not, and social dominance was associated with increased D_2 dopamine receptor numbers, measured with positron emission tomography (PET) imaging (Morgan et al. 2002).

The neurobiology of addiction is complex, but several clear underpinnings include a *desensitization of the brain reward system,* with the result that the strong rewarding stimuli that deliver drugs of abuse overshadow natural rewards. This can be measured at the preclinical level in a variety of models, including the threshold for brain-stimulation reward, which suggests blunting of the responsiveness of the brain reward system after chronic drug administration. Among clinical populations of drug-dependent and alcohol-dependent patients, deficits in the brain dopamine system have been documented with brain imaging, including decreased density of dopamine D_2 receptors and decreased release of dopamine in response to dopamine-releasing drugs, such as dextroamphetamine or methylphenidate (Martinez et al. 2005, 2007).

Another central pathophysiological feature of the neurobiology of addiction is the phenomenon of *cue-elicited drug seeking,* often manifested clinically as drug or alcohol craving. Neuroimaging studies across PET and magnetic resonance imaging platforms have yielded convergent results, suggesting that drug or alcohol cues result in activation of brain regions associated with the brain reward system, including the anterior cingulate and amygdala, regions innervated by mesolimbic and mesocortical dopamine fibers. The phenomenon of cue-elicited drug responding or craving is consistent with Pavlovian conditioning and is reminiscent of the fear-conditioning circuitry, on which other chapters of this monograph that discuss anxiety disorders have focused. This similarity suggests that both anxiety and substance use disorders may be viewed as disorders of learning and memory.

Neurobiological commonalities of anxiety and substance abuse are also suggested by studies of the HPA axis, which mediates the stress response. Disorders of fear conditioning prominently involve overactivation and dysregulation of corticotropin-releasing factor (CRF) and the HPA axis. Similarly, chronic drug self-administration in animals and chronic use of abusable drugs in humans has been shown to be associated with dysregulation of CRF and the HPA axis. Some evidence suggests that CRF may mediate the relationship between environmental stress and increased drug self-administration. This may set up a vicious circle in which activation of the HPA axis and CRF by drug use and withdrawal increases susceptibility to stress and fear conditioning, which, in turn, continue to drive elevated stress hormone levels, thereby promoting susceptibility to chronic drug taking.

Neuropsychological Deficits in Addictions and Anxiety Disorders

A growing literature now documents the presence and high prevalence of neuropsychological deficits—including subtle decrements in verbal IQ and deficits in attention, memory, decision making, and executive functioning—among alcohol-dependent and drug-dependent patients. The extent to which these deficits may represent toxic effects of drugs and alcohol or premorbid deficits that may function as risk factors is unclear. However, considerable evidence supports these deficits as premorbid risk factors. For example, school-aged children of parents with drug dependence have been shown to have decrements in verbal IQ. These children are at risk for substance dependence but have not yet passed into the age of risk.

A well-known association of conduct disorder, impulsivity, and inattention as early risk factors for addiction has been highlighted in longitudinal studies. Indeed, school failure and early dropout from school are potent risk factors in the development of drug and alcohol problems in adolescence and likely effect conduct and learning deficits. Experimental paradigms that reflect impulsivity and decision making have been studied in alcohol-dependent and drug-dependent populations as well as normal control populations. Relatively consistently, these studies found increased impulsivity and deficits in decision making among substance-dependent individuals compared with control subjects. Neuroimaging studies also have shown reduced activation of frontal brain regions, measured during the performance of decision-making tasks.

These findings are reminiscent of the failure of "top-down modulation" in the anxiety disorders. In this model, frontal brain regions that are responsible for executive functioning fail to modulate or extinguish fear-conditioned responses in a timely manner, thereby permitting the continuation or exacerbation of a clinical anxiety disorder. Thus, failure of executive functioning in substance dependence and of top-down regulation in anxiety may represent another shared etiological mechanism between anxiety and substance use disorders.

Neurobiology of Acute Substance Effects

Drug intoxication is often described as anxiolytic. This is clearly the case with alcohol, benzodiazepines, other sedatives, and opiates, although the stimulatory effects of cocaine, other stimulants, and even cannabis also can be experienced as anxiolytic. This has led to the tension-reduction hypothesis of the relationship between substance abuse and mood or anxiety disorders, in which intoxicating substances become habit forming to the extent that they help patients to experience a reduction in anxiety symptoms. The self-medication model is a related conceptualization that grew out of clinical work.

However, intoxication may also be *anxiogenic,* particularly with cocaine, other stimulants, or cannabis. In addition, withdrawal syndromes are prominently anxiogenic, especially with alcohol, sedatives, and opiates. The anxiety generated by withdrawal may become a basis for continued drug taking and addiction through a negative-reinforcement mechanism.

In addition to highlighting potential relationships between anxiety and addiction, the anxiolytic or anxiogenic effects of intoxication or withdrawal may be viewed as "windows" into the neurobiology of anxiety. The pharmacology of each of the different classes of addictive drugs is well understood, to varying degrees. For example, the anxiogenic effects of opiate withdrawal have been traced to overactivity of the locus coeruleus and to dysregulation of intracellular physiology within the locus neurons. In another example, studies of models of anxiety in young primates have shown that separation anxiety is relieved preferentially by opiates, whereas anxiety provoked by aggressive threats is relieved preferentially by benzodiazepines. These studies suggest that the effects of substances of abuse can be used as tools to pharmacologically dissect different brain mechanisms of anxiety.

In the clinical realm, the acute toxic and withdrawal effects of substances of abuse are a nuisance when trying to make a diagnosis because it can be difficult to distinguish those particular anxiety symptoms which represent toxic or withdrawal effects, and would be expected to subside with abstinence or appropriate treatment for the addiction, from anxiety symptoms that represent underlying or independent disorders that are in need of specific treatment.

Conclusion and Recommendations for DSM-V

This brief review suggests there is a complex interplay between the substance use disorders and the disorders of anxiety or fear conditioning. The highlights of the review are summarized in Table 14–2 according to the three types of relationships that could hold between anxiety and substance abuse (illustrated in Figure 14–1). Briefly, existing anxiety disorders may function as causative risk factors for the subsequent development of substance use disorders (for which there is evidence in the epidemiological literature), perhaps through a tension reduction or self-medication model in which relief of anxiety symptoms by substances of abuse sets up a pattern of habitual use and dependence.

Conversely, substance abuse may function as a causative risk factor for the development of anxiety disorders in several ways: 1) substances can induce anxiety as toxic or withdrawal effects; 2) chronic substance use or cycles of intoxication and withdrawal may increase the activity and sensitivity of the HPA axis, predisposing individuals to excess anxiety under stress; 3) intoxication may increase the risk of experiencing trauma, thereby predisposing individuals to anxiety disorders; and 4) stress, trauma, and neuropsychological deficits, which result in failure of top-down regulatory mechanisms, likely function as common etiological factors that predispose individuals to anxiety disorders and substance use disorders.

Common genetic risk factors for depression and substance use disorders have been suggested by shared variance in twin studies and by a chromosomal locus for a phenotype of alcoholism and depression. Similar investigations that seek shared genetic underpinnings of anxiety and substance use disorders might be undertaken.

This review suggests that any attempt to develop a nosology of anxiety disorders based on pathophysiology would benefit from consideration of the relationships between substance use disorders and anxiety. Neurobiological effects of

TABLE 14–2. Likely etiological relationships between substance use disorders and anxiety disorders

Relationship	Model or mechanism of relationship
Anxiety is a causative risk factor for development or maintenance of substance use disorders.	Tension-reduction model Self-medication model Anxiety as a conditioned cue triggering substance use
Substance use disorders are a causative risk factor for development or maintenance of anxiety disorders.	Anxiety as a toxic or withdrawal effect of substances Chronic substance use or episodes of intoxication and withdrawal activate corticotropin-releasing factor and the hypothalamic-pituitary-adrenal axis, increasing sensitivity to environmental stress Intoxication increases risk of traumatic events
Common risk factors contribute to both anxiety and substance use disorders.	Acute stress (trauma, abuse) or chronic stress (e.g., social) Neuropsychological deficits in "top-down" regulatory mechanisms modulating conditioned responses (fear conditioning or drug cues) Common genetic factors?

addictive substances and mechanisms of the development of addiction may shed light on the mechanisms of anxiety disorders and vice versa.

In terms of pragmatic recommendations for DSM-V, perhaps the most salient problem for clinicians is the problem of separating anxiety symptoms that are toxic or withdrawal effects of substances from independent anxiety disorders. DSM-IV realized a substantial advance in the diagnosis of co-occurring substance use and depression by dividing depressive disorders in the setting of substance abuse into primary or independent major depression, substance-induced depression, or expected effects of substances. Whereas the diagnosis of depression among substance-dependent patients had previously been a source of confusion and controversy among clinicians, this new conceptualization provided clarity. In particular, inclusion of the category of substance-induced depression marked a recognition that depressive symptoms among substance-dependent patients may appear, upon examination of the patient's history, to occur only in the context of substance abuse and yet still be of clinical or prognostic significance. These new criteria provide clinicians with a systematic way of classifying these patients. Recently emerging lines of clinical and epidemiological evidence support the predictive validity of substance-induced depression.

Thus, further effort in DSM-V might be exerted toward the elaboration of criteria for independent versus substance-induced anxiety disorders. *Substance-induced depression* is defined as depression that occurs only in the setting of ongoing substance use, but wherein the depressive symptoms exceed what would be expected from the usual toxic or withdrawal effects of substances. In considering the symptoms of anxiety disorders, it is clear that some symptoms and syndromes, particularly the phobias, do not overlap with symptoms of drug intoxication or withdrawal. Fear of social situations or fear of public places is not typical of drug intoxication or withdrawal. On the other hand, panic attacks, the arousal and numbing symptoms of PTSD, and many of the symptoms of GAD have substantial overlap with the intoxication and withdrawal syndromes of various substances. Thus, these different degrees of symptom overlap for the various anxiety and substance disorders could be considered in the DSM-V. Clarified criteria would encourage further clinical research on the relationships between anxiety and substance use disorders, which would further inform the ultimate goal of a pathophysiologically based nosology.

References

American Psychiatric Association: Diagnostic and Statistical Manual of Mental Disorders, 3rd Edition. Washington, DC, American Psychiatric Association, 1980

American Psychiatric Association: Diagnostic and Statistical Manual of Mental Disorders, 4th Edition. Washington, DC, American Psychiatric Association, 1994

American Psychiatric Association: Diagnostic and Statistical Manual of Mental Disorders, 4th Edition, Text Revision. Washington, DC, American Psychiatric Association, 2000

Angst J: Comorbidity of mood disorders: a longitudinal prospective study. Br J Psychiatry Suppl 30:31–37, 1996

Brady KT, Dansky BS, Back SE, et al: Exposure therapy in the treatment of PTSD among cocaine-dependent individuals: preliminary findings. J Subst Abuse Treat 21:47–54, 2001

Brady KT, Sonne S, Anton RF, et al: Sertraline in the treatment of co-occurring alcohol dependence and posttraumatic stress disorder. Alcohol Clin Exp Res 29:395–401, 2005

Breslau N, Kilbey MM, Andreski P: Nicotine dependence and major depression: new evidence from a prospective investigation. Arch Gen Psychiatry 50:31–35, 1993

Brook DW, Brook JS, Zhang C, et al: Drug use and the risk of major depressive disorder, alcohol dependence, and substance use disorders. Arch Gen Psychiatry 59:1039–1044, 2002

Burns L, Teesson M, O'Neill K: The impact of comorbid anxiety and depression on alcohol treatment outcomes. Addiction 100:787–796, 2005

Crum RM, Juon HS, Green KM, et al: Educational achievement and early school behavior as predictors of alcohol-use disorders: 35-year follow-up of the Woodlawn Study. J Stud Alcohol 67:75–85, 2006

Ensminger ME, Juon HS, Fothergill KE: Childhood and adolescent antecedents of substance use in adulthood. Addiction 97:833–844, 2002

Feighner JP, Robins E, Guze SB, et al: Diagnostic criteria for use in psychiatric research. Arch Gen Psychiatry 26:57–63, 1972

Fergusson DM, Horwood LJ, Swain-Campbell N: Cannabis use and psychosocial adjustment in adolescence and young adulthood. Addiction 97:1123–1135, 2002

Furr-Holden CD, Ialongo NS, Anthony JC, et al: Developmentally inspired drug prevention: middle school outcomes in a school-based randomized prevention trial. Drug Alcohol Depend 73:149–158, 2004

Goeders NE: The impact of stress on addiction. Eur Neuropsychopharmacol 13:435–441, 2003

Grant BF, Stinson FS, Dawson DA, et al: Co-disorders of 12-month alcohol and drug use disorders and personality disorders in the United States: results from the National Epidemiologic Survey on Alcohol and Related Conditions. Arch Gen Psychiatry 61:361–368, 2004a

Grant BF, Stinson FS, Dawson DA, et al: Prevalence and co-occurrence of substance use disorders and independent mood and anxiety disorders: results from the National Epidemiologic Survey on Alcohol and Related Conditions. Arch Gen Psychiatry 61:807–816, 2004b

Hasin D, Nunes E, Meydan J: Comorbidity of alcohol, drug and psychiatric disorders: epidemiology, in Dual Diagnosis and Psychiatric Treatment: Substance Abuse and Comorbid Disorders. Edited by Kranzler HR, Tinsley JA. New York, Marcel Dekker, 2004, pp 1–34

Hien DA, Cohen LR, Miele GM, et al: Promising treatments for women with comorbid PTSD and substance use disorders. Am J Psychiatry 161:1426–1432, 2004

Juon HS, Ensminger ME, Sydnor KD: A longitudinal study of developmental trajectories to young adult cigarette smoking. Drug Alcohol Depend 66:303–314, 2002

Kellam SG, Brown CH, Fleming JP: Developmental epidemiological studies of substance use in Woodlawn: implications for prevention research strategy. NIDA Res Monogr 41:21–33, 1982

Kessler RC, Sonnega A, Bromet E: Posttraumatic stress disorder in the National Comorbidity Survey. Arch Gen Psychiatry 52:1048–1060, 1995

Kessler RC, Crum RM, Warner LA, et al: Lifetime co-occurrence of DSM-III-R alcohol abuse and dependence with other psychiatric disorders in the National Comorbidity Survey. Arch Gen Psychiatry 54:313–321, 1997a

Kessler RC, Zhao S, Blazer DG, et al: Prevalence, correlates, and course of minor depression and major depression in the National Comorbidity Survey. J Affect Disord; 45:19–30, 1997b

Kranzler HR, Burleson JA, Del Boca FK, et al: Buspirone treatment of anxious alcoholics: a placebo-controlled trial. Arch Gen Psychiatry 51:720–731, 1994

Kushner MG, Abrams K, Thuras P, et al: Follow-up study of anxiety disorder and alcohol dependence in comorbid alcoholism treatment patients. Alcohol Clin Exp Res 29:1432–1443, 2005

Magee WJ, Eaton WW, Wittchen HU, et al: Agoraphobia, simple phobia, and social phobia in the National Comorbidity Survey. Arch Gen Psychiatry 53:159–168, 1996

Malanga CJ, Kosofsky BE: Does drug abuse beget drug abuse? Behavioral analysis of addiction liability in animal models of prenatal drug exposure. Brain Res Dev Brain Res 147:47–57, 2003

Martinez D, Gil R, Slifstein M, et al: Alcohol dependence is associated with blunted dopamine transmission in the ventral striatum. Biol Psychiatry 58:779–786, 2005

Martinez D, Narendran R, Foltin RW, et al: Amphetamine-induced dopamine release: markedly blunted in cocaine dependence and predictive of the choice to self-administer cocaine. Am J Psychiatry 164:622–629, 2007

McRae AL, Sonne SC, Brady KT, et al: A randomized, placebo-controlled trial of buspirone for the treatment of anxiety in opioid-dependent individuals. Am J Addict 13:53–63, 2004

Morgan D, Grant KA, Gage HD, et al: Social dominance in monkeys: dopamine D2 receptors and cocaine self-administration. Nat Neurosci 5:169–174, 2002

Najavits LM, Weiss RD, Shaw SR, et al: "Seeking safety": outcome of a new cognitive-behavioral psychotherapy for women with posttraumatic stress disorder and substance dependence. J Trauma Stress 11:437–456, 1998

Nunes EV, Levin FR: Treatment of depression in patients with alcohol or other drug dependence: a meta analysis. JAMA 291:1887–1896, 2004

Nunes EV, Raby WN: Comorbidity of depression and substance abuse, in Biology of Depression: From Novel Insights to Therapeutic Strategies, Vol 1. Edited by Licinio L, Wong M-L. Weinheim, Germany, Wiley-VCH, 2005, pp 341–364

O'Leary TA, Rohsenow DJ, Martin R, et al: The relationship between anxiety levels and outcome of cocaine abuse treatment. Am J Drug Alcohol Abuse 26:179–194, 2000

Patton GC, Coffey C, Carlin JB, et al: Cannabis use and mental health in young people: cohort study. BMJ 325:1195–1198, 2002

Randall CL, Johnson MR, Thevos AK, et al: Paroxetine for social anxiety and alcohol use in dual-diagnosed patients. Depress Anxiety 14:255–262, 2001

Regier DA, Farmer ME, Rae DS, et al: Comorbidity of mental disorders with alcohol and other drug abuse: results from the Epidemiologic Catchment Area (ECA) Study. JAMA 264:2511–2518, 1990

Rickels K, DeMartinis N, García-España F, et al: Imipramine and buspirone in treatment of patients with generalized anxiety disorder who are discontinuing long-term benzodiazepine therapy. Am J Psychiatry 157:1973–1979, 2000

Schade A, Marquenie LA, van Balkom AJ, et al: The effectiveness of anxiety treatment on alcohol-dependent patients with a comorbid phobic disorder: a randomized controlled trial. Alcohol Clin Exp Res 29:794–800, 2005

Schneider U, Altmann A, Baumann M, et al: Comorbid anxiety and affective disorder in alcohol-dependent patients seeking treatment: the first Multicentre Study in Germany. Alcohol Alcohol 36:219–223, 2001

Wolffgramm J, Heyne A: Social behavior, dominance, and social deprivation of rats determine drug choice. Pharmacol Biochem Behav 38:389–399, 1991

15

CONCLUDING REMARKS

Gavin Andrews, M.D.
Peter McEvoy, Ph.D.
Tim Slade, Ph.D.

Common Characteristics of Disorders

Do posttraumatic stress disorder (PTSD), panic/agoraphobia, social phobia/social anxiety disorder (SocAD), and specific phobia constitute a coherent group? It appears that they might, within the present framework, given that—for the purposes of developing a DSM-V research agenda—general anxiety disorder (GAD) was included for consideration by the mood disorders committee and obsessive-compulsive disorder (OCD) was allocated to its own committee of OCD spectrum disorders.

At a more conceptual level, these four disorders could be defined as *fear and avoidance* of 1) situations invoking memories of personal trauma; 2) situations invoking sudden panic or other dysphoric symptoms; 3) situations invoking social embarrassment; and 4) situations of minor danger invoking disabling anxiety, in which case these disorders could constitute a group. The key question is why most people exposed to trauma, panic, social embarrassment, or childhood fear do not succumb. Most individuals shrug off the experiences and proceed normally; they do not develop a disorder.

These four disorders begin early in life. In the National Comorbidity Survey Replication (Kessler et al. 2005a), the median (and twenty-fifth percentile) ages at onset were 23 (15) for PTSD, 24 (16) for panic disorder with or without agoraphobia, 20 (13) for agoraphobia without panic, 13 (8) for SocAD, and 7 (5) for specific phobia. The median ages at onset for the two other anxiety disorders,

OCD and GAD, were 19 and 31 years, respectively. Other surveys are in agreement with these estimates (Oakley Browne et al. 2006). These findings are consistent with a preexisting vulnerability that is affected by the requisite stressor. They are even more consistent with genetic and early environmental contributions that prime an individual to react to difficult situations with fear and avoidance and to not be able to adjust to the threat (Hettema et al. 2006; see also Alter and Hen, Chapter 9, "Serotonin, Sensitive Periods, and Anxiety," this volume).

Rauch and Drevets, in Chapter 12 ("Neuroimaging and Neuroanatomy of Stress-Induced and Fear Circuitry Disorders"), select several functional domains to illustrate the underlying concepts that should be researched in order to better understand onsets of these disorders: 1) persistent or indelible learning about threat-related stimuli; 2) exaggerated fear responses; 3) impaired extinction capacity; 4) deficient ability to suppress attention/response to disorder-relevant stimuli; 5) excessive contextual conditioning and/or inability to appreciate safe contexts; 6) exaggerated interoceptive/anxiety sensitivity; and 7) perceptual hypersensitivity to threat-related stimuli. Huppert and colleagues (Chapter 10, "Role of Cognition in Stress-Induced and Fear Circuitry Disorders") and Yehuda (Chapter 13, "Role of Neurochemical and Neuroendocrine Markers of Fear in Classification of Anxiety Disorders") take similar positions in respect to particular domains.

Unique Aspects of Disorders

It is important to identify facts that are specific to one, some, or all of the four disorders. A *fact* is a finding that has been independently replicated and not challenged by any methodologically incontestable failure to replicate. In terms used by Cook and Leviton (1980), facts are "the stubborn findings that regularly occur." There are a number of ways that facts could inform classifications of our disorders:

- Facts could inform the reliability and critical importance of any of the current diagnostic criteria.
- Facts that are independent of current clinical status could inform a diagnostic test.
- Facts might identify risk factors for the subsequent development of a disorder.

Facts about demographic correlates seem to be of little use in informing diagnostic criteria for our disorders. To show that childhood neglect and abuse are associated with these four disorders is of little use, because the finding is not specific to these disorders alone. Indeed, abuse and neglect are associated with most mental disorders. Likewise, other facts, such as poor education and poor workforce participation rates, are not specific to these four disorders. These facts apply to most mental disorders and could be a cause and/or a consequence of the early onset of these disorders.

In reflecting on the contributions to the meeting on which this book is based, in which the participants aimed to refine a research agenda for these disorders, we began by asking about the evidence of continuities across the life span. This discussion helped frame, and served as a point of departure for, the insights and recommendations of all participants in this workgroup, which are the basis for their chapters and are summarized here.

Posttraumatic Stress Disorder

FRIEDMAN AND KARAM

Friedman and Karam (Chapter 1) suggest that PTSD may be the prototypical stress-related fear circuitry disorder. They argue that stimulus-driven paradigms and pharmacological probes have shown promise in identifying psychophysiological markers of PTSD. Moreover, they discuss several biological risk factors, including the serotonin transporter gene, hippocampal volume, capacity to mobilize and sustain elevated levels of neuropeptide Y, and startle responses. They outline differences in diagnostic criteria between DSM-IV (American Psychiatric Association 1994) and ICD-10 (World Health Organization 1992) and review the validity of each criterion, finding much inconsistency in the literature. The requirements for exposure to a traumatic event, involving actual or threatened death or serious injury, or a threat to the physical integrity of self or others (Criterion A1) and for the person's response to involve intense fear, helplessness, or horror (Criterion A2) are under-researched and to date have not been validated. The authors argue that these criteria may, in fact, be unnecessary if clearer guidelines relating to functional impairment (Criterion F) are developed. Evidence for reexperiencing (Criterion B), avoidance (Criterion C), and arousal (Criterion D) symptoms is somewhat inconsistent, but there is some support for a fourth "numbing" symptom cluster. DSM-IV's requirement that symptoms endure for at least 1 month (Criterion E) allows for delayed-onset PTSD, which is supported by the evidence. The authors suggest that ICD-10's criterion of symptom onset within 6 months of exposure to the trauma is, therefore, overly restrictive. The presence of clinically significant distress or impairment (Criterion F) in DSM-IV, and its absence in ICD-10, results in large discrepancies in prevalence between ICD and DSM, which the authors argue needs to be addressed in DSM-V and ICD-11.

Karam argues that although impairment is likely to be a dimensional construct, there is value in determining a clinically significant cutoff that provides clearer guidelines for establishing functional capacity. This author further argues that a diagnosis of PTSD could occur separately from impairment. In contrast, Friedman argues that it is essential for impairment to be a prerequisite for a positive diagnosis and thus is not separable from symptoms. This issue therefore appears to be unresolved.

Together, these authors provide an argument for a spectrum of diagnostic categories from partial or subsyndromal PTSD (for those not meeting full criteria but who nonetheless experience a degree of incapacitation) to complex PTSD, involving debilitating symptoms in addition to standard PTSD symptoms. They also suggest that the association between chronic stress and medical illnesses may warrant additional diagnoses, specifically posttraumatic medical disorder and chronic stress disorders that are unrelated to external trauma.

Research into independent nonverbal diagnostic assessment via stimulus-driven paradigms and pharmacological probes (genotype, dexamethasone suppression test, α_2 receptor antagonists) would be useful to translate laboratory protocols into practical, clinical diagnostic tests.

Panic Disorder

FARAVELLI, FURUKAWA, AND TRUGLIA

In Chapter 2, Faravelli and colleagues point out that there is consensus regarding the symptoms that constitute a panic attack and that, although there is evidence that the requirement of four symptoms is associated with work disability, the number of symptoms required for diagnosis of the disorder is arbitrary. The finding that panic disorder is preceded by anxiety sensitivity or a "phobic attitude" (cognition, temperament, traits) has been consistent. Diagnostic classifications have generally been consistent with this notion, allowing for panic disorder with or without agoraphobic avoidance or agoraphobia without panic. Anxiety sensitivity is a risk factor both for the onset of panic attacks and for nonremission of panic disorder. There is evidence that a panic/agoraphobia spectrum can identify individuals who have clinically significant features without meeting diagnostic criteria and also predict the development of panic disorder.

Consistent evidence indicates that the amygdala is related to the detection, evaluation, and avoidance of environmental dangers and that serotonin has an important regulatory role in the fear network. Other specific neuroanatomical and neurochemical mechanisms have been found to be associated with panic disorder, although evidence is often inconsistent or nonspecific to panic disorder. Likewise, there is some evidence that stressful life events can contribute to the onset of panic disorder, but this relationship may also be reciprocal.

Research to determine separable operational definitions of panic attacks, phobic cognitions, and agoraphobia is required.

Social Phobia

BÖGELS AND STEIN

Bögels and Stein (Chapter 3) argue that although SocAD is one of the most prevalent anxiety disorders, little is known about its etiology or specific risk or protective factors. In more generalized forms of social phobia, individuals cannot avoid triggers but rather endure them with distress. Evidence for qualitative differences between circumscribed and more generalized social anxiety is limited and rather suggests a continuum of severity, from subthreshold symptoms to avoidant personality disorder. These authors call for more research on a generalized "interpersonal" subtype, which is rooted in early schema of the self being unlovable, boring, or weak and is characterized by a more neurotic and less extraverted early personality development that may have resulted from lack of closeness with an adult.

There is also some evidence for a performance-anxiety subtype. The authors review evidence that fear of showing bodily sensations may be a nongeneralized subtype. The overlap between a social-physique anxiety subtype and body dysmorphic disorder is perhaps too great at this stage to consider the former as a distinct entity.

The authors make a strong argument for excluding Criterion C, which requires that adults recognize that their fear is irrational or exaggerated. Specifically, this criterion is not included for some anxiety disorders (e.g., panic disorder), whereas others are less stringent (e.g., OCD diagnosis requires that *at some stage* the person recognizes the irrationality); persons with less insight may still benefit from treatment and thus the distinction may be unhelpful, because insight is changeable. A qualitative distinction between SocAD and avoidant personality disorder cannot be sustained from the evidence. However, the authors argue that only a qualitative subtyping is likely to add to our knowledge of etiology and suggest that performance fear, fear of showing bodily symptoms, social physical fear, and interpersonal anxiety are possible subtypes.

Research examining differential risk factors across these subtypes has a potential to increase our knowledge. Neuroimaging studies that examine heightened amygdala activation to emotional processing demands as an endophenotype for social phobia and related disorders such as behavioral inhibition are also indicated.

Specific Phobias

EMMELKAMP AND WITTCHEN

In Chapter 4, Emmelkamp and Wittchen recognize that although specific phobias alone appear to be less debilitating than the other disorders, they most often precede the other anxiety disorders and other psychopathology. The hypothesis that specific phobias may serve as risk factors for later psychopathology is important. Neuroticism appears to be a common factor among anxiety and depressive disorders, and it is not clear that specific phobias add predictive power. There is some evidence for subtypes, but there are a number of inconsistencies in the literature. Most identified risk factors, such as neuroticism and behavioral inhibition, are nonspecific, although there is evidence for both common and specific general vulnerability. Genetic effects are stronger than environmental effects. Although specific phobias clearly belong in the fear circuitry disorders, there is a dearth of robust evidence to guide diagnostic criteria. There is, however, some evidence that criteria should be different for children younger than 14 years versus adults. A more dimensional approach is suggested for children. Evidence for subtyping separates blood–injury from other situational fears.

Research into the neuropsychological, cognitive, and neurobiological interface of specific phobias is indicated.

Continuity and Etiology of Anxiety Disorders: Are They Stable Across the Life Course?
POULTON, PINE, AND HARRINGTON

Poulton and colleagues (Chapter 5) review five studies and conclude that continuities exist between childhood/juvenile anxiety disorder and adult anxiety diagnoses. They argue that a means for characterizing the developmental history of symptomatology should be developed for DSM-V. There is evidence for both homotypic (most strongly for social phobia) and heterotypic continuity, the strength of which appears to vary among the disorders. Follow-back analyses of adult anxiety disorder (any of panic disorder, agoraphobia, specific phobia, SocAD, PTSD, GAD, and OCD) showed evidence of homotypic continuity; that is, adults with anxiety disorders had also had anxiety disorders in childhood or adolescence. In addition, adults with anxiety disorders were also at elevated risk of having had juvenile externalizing-spectrum diagnoses of attention-deficit/hyperactivity disorder and conduct disorder/oppositional defiant disorder.

Areas flagged for further research by these contributors are the processes that promote homotypic continuity in panic disorder and social phobia and the process that underlies sequences in heterotypic continuity. The major challenge here is to describe *how, when, why,* and *for whom* continuity exists.

Stress-Induced and Fear Circuitry Anxiety Disorders: Are They a Distinct Group?
FYER AND BROWN

Returning to our earlier question of group coherence for these disorders, Fyer and Brown, in Chapter 6, discuss the available genetic/epidemiological data that provide clear evidence of both commonalities and distinctions among the DSM-IV anxiety disorders. In addition, the pattern of interrelationships between the categories is not consistent. Findings vary across studies, and the groupings themselves change depending on which type of data are used as the criterion. For example, categorizing by genetic data creates one set of groupings; using age at onset creates a second set, and sorting by latent-class analysis results in a third set. For all groupings, considerable within-disorder heterogeneity exists.

These observations suggest that the DSM anxiety categories do not map neatly onto simple, consistent, and distinct etiological pathways. Instead, it seems most likely that many different specific developmental trajectories (each of which incorporates a variety of influences: genetic, environmental, interpersonal, and so on) can lead to the final common pathway that is a particular DSM anxiety diagnosis. Given this complexity, and our current extremely incomplete stage of knowledge, we are unlikely at this point in time to define a significantly "truer" anxiety nosology. Plans to make major modifications in the classification should probably be undertaken with some degree of caution.

Anxiety Disorders in African Americans and Other Ethnic Minorities

LAWSON

Lawson (Chapter 7) details important dynamics between race and distress that may help to explain discrepancies in the prevalence of anxiety disorders in minority versus majority populations, and particularly African Americans. Anxiety disorders, including panic disorder, phobias, obsessive-compulsive disorder, and posttraumatic stress disorder (PTSD), may be frequently underdiagnosed or incorrectly diagnosed in African Americans despite evidence that there may actually be a greater prevalence of some of these disorders (e.g., PTSD) in this population. Lawson contends that prevalence gaps are likely a reflection of several converging factors, including clinician bias and under-recognition, differences in core and/or secondary symptom presentation, and cultural factors specific to symptom manifestation and the clinical setting. Unfortunately, interpreting these discrepancies continues to be an intricate and ongoing process due to the availability of confounding research data, such as differences in combat exposure by African Americans; the interaction between race and environmental stress (e.g., living in urban dwellings) as a trigger for symptoms; and an increased likelihood for African Americans to receive diagnoses with psychotic features. Refined assessment tools and greater attention in the research literature would assist in our ability to detect and understand actual differences in prevalence rates, rather than accepting the available data at face value.

The Genetic Basis of Anxiety Disorders
ELEY

Eley (Chapter 8) provides a tutorial on the role of genetic research in understanding the mental disorders. In respect to the four disorders in question, the genetic influences on anxiety were best explained by two additive genetic factors common across the disorders. The first loaded most strongly in GAD, panic disorder, and agoraphobia, whereas the second loaded primarily in the two specific phobias studied. SocAD was intermediate in that it was influenced by both genetic factors (Hettema et al. 2005).

There is substantial, but not complete, overlap between the genetic factors that influence individual variation in neuroticism and those that increase liability across the internalizing disorders, which helps to explain the high rates of comorbidity among the latter. This may have important implications for identifying the susceptibility genes for these conditions (Hettema et al. 2006). Although there is substantial genetic overlap between differing aspects of anxiety and depression, it is clear that we should research *how* genes influence anxiety. One approach to this question is to examine cognitive biases as potential mediators of genetic risk.

Serotonin, Sensitive Periods, and Anxiety
ALTER AND HEN

Alter and Hen (Chapter 9) emphasize that both genetic variation and experience impact the formation of neural circuits during a developmentally sensitive period and that disruptions of neural circuit formation during this sensitive period are mediators of increased risk of psychopathology later in life. In their review the authors discuss the evidence for this hypothesis and address, in depth, the role of serotonin in neural circuit formation and how changes in the genetics of the serotonin system can lead to disruptions of this process and an increased risk of psychiatric disorders, in particular, anxiety. The pressing research issue in this area involves identification of the neural circuit differences specific to these four disorders.

Role of Cognition in Stress-Induced and Fear Circuitry Disorders
HUPPERT, FOA, McNALLY, AND CAHILL

Huppert and colleagues (Chapter 10) point out that, with some exceptions, the general pattern emerging is that patients with anxiety disorders are biased toward negative or threat aspects of content-specific concerns in evaluations, interpretation, attention, and memory and that these biases tend to decrease with successful treatment. Future research should examine the effects of directly reducing these negative biases among individuals with anxiety disorders or whether such training can prevent individuals from developing an anxiety disorder.

Although research on the neurobiological correlates of these disorders has already begun, much more needs to be learned about the interplay of neuroendocrine response and cognition, neuroimaging and cognition, neurophysiology and cognition, and genetics and cognition. The question of whether cognitions and cognitive processes are constitutive (essential aspects of the disorder that are not etiological in nature) or causal (distinct processes that precede the disorder and inevitably lead to it) needs further examination. Regardless of their etiological role, cognitions and cognitive processes constitute a central aspect of stress and fear-related disorders.

Stress and Psychosocial Factors in Onset of Fear Circuitry Disorders

RAPEE AND BRYANT

Rapee and Bryant, in Chapter 11, remind us that the majority of fear-based disorders appear to have their onsets in early to mid-adolescence. Thus, environmental factors important to the onset of anxiety disorders are likely to be those that are present during the early years of life. It is highly unlikely that anxiety is a purely genetic condition. Hence, some influence from the environment must be assumed, and this is supported by behavior genetic research.

The form of this environmental influence is unclear from twin studies but may differ across the developmental span, with a greater influence from shared environmental factors earlier in development and a dominant influence from individual environmental factors in the expression of adult anxiety. Twin studies are also largely consistent with a general neurotic influence, attributed to genetic factors, and hence it is logical to suggest that differentiation between anxiety disorders may be more attributable to environmental influence. Although evidence is building to support the roles of several environmental factors, it is still far too early either to assign causality to any specific factors or to determine specific links between environmental factors and specific disorders. From a DSM perspective, it is clearly too soon to determine diagnostic criteria based on causal environmental factors. This should be a focus of research.

Neuroimaging and Neuroanatomy of Stress-Induced and Fear Circuitry Disorders

RAUCH AND DREVETS

Rauch and Drevets, in Chapter 12, build on the foundation of extant data regarding the neurocircuitry of PTSD, panic disorder, specific phobia, and SocAD to outline a future agenda for research in this domain. The convergence of physiological and anatomical data, obtained from basic studies in experimental animals, with the neuroscience data obtained from human neuroimaging studies has contributed to the development of tentative neurocircuitry models of anxiety disorders. In particular, human neuroimaging studies of PTSD, panic disorder, specific phobia, and SocAD versus control groups have provided support for amgydalocentric models of disease, with varying involvement of medial prefrontal cortex subterritories and the hippocampus. Interestingly, anterior insular involvement may be another universal feature of these conditions. Thus, commonalities and differences in brain imaging profiles for these four syndromes offer support for maintaining these as distinct diagnoses categorized together as "stress-induced and fear circuitry disorders." Although this line of inquiry appears quite promising, the reliability, sensitivity, and specificity of the extant human neuroimaging findings have been limited. In addition to a critical review of the relevant human neuroimaging data, these authors provide suggestions, mentioned in the introduction to this chapter, regarding key considerations for the future research agenda in this domain.

Role of Neurochemical and Neuroendocrine Markers of Fear in Classification of Anxiety Disorders

YEHUDA

In Chapter 13, Yehuda suggests that anxiety disorders could be reconceptualized in terms of abnormal expressions of stress and fear. If this were to occur, the emphasis of biological research would shift from trying to find similarities with normal fear, experienced in appropriate contexts, to delineating the biological processes that differentiate responses in disorders. This shift could potentially support a reclassification based on disorders representing abnormal manifestations of fear responses. In such cases, observed biological *differences*—not similarities—between fear responses, as they occur in anxiety disorders and those described in the preclinical or normal human literature, could constitute important targets for drug development. Neurochemical and neuroendocrine studies would therefore be potentially relevant to pathophysiology, whereas imaging findings would be reflections of physiology.

Anxiety and Substance Abuse: Implications for Pathophysiology and DSM-V
NUNES AND BLANCO

Nunes and Blanco (Chapter 14) describe neurobiological aspects common to addiction and anxiety disorders in an attempt to elucidate possible shared etiologies. Large scale epidemiological and longitudinal studies have upheld the comorbidity between anxiety disorders and substance use disorders. Trauma and stress may represent the most prominent shared pathway between anxiety and addiction, and neurobiological models from animal studies consistently implicate overactivation of the HPA axis. The cue-elicited model of addiction echoes behavioral models of Pavlovian conditioning, which in turn mirrors the fear-conditioning that exists in many anxiety and stress-related disorders. Results from neuropsychological testing have implicated frontal lobe deficits, and particularly executive dysregulation, as another shared factor between anxiety and addiction. Further, Nunes and Blanco point out that substance use and intoxication may induce anxiolytic effects (e.g., self-medication models), but may also serve as a springboard for anxiety through substance withdrawal, HPA hyperactivation, increased vulnerability to trauma, and failed self-regulatory mechanisms. Our understanding of the interrelationship between anxiety and substance use would likely benefit from development of a nosology based on pathophysiology. This in turn may necessitate conceptualization of anxiety disorders as both independent and substance-induced phenomena.

Discussion

People can become anxious in response to many threats, but the manifestations of being anxious are very limited: fear and avoidance of the situation—whether it be real, remembered, or symbolic—and physical symptoms of the flight-or-fight response. The surprising thing about the anxiety disorders, as presently characterized, is the very limited range of triggers and manifestations. Whenever we establish a treatment group of people with a phobia, with panic, or with PTSD, the similarities between the individuals are much greater than the differences. Most patients are amazed that there are other people who have exactly the same fears, avoidances, and physical symptoms. What seemed personal and idiosyncratic is actually a class of responses. This is what is known as a *syndrome*—a set of responses that tend to co-occur and that share antecedents and consequences.

Syndrome recognition simplifies clinical practice; one quickly knows what questions to ask to confirm the diagnosis, what treatments are likely to be effective, and what impediments are likely to stand in the way of a successful outcome. The ability to identify syndromes (when you know the causes you can call them diseases) is central to research, whether in epidemiology, genetics, information processing, environmental stressors, treatment, or outcome. The key issue is the boundaries of the syndrome.

This American Psychiatric Association DSM-V workgroup focused on four disorders: PTSD, panic/agoraphobia, social anxiety disorder, and specific phobia. Should they have been asked to specify pathognomonic symptoms unique to a disorder? Should they have also looked at OCD and GAD (and, for that matter, major depression)? Should somatoform disorder, body dysmorphic disorder, and hypochondriasis have been added to make the list of internalizing disorders complete?

Deciding which goes with what is, we hope, no longer a matter of clinical opinion. Is there research evidence from epidemiology (e.g., age at onset, patterns of comorbidity), genetics, brain function, information processing, environmental stressors, treatments that work, or outcome that is independent of the symptom picture and could inform the discussion?

AGE AT ONSET

Kessler et al. (2005a) reported, on the basis of data from the U.S. World Mental Health Survey (National Comorbidity Survey Replication), that the median age at onset varies from 7 years for specific phobias to 32 years for major depressive disorder. Kessler et al. (2007) argued, on the basis of the consolidated data from 15 World Mental Health Surveys, that there are two major distribution patterns: a linear pattern, seen in mood disorders and GAD, PTSD, and panic disorder, and a curvilinear distribution for the other phobias. However, the data from the U.S. and New Zealand sites do not confirm this finding in respect to panic/agoraphobia and OCD, although they do confirm the finding for GAD and major depressive disorder. PTSD has an intermediate pattern, but the onset of PTSD depends on exposure to trauma, which is age related.

COMORBIDITY

There are two ways of approaching the comorbidity problem. The rates of co-occurrence among the mental disorders are higher than would be expected by chance (Andrews 1996; Andrews et al. 2002). It has been suggested that such rates could reflect the existence of higher-order dimensions of psychopathology. A number of studies have examined this suggestion and found consistent and meaningful groupings of mental disorders (Kessler et al. 2005b; Krueger 1999).

In the most recent of these studies, Slade and Watson (2006), using methodology originally outlined in Krueger (1999), identified a hierarchical three-factor structure as the best fit to 10 common DSM-IV and 11 common ICD-10 mental disorders. This structure was characterized by a distress and a fear factor (which were best considered lower-order facets of a broader internalizing factor) as well as an externalizing factor. As can be seen in Figure 15–1, the individual mental disorders that were characteristic of the distress factor were major depression, dysthymia, GAD, PTSD, and neurasthenia (in the ICD-10 model). The mental disorders that were characteristic of the fear factor were SocAD, agoraphobia, panic disorder, and OCD (specific phobias were not included in this survey). The externalizing factor was best characterized by drug and alcohol dependence.

Expanding on these analyses, Krueger and Markon (2006) proposed that comorbidity among individual mental disorders can be explained by latent liability factors that exist along a continuous, graded range and that each factor has an impact on multiple disorders. Thus, the finding that major depression, dysthymia, GAD, and PTSD are all highly comorbid suggests the existence of a latent continuous liability to a distress-based form of psychopathology. The authors argued for the need to carry out model-based analyses of comorbidity (i.e., using empirical data to confirm or refute alternative theoretically derived models of comorbidity) and proposed that these analyses have significant implications for the organization of mental disorders within a nosological system.

GENETICS

For 20 years, Kendler and colleagues have studied the subjects in the Virginia Twin Registry and used structural equation modeling to estimate the salience of genetic vulnerability to various diseases. Hettema et al. (2005) obtained lifetime diagnoses for six anxiety disorders (GAD, panic disorder, agoraphobia, SocAD, animal phobia, and situational phobia) during personal interviews from a population-based twin registry. Multivariate structural equation modeling that allowed for sex differences was performed. The underlying structure of the genetic and environmental risk factors for the anxiety disorders was similar between men and women. Genes predisposed to two broad groups of disorders, dichotomized as panic, generalized-agoraphobic anxiety versus the specific phobias. The remaining associations between the disorders are largely explained by a unique environmental factor shared across the disorders and, to a lesser extent, a common shared environmental factor.

Hettema et al. (2006) subsequently added lifetime major depression and neuroticism to these six anxiety disorders. Multivariate structural equation models were again used to decompose the correlations between these phenotypes into genetic and environmental components, allowing for sex-specific factors. The genetic factor for neuroticism significantly affected all of the internalizing disorders, whereas a common genetic factor, independent of neuroticism, accounted for degrees of variance and covariance among major depression, GAD, and panic disorder that were similar to those for the common genetic factor shared with neuroticism. Disorder-specific genetic factors were substantial for the phobias but not

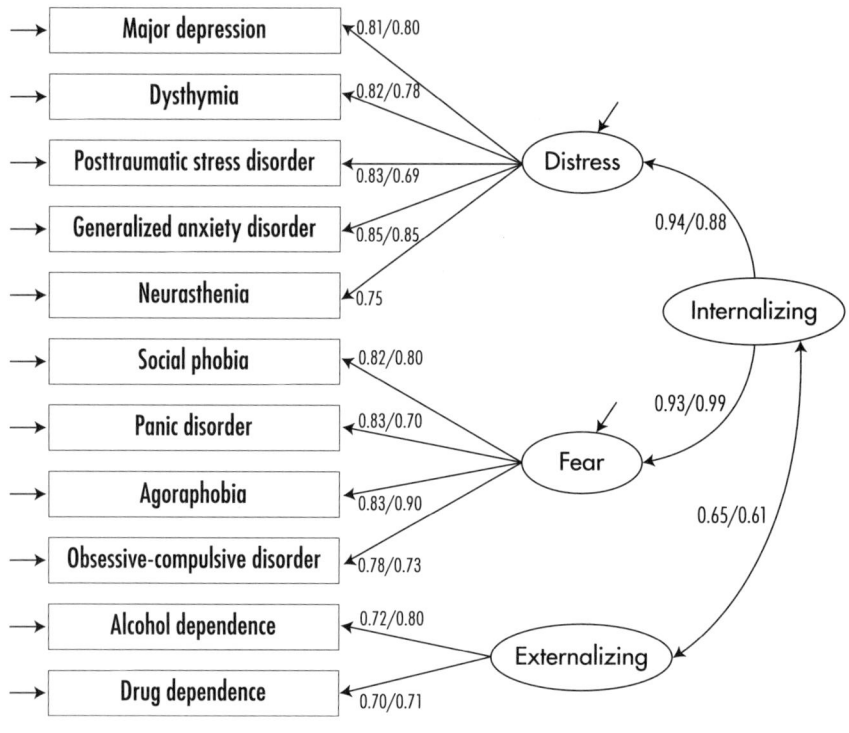

FIGURE 15–1. Best-fitting model of the structure of 10 common DSM-IV and 11 common ICD-10 mental disorders from the 1997 Australian National Survey of Mental Health and Well-Being.

All parameter estimates (DSM-IV/ICD-10) are standardized and significant at $P<0.05$. All parameter estimates, except for neurasthenia, relate to DSM-IV/ICD-10. The single parameter estimate for neurasthenia relates to ICD-10 only.
Source. Reprinted from Slade T, Watson D. "The Structure of Common DSM-IV and ICD-10 Mental Disorders in the Australian General Population." *Psychological Medicine* 2006; 36: 1593–1600, with permission of Cambridge University Press. Copyright © 2006, Cambridge University Press.

for the other phenotypes in this model. There was substantial, but not complete, overlap between the genetic factors that influence individual variation in neuroticism and those that increase liability, across the internalizing disorders, helping to explain the high rates of comorbidity among the latter. This overlap may have important implications for identification of the susceptibility genes for these conditions, which raises the possibility that the genetic vulnerability, with respect to many internalizing disorders, may be subsumed by genetic influences in preexisting personality and temperament vulnerabilities (Martin et al. 1988).

BRAIN STRUCTURE AND FUNCTION

Neuroimaging studies with positron emission tomography (PET) and functional magnetic resonance imaging (fMRI) have begun to describe the functional neuroanatomy of emotion. Phan et al. (2002) reported that, taken separately, specific studies vary in task dimensions and in type(s) of emotion studied and are limited by statistical power and sensitivity. By examining findings across studies, these investigators sought to determine if common or segregated patterns of activations exist across various emotional tasks. They reviewed 55 PET and fMRI activation studies (yielding 761 individual peaks) that investigated emotion in healthy subjects. This review yielded the following summary observations:

1. Medial prefrontal cortex had a general role in emotional processing.
2. Fear specifically engaged the amygdala.
3. Sadness was associated with activity in the subcallosal cingulate.
4. Emotional induction by visual stimuli activated the occipital cortex and amygdala.
5. Induction by emotional recall/imagery recruited the anterior cingulate and insula.
6. Emotional tasks with cognitive demand also involved the anterior cingulate and insula.

This review provides a critical comparison of findings across individual studies and suggests that separate brain regions are involved in different aspects of emotion. Mental disorders are increasingly being conceptualized as dimensional. It would be surprising if these findings were not to be found to transfer to the internalizing disorders of fear and sadness.

INFORMATION PROCESSING

Information processing biases in attention, interpretation, and memory have been examined across the emotional disorders using a variety of paradigms. In Chapter 10, Huppert and colleagues review cross-sectional, longitudinal, treatment, and experimental studies for each of the so-called stress-induced and fear circuitry disorders. There are some similarities and differences across the emotional disorders that may inform classification, although methodological limitations prevent firm conclusions from being drawn in many cases. There is consistent evidence for attentional biases at the strategic level for panic disorder, SocAD, and specific phobias. The evidence is mixed for an automatic attentional bias in PTSD because of the use of different paradigms, different types of trauma, and the dearth of studies. However, there have been multiple replications across trauma types of an attentional bias at the strategic level of processing for trauma-related words (Buckley et al. 2000). It is noteworthy that there is evidence for an automatic attentional bias for OCD (contamination type; Summerfeldt and Endler 1998) and GAD (MacLeod and Rutherford 2004), whereas depression only shows a bias at the strategic level of processing (Mathews and MacLeod 2005).

Diagnosis-related interpretation biases have been found reliably across all of the emotional disorders, not just the stress and fear circuitry disorders. However, there has been very limited research on interpretation biases in OCD, and the heterogeneity of OCD subtypes has resulted in many inconsistencies within the information processing literature more broadly.

Research on memory biases in the anxiety disorders is also rife with inconsistencies. Evidence for explicit memory biases is probably strongest for panic disorder. Although there is limited support for a general memory bias in SocAD, there is evidence of a bias toward recognizing faces perceived as critical (Lundh and Öst 1996). Few studies have investigated explicit memory biases in PTSD, and currently the weight of evidence is against an explicit memory bias in GAD. The evidence for implicit memory biases is limited for PTSD and SocAD and equivocal for GAD. The weight of evidence for panic disorder does not support an implicit memory bias (Coles and Heimberg 2002). No firm conclusions can be drawn from the memory literature for OCD, probably with the exception of visual or visuospatial memory deficits (Coles and Heimberg 2002). In contrast, depression is reliably associated with a memory bias (Mathews and MacLeod 2005).

In general, there seem to be more similarities than differences across the anxiety disorders in terms of the cognitive-processing biases, at least relative to mood disorders. However, few studies have compared information processing biases across disorders directly or used nonanxious and high-trait anxious control subjects. Therefore, it is unclear whether such biases reliably distinguish between the anxiety disorders or reflect common underlying processes. At this stage, it appears that although the content of cognitions reliably distinguishes between the disorders, our knowledge of underlying cognitive processes cannot robustly inform classification.

ENVIRONMENTAL STRESSORS

As Rapee and Bryant note in Chapter 11, although a number of environmental stressors raise the probability of a fear disorder occurring, there is little specificity between a particular stressor and the onset of a particular disorder. Even in PTSD, in which it appears that the range of candidate events is increasingly large, the issue remains: why did this person develop the disorder, when four out of five people who encountered the same stressor did not? Adverse life events also are implicated in the onset of depression, and there may be little specific in the environmental stressor, only in the person's response to the stressor.

Treatments That Work

Identifying a diagnosis based on response to treatment has always been hazardous. Both selective serotonin reuptake inhibitor (SSRI) antidepressant drugs and cognitive-behavioral therapy (CBT) are efficacious in internalizing disorders. The evidence is slight with respect to the efficacy of SSRIs in specific phobia or mild depression and, with respect to CBT, in severe depression, but otherwise there is little evidence of specific relations between a particular drug or form of CBT and one of the four fear circuitry disorders.

Conclusion

At the simplest level, PTSD, panic/agoraphobia, SocAD, and specific phobia form a coherent group that is distinct from the other internalizing disorders. This group is characterized by fear and avoidance of certain situations, attentional bias at the strategic level of processing for threat-related words, and amgydalocentric processing of this information. Disorder-specific genetic factors are considered to be substantial for the phobias, but some of these may be shared with personality variables that are germane to other internalizing disorders. The contributors to this book have defined a program of research to advance these propositions.

References

American Psychiatric Association: Diagnostic and Statistical Manual of Mental Disorders, 4th Edition. Washington, DC, American Psychiatric Association, 1994

Andrews G: Comorbidity and the general neurotic syndrome. Br J Psychiatry 168(suppl):76–84, 1996

Andrews G, Slade T, Issakidis C: Deconstructing current comorbidity: data from the Australian National Survey of Mental Health and Well-being. Br J Psychiatry 181:306–314, 2002

Buckley TC, Blanchard EB, Neill WT: Information processing and PTSD. Clin Psychol Rev 20:1041–1065, 2000

Coles ME, Heimberg RG: Memory biases in the anxiety disorders. Clin Psychol Rev 22:587–627, 2002

Cook TD, Leviton LC: Reviewing the literature: a comparison of traditional methods with meta-analysis. J Pers 48:472–499, 1980

Hettema JM, Prescott CA, Myers JM, et al: The structure of genetic and environmental risk factors for anxiety disorders in men and women. Arch Gen Psychiatry 62:182–189, 2005

Hettema JM, Neale MC, Myers JM, et al: A population-based twin study of the relationship between neuroticism and internalizing disorders. Am J Psychiatry 163:857–864, 2006

Kessler RC, Berglund P, Demler O, et al: Lifetime prevalence and age-of-onset distributions of DSM-IV disorders in the National Comorbidity Survey Replication. Arch Gen Psychiatry 62:593–602, 2005a

Kessler RC, Chiu WT, Demler O, et al: Prevalence, severity, and comorbidity of 12-month DSM-IV disorders in the National Comorbidity Survey Replication. Arch Gen Psychiatry 62:617–627, 2005b

Kessler RC, Angermeyer M, Anthony JC, et al: Lifetime prevalence and age-of-onset distributions of mental disorders in the World Health Organization's World Mental Health Survey Initiative. World Psychiatry 6:168–176, 2007

Krueger RF: The structure of common mental disorders. Arch Gen Psychiatry 56:921–926, 1999

Krueger RF, Markon KE: Reinterpreting comorbidity: a model-based approach to understanding and classifying psychopathology, in Annual Review of Clinical Psychology, Vol 2. Palo Alto, CA, Annual Reviews, 2006, pp 111–133

Lundh LG, Öst LG: Recognition bias for critical faces in social phobics. Beh Res Ther 34:787–794, 1996.

MacLeod C, Rutherford EM: Information processing approaches, in Generalized Anxiety Disorder. Edited by Heimberg RG, Turk CL, Mennin DS. New York, Guilford, 2004, pp 109–142

Martin NG, Jardine R, Andrews G, et al: Anxiety disorders: are there genetic factors specific to panic? Acta Psychiatr Scand 77:698–706, 1988

Mathews A, MacLeod C: Cognitive vulnerability to emotional disorders, in Annual Review of Clinical Psychology, Vol 1. Palo Alto, CA, Annual Reviews, 2005, pp 167–195

Oakley Browne MA, Wells JE, Scott KM, et al: Lifetime prevalence and projected lifetime risk of DSM-IV disorders in Te Rau Hinengaro: the New Zealand Mental Health Survey. Aust N Z J Psychiatry 40:865–874, 2006

Phan KL, Wager T, Taylor SF, et al: Functional neuroanatomy of emotion: a meta-analysis of emotion activation studies in PET and fMRI. Neuroimage 16:331–348, 2002

Slade T, Watson D: The structure of common DSM-IV and ICD-10 mental disorders in the Australian general population. Psychol Med 36:1593–1600, 2006

Summerfeldt LJ, Endler NS: Examining the evidence for anxiety-related cognitive biases in obsessive compulsive disorder. J Anxiety Disord 12:579–598, 1998

World Health Organization: International Statistical Classification of Diseases and Related Health Problems, 10th Revision. Geneva, Switzerland, World Health Organization, 1992

INDEX

Page numbers printed in **boldface** *type refer to tables or figures.*

Active gene-environment correlation, 149
Acute stress disorder, 7, 200
Adjustment disorder, 17–18
Adolescents and adolescence. *See also* Age; Children and childhood
    continuity of anxiety disorders in, 107–108, **109**
    genetics of anxiety disorders and, 145–154
    onset of specific phobias and, 80
    panic disorder and, 34
    specific phobias and, 83
    substance use disorders in, 270
Adrenocorticotropic hormone (ACTH), and panic disorder, 45
Affect. *See* Negative affectivity; Positive affectivity
Affective disorders, and substance abuse, **268**
African Americans, and anxiety disorders, 79, 139–142, 289
Age, and prevalence of specific phobias, 79–80. *See also* Adolescents and adolescence; Age of onset; Children and childhood
Age of onset
    of anxiety disorders, 126–127, 195–196, 283–284, 294
    of social phobia, 59
    of specific phobias, 79–80
    of substance use disorders, 270
Agoraphobia
    classification of panic disorder and, 36–37

    comorbidity and, 127
    continuity of, 107, **109**, 110
    epidemiology of, 39–41
    future research on, 46
    panic attacks and, 31–32
    subtypes of panic disorder and, 38
    without panic, 39–41, **40**
Allostatic load model, of PTSD, 19
American Heart Association, 118
American Psychiatric Association, 294
American view, of panic disorder, 32
Amygdala. *See also* Brain; Neuroimaging
    cognitive activation probes of function, 224–225
    commonalities among anxiety disorders and, 237, 238
    fear conditioning and, 219
    panic disorder and, 42–43, 233, 286
    PTSD and, 227–228
    serotonin system and, 167
    social phobia and, 69, 236, 237
Animal models
    for development of anxiety phenotype, 164–165
    for neurocircuitry of relevant functional domains, 218–220, 242
    for panic disorder, 42–43, 44, 45–46
    for PTSD, 4
    for substance use disorders, 271, 273
Animal phobias, 78, 79, 80, 82, 84, 88, 235
Anterior cingulate cortex (ACC), 225, 239
Anthropology, and cross-cultural issues in PTSD, 21

Anticipatory panic attacks, 38, 39
Antisocial behavior, 110
Antisocial personality disorder, **268**
Anxiety. *See also* Anxiety disorders; Anxiety sensitivity
  development of phenotype in early life, 164–165
  neural circuits and development of, 165–167
  role of serotonin in development of, 161–162, 167–168, 290
Anxiety Disorder Interview Schedule, 68
Anxiety disorders. *See also* Anxiety; Generalized anxiety disorder; Panic disorder; Posttraumatic stress disorder; Social phobia; Specific phobia; Stress-induced and fear circuitry disorders
  in African Americans and ethnic minorities, 139–142, 289
  age at onset of, 126–127, 195–196, 283–284, 294
  behavioral genetic methodology and, 145–147
  children with behavioral inhibition and, 87
  cognition and, 175–187
  cognitive-behavioral therapies for, 182
  common characteristics of, 283–284, 288–289
  comorbidity and, 41–42, 127, 294–295
  continuity of, 106–111, 288
  demographic factors and, 197–200
  depression and, 82–83
  developmental perspective for DSM-V and, 118
  epidemiology of, 116–118, 126–127
  etiology of, 111–116, 288
  extreme analyses and, 149
  family factors in onset of, 203–207
  follow-up studies of children with, **89**
  genetic-environment interaction and, 147, 150–152, **153**
  genetics of, 90, 91, 128–129, 145–154, 196–197, 290, 295–296

  identification of common underlying diatheses, 129–131
  information processing and, 115–116, 297–298
  molecular biology and epidemiology of, 116–118
  multivariate genetic analyses and, 148
  neurochemical and neuroendocrine findings in, 255–257, 259–260, 292
  neurocircuitry of functional domains relevant to, 222–225
  neuroimaging studies of, 226–244, 292, 297
  prevalence of, 126–127, 139–142
  reconceptualizing role of fear and stress in, 261–262
  social phobia as, 61–62
  stressors and onset of, 200–202, 291, 298
  substance use disorders and, 265–278, 293
  unique aspects of, 284–288, 289
Anxiety sensitivity
  panic disorder and, 37, 181, 182
  social phobia and, 64
Anxiety Sensitivity Inventory, 181
Anxiogenic intoxication, 275
Associative-conditioning processes, and dysfunctional fear, 112
Assortative mating, and twin studies, 147
Asthma, and specific phobias, 81
Attachment styles, and parent-child interaction, 205
Attentional bias, 176–177, 186, 297–298
Attention-deficit/hyperactivity disorder (ADHD), 108, 117
Auditory startle response, 7
Australia, research on PTSD in, 7, 14, 200
Australian National Survey of Mental Health and Well Being, 42, **296**
Automatic cognitive processes, 176
Autonomic symptoms, of panic disorder, 33
Avoidance. *See also* Avoidant personality disorder

common characteristics of anxiety
  disorders and, 283
 PTSD and, 13–15
 social phobia and, 63–64
Avoidant personality disorder, 61, 62, 69

Baltimore Epidemiologic Catchment Area
  Follow-up Study, 83
Behavioral genetic methodology, and
  anxiety disorders, 145–147
Behavioral inhibition
 anxiety disorders and, 116, 127, 131
 neuroimaging studies and, 241
 social phobia and, 60
 specific phobias and, 86, 87
Behavior genetic data, on anxiety
  disorders, 196–197
Behavior therapy paradigm, for specific
  phobias, 92
Benzodiazepines, 232–233, 272
BiDil (drug), 140
Bipolar disorder, 42, **268**
Blood-injection-injury phobias, 78, 79,
  80, 82, 84, 88, 94
Bodily sensations
 panic disorder and, 178, 181, 287
 social phobia and, 66–67, 70
Body dysmorphic disorder, 67
Body image, and social phobia, 67
Brain. See also Amygdala; Hippocampus;
  Hypothalamic-pituitary-adrenal axis;
  Neural circuits; Neurobiology;
  Neuroimaging
 addiction and desensitization of
   reward system, 273–274
 anxiety disorders and structure and
   function of, 297
 sensitive period of development, **161**
Brain activation, and specific phobias,
  92–93
Brain imaging. See Neuroimaging
Brazil, and prevalence of specific phobias,
  79
Buspirone, 271–272

Cannabis use, and development of
  psychosis, 116
Carbon dioxide challenge, 185, **256**
Cardio-respiratory symptoms, of panic
  disorder, 38, 39
Cardiovascular risk factors, for anxiety
  disorders, 118
Catecholamine, **256**
Categorical issues, in PTSD, 17–20
Causal cognitive processes, 187
Child Behavior Checklist, 106
Children and childhood. See also
  Development; Parents and parenting
 continuity of anxiety disorders in,
   106–107
 depression in compared to adult-onset,
   114–115
 early life stress and development of
   mental health problems in,
   159–160
 follow-up studies of anxiety disorders
   in, **89**
 genetic research on anxiety disorders
   in, 145–154
 life events and anxiety disorders in,
   201
 panic disorder in, 34, 45
 sexual abuse and anxiety disorders in,
   203–204
 social phobia and, 59, 62, 63, 64–65,
   66
 specific phobias and, 79, 87
 transmission of psychopathology from
   parents to, 117–118
Cholecystokinin, **256**
Chorionicity, and twin studies, 146–147
Christchurch Health and Development
  Study, 107, 111
Chronic fatigue syndrome, 19
Chronic stress, 19–20
Classification
 of panic disorder, 36–37
 of specific phobias, 93–94
Claustrophobia, 80

Clinical studies, of panic disorder and agoraphobia, **40**, 46
Clinician Administered PTSD Scale, 14
Cognition
　assumptions on, 177
　commonalities among anxiety disorders and, 290–291
　cross-sectional studies of, 178–180
　definition of, 175–177
　experimental studies of, 176–177, 185–187
　genetic and environmental risk of anxiety disorders and, 153–154
　longitudinal studies of, 180–182
　phobic attitudes in panic disorder and, 37–38
　risk factors for PTSD and, 6
　training of biases, 186–187
　treatment studies of, 182–184
Cognitive activation probes, and neuroimaging studies, 224–225
Cognitive-behavioral activation paradigms, of neuroimaging, 222
Cognitive-behavioral therapies (CBT). *See also* Exposure therapy
　diagnosis and effectiveness of, 299
　panic disorder and, 183
　PTSD and, 183
　social phobia and, 184
　substance use disorders and, 272
Cognitive processes, 176
Comorbidity
　of anxiety disorders, 127, 294–295
　panic disorder and, 41–42
　PTSD and, 17, 20–21
　social phobia and, 68
　specific phobias and, 82–83, 84
Complex PTSD/Disorders of Extreme Stress Not Otherwise Specified (DES-NOS), 18–19, 286
Composite International Diagnostic Interview (CIDI), 10, 39, 106
Conditioned stimulus
　research on neurocircuitry and, 218
　specific phobias and, 85–87

Conduct disorder (CD), 108, 275
Constitutive cognitive processes, 187
Continuity, of anxiety disorders, 106–111, 288
Corticotropin-releasing hormone (CRH), 45, 255, **256**, 257, 274
Cortisol concentration, **256**, 257
Cross-sectional studies, of cognition, 178–180
Cue-elicited drug seeking, 274
Culture and cross-cultural issues
　anxiety disorders in ethnic minorities and, 141
　PTSD and, 21, 200
　social phobia and, 62, 65, 67, 199–200
Cyclic adenosine monophosphate (cAMP), 46

Decision making, and substance abuse, 275
Delayed-onset PTSD, 7, 15
Demographic factors, and anxiety disorders, 197–200. *See also* Age; Gender; Ethnic minorities
Depression. *See also* Major depressive disorder
　comorbidity of with PTSD, 17
　development and, 110
　genetic association between parenting and, 150, 151
　genetic vulnerability to, 148
　juvenile vs. adult-onset cases of, 114–115
　life events and serotonin system, 152, **153**
Development. *See also* Children and childhood; Prospective-developmental studies
　of anxiety phenotype in early life, 164–165
　disruption of serotonin homeostasis during, 163–164
　life course stability of etiology of anxiety disorders, 113–114
　multiple roles of serotonin in, 162
　neural circuits and anxiety, 165–167
　neuroimaging studies for risk and, 241

perspective for anxiety disorders in DSM-V and, 118
PTSD and issues of, 21–22
serotonin and sensitive periods of, 160–162, 167–168
specific phobias and, 88, 90
Dexamethasone suppression test (DST), 5, **256**
Diagnosis
of anxiety disorders in ethnic minorities, 140, 141
effectiveness of treatment and, 299
nonverbal implications of stress-related fear circuitry model for PTSD, 5–6
of social phobia, 60–62
of specific phobias, 93–94
Diagnostic Interview Schedule, 39, 199
Dimensional issues, in PTSD, 17–20
Discomfort, and panic attacks, 39
Dissociation, and PTSD, 21
Distal causes, of anxiety disorders, 206–207
Dot probe studies, 176–177, 179, 186
DSM-I, and depression diagnoses, 17
DSM-III
panic disorder and, 31, 35, 36, 39
PTSD and, 10
social phobia and, 60–62, 63, 69
standardization of definition and diagnosis, 113
DSM-III-R
panic disorder and, 31, 35, 36, 39
PTSD and, 10
social phobia and, 61, 63, 69
DSM-IV
definitional problems in, 259
diagnostic criteria for PTSD, 3, 7–17, 22
model for structure of anxiety disorders, **296**
panic disorder and, 31, 35, 36, 39
social phobia and, 60–62, 63
specific phobias and, 77, 93
substance use disorders and, 272, 278
DSM-IV-TR
etiology of anxiety disorders and, 112

heterogeneity of diagnoses and, 116
panic disorder and, 39
social phobia and, 61
specific phobias and, 77, 78, 81, 93, 94
substance use disorders and, 272
DSM-V
developmental perspective for anxiety disorders in, 118
social phobia and, 64
substance use disorders and, 265, 276, 278, 293
Dunedin birth cohort study, 108
Duration, of symptoms in PTSD, 15
Dyspnea, 38
Dysthymia, and substance abuse, **269**

Early Developmental Stages of Psychopathology sample, 82
Early-onset panic, 38
Emotional faces paradigm, 239
Emotional lability, and specific phobias, 86–87
Emotional Stroop paradigm, 85, 176, 179, 180
Endophenotypes, 153
Environment. *See also* Gene-environment interactions; Life events
nonclinical models of stress and fear, 261
onset of anxiety disorders and specific events in, 201–202, 298
Epidemiological Catchment Area (ECA) study, 38, 83, 139, 141, 267, **268–269**
Epidemiology. *See also* Prevalence of anxiety disorders, 116–118, 126–127
of panic disorder, 39–41
of specific phobias, 78–87
of substance abuse, 266–270
Ethnic minorities, and anxiety disorders, 139–142, 289
Etiology
of anxiety disorders, 111–116, 288
of panic disorder, 42–46, 112–113
of PTSD, 216

Etiology *(continued)*
  relationships between anxiety and substance use disorders, 265–266, 277
  of social phobia, 59–60
  of specific phobias, 95
European view, of panic disorder, 32
European-wide Size and Burden of Disorders of the Brain Project, 79
Evocative gene-environment correlations, 149
Experimental studies, of cognition, 176–177, 185–187
Explicit memory tasks, 177
Exposure therapy
  specific phobias and, 88, 184
  substance use disorders and, 272
Extinction, and neuroimaging studies of fear conditioning, 222–224
Extraversion, and anxiety disorders, 130
Extreme analyses, and genetics of anxiety disorders, 149
Eye-tracking paradigms, 180

Fact, definition of, 284
Factor-analysis studies, of specific phobias, 83–84
Factor structure, of PTSD, 13–15
Family. *See also* Family studies; Parents and parenting
  links between psychopathology and environment of, 150
  onset of anxiety disorders and, 197–198, 203–207
  specific phobias and, 90
Family studies, of anxiety disorders, 128–129, 196–197
Fear. *See also* Fear conditioning; Irrationality
  common characteristics of anxiety disorders and, 283
  as diagnostic criterion for PTSD, 12–13
  fearful vs. nonfearful panic attacks, 38
  reconceptualizing role of in anxiety disorders, 261–262
  social phobia and irrationality of, 67–68
  specific phobias and structure of, 83–85
Fear conditioning, and research on neurocircuitry, 218–219, 222–224
Fibromyalgia, 19
Filial imprinting, 160
Florida, and research on PTSD, 11
Flumazenil, 233
Fluoxetine, 164
Follow-up studies, and neuroimaging research, 243
Food and Drug Administration, 140
Four-factor model, of PTSD, 13, 14
Frequency, of occurrence of symptoms in PTSD, 15
Functional impairment. *See* Impairment
Functional magnetic resonance imaging (fMRI), 221, 223, 231, 235, 236, 297. *See also* Neuroimaging
Future research
  on continuity of anxiety disorders, 110–111
  on molecular biology and epidemiology of anxiety disorders, 116–118
  neuroimaging studies and agenda of, 241–244
  on panic disorder and agoraphobia, 46
  on social disorder, 69–70
  on specific phobias, 93–95
  on stability of etiology of anxiety disorders, 114–116

Gender, and prevalence
  of anxiety disorders, 126–127, 199
  of specific phobias, 80
Gene-environment interactions. *See also* Environment; Genetics
  anxiety disorders and, 116–118, 147, 150–152, **153**
  sensitive period in development of anxiety and, 167–168
General adaptation syndrome, and panic disorder, 46

Generalized anxiety disorder
    age at onset of, 195
    comorbidity with panic disorder, 41
    continuity of, **109**, 110
    demographic factors in, 199
    family disruption and, 203
    family studies of, 129
    genetics of, 148
    neurochemical and neuroendocrine findings in, 255, **256**, 257, 260
    prevalence of, 126–127
    substance abuse and, 267, **268**
Generalized social anxiety disorder, 64–65, 127
Genetics. *See also* Gene-environment interactions
    anxiety disorders and, 90, 91, 128–129, 145–154, 196–197, 290, 295–296
    neuroimaging studies and, 244
    risk factors for PTSD and, 6
    serotonin system and, 162
    social phobia and, 60, 69–70, 129
    specific phobias and, 86, 90–91
    variability of responses to stress, 160
Germany, and research on panic disorder, 34
Global Assessment of Function (GAF) scale, 16
Great Smoky Mountains Study, 111

Helplessness, and diagnostic criteria for PTSD, 12
Heterotypic continuity, of anxiety disorders, 106, 108, 110
Hippocampus
    anxiety and anxiety-related behavior, 165–166
    commonalities among anxiety disorders and, 237
    contextual conditioning and, 219
    neuroimaging studies and cognitive activation probes of, 225
    panic disorder and, 233
    PTSD and, 7, 227, 228, 229

Homeostasis, disruption of serotonin, 163–164
Homotypic continuity, of anxiety disorders, 106, 108, 110
Horror, and diagnostic criteria for PTSD, 12
Hydralazine, 140
Hyperarousal, and PTSD, 13–15
Hyperventilation, and panic disorder, 232
Hypochondriasis, 94
Hypothalamic-pituitary-adrenal (HPA) axis, 44–45, 273, 274

ICD-10
    diagnostic criteria for PTSD in, 3, 7–17, 22
    model for structure of anxiety disorders, **296**
    panic disorder and, 36
    specific phobia and, 78
Illness phobia, 94
Imipramine, 232, 272
Impairment
    PTSD and, 16–17, 285
    specific phobias and, 80–81
Implicit memory tasks, 177
Impulsivity, and substance abuse, 275
Information processing
    anxiety disorders as perturbations of, 115–116, 297–298
    onset of anxiety disorders and transmission of, 206
    specific phobias and, 85–87
Insight, and social phobia, 67–68
Insular cortex, and neuroimaging, 225
International Affective Picture System, 224–225
Interoceptive function, and neuroimaging, 225
Interpretation biases, 186–187
Irrationality, of fear
    in panic disorder, 287
    in social phobia, 67–68
Isosorbide dinitrate, 140

Japan
   prevalence of specific phobias in, 79
   research on social phobia in, 65, 66, 199, 200

Kenya, and research on PTSD, 21
Klein, Donald, 31, 32
Korea, and social phobia, 199, 200

Lactate/carbon dioxide, **256**
Late-onset panic, 38
Latinos, and anxiety disorders, 139, 142. *See also* Mexican Americans
Learning
   onset of anxiety disorders and, 202
   specific phobias and, 85
Life events. *See also* Stress
   anxiety disorders and nonspecific, 200–201
   depressive symptoms in adults and, 152, **153**
   panic disorder and, 45–46
   social phobia and, 60
Limited symptom panic attacks, 33
Longitudinal studies
   cognition in anxiety disorders and, 180–182
   continuity of anxiety disorders and, 106
   future research in neuroimaging and, 243
   of substance use disorders, 270–271
Los Angeles Symptom Checklist, 14

Magnetic resonance imaging (MRI), 220–221, 229, 236. *See also* Neuroimaging
Magnetic resonance spectroscopy (MRS), 222
Major depressive disorder (MDD). *See also* Depression
   comorbidity with anxiety disorders, 20–21, 41, 295
   neuroimaging studies of, 238–239
   substance abuse and, 267, **269**

Masked Stroop effect, 85–86
Medical illness, and chronic stress, 19–20
Memory bias, 177, 298
Mexican Americans, and specific phobias, 79. *See also* Latinos
Michigan, and research on PTSD, 11
Minnesota Multiphasic Personality Inventory (MMPI), 142
Mobility Inventory for Agoraphobia, 40
Modeling, and parent-child interaction, 206
Molecular biology
   epidemiology of anxiety disorders and, 116–118
   panic disorder and, 44
Monoamine oxidase A gene (*MAOA*), 160, 163, 167
Mood disorders, and African Americans, 142
Multidimensional Personality Questionnaire, 113
Multimodel imaging, 243
Multivariate genetic analyses, and anxiety disorders, 148
Munich-CIDI, 39

National Comorbidity Survey (NCS), 13, 20, 38, 81, 83, 114, 126, 127, 130, 139, 267, 283, 294
National Epidemiologic Survey of Alcohol and Related Conditions (NESARC), 267
National Institute of Mental Health Diagnostic Interview Schedule, 14
Natural environment phobias, 78, 79, 82, 84
Negative affectivity. *See also* Positive affectivity
   anxiety disorders and, 130
   specific phobias and, 86, 87
Negative imagery, and social phobia, 185
Netherlands, and research
   on PTSD, 11
   on social phobia, 66
   on specific phobias, 84

Neural circuits. *See also* Neuroimaging
  animal models of relevant functional domains in, 218–220
  development of anxiety and, 165–167
  fear conditioning and extinction, 222–224
  models of stress-induced and fear circuitry disorders and, 217–218
  sensitive period of development and, 161
Neurasthenia, 295, **296**
Neurobiology
  of acute substance effects, 275–276
  specific phobias and, 88, 90
  of stress, social anxiety, and substance addiction, 273–274
Neurochemical and neuroendocrine findings, in anxiety disorders, 255–257, 259–260, 292
Neuroimaging.
  anatomical correlates of anxiety disorders and, 226–237, 292, 297
  cognitive activation probes and, 224–225
  commonalities and specificity across anxiety disorders and, 237–239
  fear conditioning and extinction, 222–224
  functional techniques and paradigms, 221–222
  future research and, 241–244
  interoceptive function and insular cortex, 225
  panic disorder and, 43
  PTSD and, 4, 5
  sensitivity, specificity, and replication in studies of anxiety disorders, 239–241
  specific phobias and, 91–93
  structural techniques of, 220–221
Neuromodulators, and serotonin, 162
Neuropeptide Y, 7
Neuropsychological deficits, in substance addictions and anxiety disorders, 274–275

Neuroscience, and risk factors for PTSD, 7
Neuroticism
  anxiety disorders and, 130, 131, 295
  social phobia and, 64
  specific phobias and, 82–83
Neurotic panic, 42
Neurotransmitters, and role of serotonin in development, 162
Neutral state paradigms, of neuroimaging, 221
New Zealand, and research
  on continuity of anxiety disorder, 107
  on social phobia, 63
Nocturnal attacks, 38
Non-fearful panic, 38–39
Nongeneralized subtype, of social anxiety disorder, 65–67
Nonmasked Stroop interference, 85
Nonshared environment, and twin studies, 146
Number of symptoms, and diagnosis of panic disorder, 33
Numbing, and PTSD, 13–15

Obsessive-compulsive disorder
  comorbidity and, 127
  continuity of, **109**, 110
  family studies of, 129
  irrationality of fear and, 67
  neuroimaging studies of, 238
  prevalence of, 126–127
  stressful life events and onset of, 201
Oklahoma City, and research on PTSD, 21
Oppositional defiant disorder (ODD), 108, **109**, 110
Overanxious disorder in childhood and adolescence, 61, 62
Overprotection, and parent-child interaction, 204–205

Panic-agoraphobic spectrum, 41
Panic attacks. *See also* Panic disorder
  in absence of panic disorder, 34
  anxiety sensitivity and, 182

Panic attacks *(continued)*
    cognition and, 181
    definition of, 33
    subtypes of, 38–39
    yohimbine and, 6
Panic disorder. *See also* Panic attacks
    agoraphobia and, 31–32, 36–37, 38, 39–41, 46
    cognition and, 178, 181, 183, 185
    comorbidity and, 41–42, 84, 127
    continuity of, 107, 108, **109**, 110
    criterion symptoms for, 33
    etiology of, 42–46, 112–113
    family disruption and, 203
    future research on, 46
    history of concept, 31–32
    life events and onset of, 200
    mode of onset of, 34
    neurochemical and neuroendocrine findings in, 255, **256**
    neuroimaging studies of, 230–234
    number of symptoms required, 33
    phenomenology of, 216–217
    phobic cognitions and attitudes in, 36, 37–38
    prevalence of, 126–127
    prodome and, 35–37
    serotonin system and, 167
    substance abuse and, **268**
    subtypes of, 34, 38–39
    underdiagnosis of in African Americans, 140
    unique aspects of, 286
Panic reaction, and diagnostic criteria for PTSD, 12
Parallel-process latent growth models, of anxiety disorders, 131
Parents and parenting. *See also* Family
    genetics of depression and, 150, 151
    onset of anxiety disorders and, 204–205
    transmission of psychopathology to children from, 117–118
Paroxetine, 272
Partial PTSD, 17–18
Passive gene-environment correlation, 149

Pavlovian fear conditioning, 4
Peer victimization, and onset of anxiety disorders, 202
Performance anxiety, 65–66, 287
Personality traits, and specific phobias, 82–83
Pervasive developmental disorder (PDD), 68
Pet-1 (transcription factor), 163
Pharmacological probes, and research on PTSD, 5–6
Pharmacotherapy. *See also* Selective serotonin reuptake inhibitors
    for social anxiety disorder, 184
    for substance use disorders, 271–272
Phenomenology, of stress-induced and fear circuitry disorders, 215–218
Phobic attitude, and panic disorder, 36, 37–38
Phobic symptoms, in panic disorder, 35–36
Population studies, of panic disorder, 46
Positive affectivity, and anxiety disorders, 130, 131. *See also* Negative affectivity
Positron emission tomography (PET), 221, 222, 226–228, 231, 232, 234–235, 236, 297. *See also* Neuroimaging
Post-severe stress syndrome, 20
Posttraumatic stress disorder (PTSD)
    African Americans and, 140, 141, 142
    age at onset of, 195
    categorical vs. dimensional issues in, 17–20
    cognition and, 179, 180, 181–182, 183
    comorbidity and, 20–21, 127
    continuity of, 108, **109**, 110
    cross-cultural factors in, 21, 200
    developmental issues and, 21–22
    differences of diagnostic criteria in DSM-IV and ICD-10, 3, 7–10
    facts supporting changes to diagnostic criteria for, 10–17
    life events and onset of, 200, 201, 202

Index 311

neurochemical and neuroendocrine findings in, 255, **256**, 257, 260
neuroimaging studies of, 226–230
nonverbal diagnostic implications of stress-related fear circuitry model of, 5–6
phenomenology of, 216
prevalence of, 126–127
reconceptualizing role of stress in, 261–262
risk factors for development of, 6–7, 112, 114
sexual abuse and, 203
as stress-related fear circuitry disorder, 4
substance abuse and, 267, **268**, 271, 272
unique aspects of, 285–286
Pregenual anterior cingulate cortex (pACC), 223
Preparedness theory, and specific phobias, 86
Prevalence. *See also* Epidemiology
of anxiety disorders, 126–127, 139–142
of mood and anxiety disorders in substance dependent patients, 267
of social phobia, 59, 63
of specific phobias, 78–80
Prodome, and onset of panic disorder, 35–37
Prospective-developmental studies, on continuity of anxiety disorders, 106–111
Prototypic panic attacks, 38
Proximal causes, of anxiety disorders, 206–207
Psychic symptoms, of panic disorder, 33
Psychophysiological reactivity, and diagnosis of PTSD, 5
Psychotic symptoms, and PTSD in African Americans, 142
PTSD Reaction Index, 14

Quality of life, and specific phobias, 81

Race, and treatment of anxiety disorders, 140–141
Re-experiencing, and PTSD, 13–15
Regional cerebral blood flow (rCBF), and specific phobias, 92
Reliability, of neuroimaging studies, 240–241, 242
Renewal, and fear response, 219
Replication, of neuroimaging studies, 242–243
Research. *See* Future research
Resilience, and vulnerability to development of PTSD, 6
Respiratory disease, and specific phobias, 81
Respiratory panic attacks, 38
Revised NEO Personality Inventory, 83
Risk factors
cardiovascular for development of anxiety disorders, 118
for development of PTSD, 6–7, 112, 114
for social phobia, 60, 64–65
for substance use disorders, 270–271, 276, **277**

Script driven imagery, 5, 231–232
Selective serotonin reuptake inhibitors (SSRIs), 272, 299
Self-medication model, and stress-addiction link, 273
Sensation-seeking hypothesis, of substance abuse, 273
Sensitive period, of development, 160–162, **161**, 167–168, 290
Separation anxiety disorder, 147, 197, 202
Serotonin
differences among anxiety disorders and, **256**
disruption of homeostasis during development, 163–164
life events and depressive symptoms in adults, 152, **153**
multiple roles of in development, 162
panic disorder and, 44
sensitive periods of development and, 160–162, 167–168, 290

Serotonin transporter gene (*SERT*), 160, 163, 167, 168
Sertraline, 272
Sexual abuse, and anxiety disorders, 203–204
Shared environment, and twin studies, 146
Single photon emission tomography (SPECT), 221, 222, 231, 236
Situational phobias, 78, 79, 80, 82, 84, 88, 94
Social anxiety disorder (SocAD). *See* Social phobia
Social phobia
  age at onset of, 50, 195
  avoidant personality disorder and, 61, 62, 69
  cognition and, 179–180, 184, 185
  comorbidity and, 41, 68, 127
  continuity of, 107, 108, **109**, 110
  cross-cultural issues and, 62, 65, 67, 199–200
  diagnosis of, 60–62
  etiology of, 59–60
  future research on, 69–70
  genetics of, 60, 69–70, 129
  modeling by parents and, 206
  neurobiology of stress, substance addiction, and, 273–274
  neurochemical and neuroendocrine findings in, 255, **256** 257
  neuroimaging studies of, 235–237
  peer victimization and, 202
  phenomenology of, 217
  prevalence of, 59, 63, 126–127
  strengths and weaknesses of current criteria for, 63–68
  substance abuse and, **268**
  unique aspects of, 286–287
Socioeconomic status, and anxiety disorders, 197
Somatization, and PTSD, 21
Specific phobias
  age at onset of, 79–80, 195
  cognition and, 180, 184, 185–186
  comorbidity and, 41, 82–83, 84, 127
  continuity of, 107, **109**, 110
  course and prognosis of, 87–93
  description of, 77–78
  epidemiology of, 78–87
  etiology of, 95
  future research on, 93–95
  neurobiological factors in, 88, 90
  neurochemical and neuroendocrine findings in, **256**
  neuroimaging studies of, 234–235
  phenomenology of, 217
  prevalence of, 126–127
  substance abuse and, **268**
  underdiagnosis of in African Americans, 140
  unique aspects of, 287–288
Spectrum
  of panic-agoraphobia, 41
  from partial or subsyndromal to complex PTSD, 285–286
Speech phobia, 65
Spider phobias, 235
Sporadic panic attacks, 34
Stability, of etiology of anxiety disorders, 111–116
Stimulus-driven paradigms, for research on PTSD, 5
Strategic cognitive processes, 176
Stress. *See also* Life events
  hypothesis for panic disorder and, 44–46
  mental health problems in children and early life, 159–160
  neurobiology of substance addiction and, 273–274
  poststress syndromes other than PTSD, 19–20
  reconceptualizing role of in anxiety disorders, 261–262
  research on PTSD and response to, 4
  role of in onset of anxiety disorders, 200–202, 291
  substance use disorders and, 271
Stress-diathesis model, for phobias, 112

Stress-induced and fear circuitry disorders.
See also Anxiety disorders; Panic
disorder; Posttraumatic stress
disorder; Social phobia; Specific
phobias
cognition and, 175–187, 290–291
neurocircuitry models of, 217–218
phenomenology of, 215–217
status of as distinct group, 288–289
Stroop interference, 85–86
Substance-induced depression, 278
Substance use disorders
comorbidity of with anxiety disorders, 127
DSM-V and, 265, 276, 278, 293
epidemiology of, 266–270
etiological relationships between anxiety disorders and, 265–266, 277
longitudinal studies of, 270–271
neurobiology of acute substance effects, 275–276
neurobiology of stress, social anxiety, and, 273–274
neuropsychological deficits in anxiety disorders and, 274–275
PTSD in African Americans and, 142
role of stress and trauma in, 271
specific phobias and, 83
treatment of, 271–273
Subsyndromal PTSD, 15, 17–18, 286
Subthreshold panic disorder, 33, 41
Subthreshold social anxiety disorder, 68
Subtypes
of panic disorder, 34, 38–39
of social phobia, 64–67
Sweden, and research on specific phobias, 84
Switzerland, and posttraumatic stress disorder, 200
Symptom provocation paradigms, of neuroimaging, 221
Syndrome, definition of, 293

Taijin Kyofusho (TK), 62, 67, 199–200
Taiwan, and research on social phobia, 63, 199
Temperament
anxiety disorders and, 131
specific phobias and, 86–87
Tension-reduction hypothesis, of substance abuse, 275
Test anxiety, 62
Three-factor models, of PTSD, 13–14
Top-down modulation, in anxiety disorders, 275
Traumatic stress, 10, 19–20
Treatment
of anxiety disorders in racial or ethnic minorities, 140–141
comorbidity in social phobia and, 68
diagnosis and effectiveness of, 299
neuroimaging studies and, 243
reconceptualizing role of fear and stress in anxiety disorders, 262
research on cognition and, 182–184
specific phobias and, 88, 94–95
of substance use disorders, 271–273
syndrome recognition and, 293–294
Tryptophan hydroxylase, 163–164
Twin studies, of anxiety disorders, 129, 146–147, 151–152, 196
Two-factor model, of PTSD, 13, 14

Unconditional stimulus
research on neurocircuitry and, 218
specific phobias and, 85–87
U.S. Special Forces troops, 7
University of Michigan-CIDI, 39

Ventromedial prefrontal cortex (vmPFC), and fear conditioning, 219, 223
Vicarious modeling, and specific phobias, 185–186
Vietnam Era Twin Registry, 6, 7, 129
Virginia Twin Registry, 129, 295
Virtual reality, and exposure therapy, 88

Withdrawal, from substances of abuse, 278
Woodlawn study, 270
Work and Adjustment Scale, 81
Work disability
 panic disorder and, 33
 specific phobias and, 81

World Health Organization survey, on PTSD, 13
World Mental Health survey, 294

Yohimbine, 5–6